Health Informatics

This series is directed to healthcare professionals leading the transformation of healthcare by using information and knowledge. For over 20 years, Health Informatics has offered a broad range of titles: some address specific professions such as nursing, medicine, and health administration; others cover special areas of practice such as trauma and radiology; still other books in the series focus on interdisciplinary issues, such as the computer based patient record, electronic health records, and networked healthcare systems. Editors and authors, eminent experts in their fields, offer their accounts of innovations in health informatics. Increasingly, these accounts go beyond hardware and software to address the role of information in influencing the transformation of healthcare delivery systems around the world. The series also increasingly focuses on the users of the information and systems: the organizational, behavioral, and societal changes that accompany the diffusion of information technology in health services environments.

Developments in healthcare delivery are constant; in recent years, bioinformatics has emerged as a new field in health informatics to support emerging and ongoing developments in molecular biology. At the same time, further evolution of the field of health informatics is reflected in the introduction of concepts at the macro or health systems delivery level with major national initiatives related to electronic health records (EHR), data standards, and public health informatics.

These changes will continue to shape health services in the twenty-first century. By making full and creative use of the technology to tame data and to transform information, Health Informatics will foster the development and use of new knowledge in healthcare.

More information about this series at http://www.springer.com/series/1114

Carlos Fernandez-Llatas

Editor

Interactive Process Mining in Healthcare

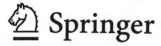 Springer

Editor
Carlos Fernandez-Llatas
Process Mining 4 Health Lab – SABIEN –
ITACA Institute
Universitat Politècnica de València
Valencia
Spain

CLINTEC – Karolinska Institutet
Sweden

ISSN 1431-1917 ISSN 2197-3741 (electronic)
Health Informatics
ISBN 978-3-030-53995-5 ISBN 978-3-030-53993-1 (eBook)
https://doi.org/10.1007/978-3-030-53993-1

This Springer imprint is published by the registered company Springer Nature Switzerland AG
The registered company address is: Gewerbestrasse 11, 6330 Cham, Switzerland

Foreword

It was on August 13, 2009, that I began my (virtual) relationship on Twitter with the SABIEN Group at ITACA Institute, Universitat Politècnica de València, in particular with my good colleague Vicente Traver. More recently, I had the pleasure of meeting Carlos Fernandez-Llatas, who is the person responsible for putting together a number of remarkable health professionals and engineers to produce this book on the use of an interactive process mining paradigm in the healthcare domain.

At that time, Carlos and Vicente were already working on ways to improve the healthcare sector through the use of technology. In addition to writing hundreds of scientific publications, they started this line of work beginning in 1998 until their team was recognized as one of the most prestigious international research groups in the application of digital solutions in the health and well-being sector, with participation in several international research projects. Therefore, I have no doubt whatsoever that the content of this book, based on wide experience from different points of view, will make a difference in the world of healthcare.

In 2009, I was a technical officer at the Ministry of Health and Consumer Affairs in Spain, where we were promoting the idea that the present and future of health information is based on digital solutions and knowledge management. After this experience, I moved to the international health sector, working for the World Health Organization (WHO), the international agency that directs and coordinates international health within the United Nations system. For the last 10 years, I have had the opportunity and great honor to lead and contribute to several projects and initiatives related to digital health, data, and health information in the health and well-being area in more than 100 countries and territories. Carlos, Vicente, and I chose different paths-academia versus government and policymaking-but we shared the same dream, to leverage the potential of data and digital solutions to improve population health.

Almost 11 years have passed since we met, and the world has dramatically changed since then. Now, we live longer and healthier lives, we are more connected, and the spread and uptake of digital solutions are a reality. However, considerable challenges in the health and well-being sector persist, including the lack of investment in the health sector where, according to WHO, the current health expenditure (percentage of gross domestic product, GDP) has only increased 0,06% since 2009, representing nowadays less than 10% of global GDP spent on health. In addition, the coronavirus (COVID-19) pandemic, the most serious public health emergency in 100 years, threatens to disrupt all the progress achieved by countries in the social and economic sectors throughout these years.

If we want to overcome the present and future health challenges, we must act together to encourage countries towards a coordinated response and investment with the target of a global impact. Hence, it is imperative for each country to strengthen its data and healthcare systems so that data gaps can be closed and every country can generate and use timely, reliable, and actionable data to ensure that decisions are data-driven.

As a response to these challenges, and in the midst of these unprecedented times, this book presents an opportunity to introduce a new paradigm for integrating health experts in the process of generating new evidence with a data-driven philosophy to enhance healthcare and overcome health threats through the use of interactive process mining.

Recent experiences have shown that we cannot predict the future, but it is true that it is possible to infer new knowledge from past actions through a combination of process mining technologies using a new machine learning paradigm. As a result, this mixture can provide accurate and personalized knowledge for future decisions and improve patient treatment and quality of life. Throughout this book, the authors guide us through a pathway to discover new ways to provide information to healthcare professionals by involving them in the complex process of generating knowledge with the idea of reducing costs and enhancing these processes. As part of this workflow, process mining algorithms are executed in a human-understandable way and high-quality data are needed to lead to the right decisions in the healthcare domain. As a consequence, methods and techniques allow for the development of new models from reality, while experts have a way to validate these models that can be applied to human behavior.

A total of 33 experts from 20 different institutions around the world have agreed to guide us through this journey across 17 chapters, and I hope that you enjoy this trip as much as I have.

We do not know what will happen tomorrow, but today we know, as the American engineer and statistician William Edwards Deming said, "Without data, you're just another person with an opinion," and this book will help us fill that gap with the use of interactive process mining.

David Novillo-Ortiz
Unit Head, Health Information, Monitoring and Analysis
World Health Organization, Regional Office for Europe

Denmark,
May 2020

The author is a staff member of the World Health Organization (WHO) and is solely responsible for the views expressed in the foreword, which do not necessarily represent the views, decisions, or policies of the WHO.

Preface

Nowadays, writing a book about the use of artificial intelligence in the medical domain is a challenge. Numerous advances in the last years have resulted in a large number of work in this area. Artificial intelligence technologies have proven highly successful in several scenarios. However, these have not yet solved some ethical and technical issues that are raising inevitable questions in the medical community: What is the role of the health professional in this scenario? Are these systems safe? This is raising suspicion among certain professionals who feel these technologies can may lose control of healthcare. This mistrust is motivating the appearance of certain works in the literature that aid in understanding the results obtained by artificial intelligence algorithms.

This book attempts to go a step further by proposing technology that involves the health professional in the process of learning. The aim of this book is to present and deepen the use of Interactive Process Mining as a new paradigm for integrating health experts in the process of generating new evidence. This paradigm combines the application of process mining technologies in healthcare using interactive machine learning for supporting health professionals in inferring new knowledge from past actions and providing accurate and personalized knowledge for future decisions and improve patients' treatments and quality of life.

This book has an eminent practical focus providing not only methodologies and technologies for the application of interactive process mining paradigm, but an important part of the book is also dedicated to presenting examples of real uses cases where this paradigm has been successfully applied in different medical domains like surgery, emergency, obesity behavior, diabetes, and human behavior modelling.

Although, inevitably, making a practical book requires tools for supporting the proposed techniques, the objective of this book is not to be tool-specific. The aim is to provide solutions, by explaining the real concepts and the engineering behind the solution, and not the tools used in detail, keeping the content timeless and independent of the tools used. The book is intended to provide a common view between health professionals and data scientists in a general way. The deep analysis of the techniques that are used is out of the scope of this book. To make it accessible for a wider audience, we have skipped the more technical parts and

Chapter 1: Introduction	
Part I: Basics	Chapter 2: Value-Driven Digital Transformation in Health and Medical Care
	Chapter 3: Medical Processes
	Chapter 4: Process Mining for Healthcare
	Chapter 5: Data Quality in Process Mining
	Chapter 6: Towards Open Process Models in Healthcare: Open Standards and Legal Issues
Part II: Interactive Process Mining in Health	Chapter 7: Interactive Process Mining Paradigm
	Chapter 8: Giving Interactive Process Mining to Health Professionals: Interactive Data Rodeos
	Chapter 9: Interactive Process Mining in Practice: Interactive Key Process Indicators
Part III: Interactive Process Mining In Action	Chapter 10: Interactive Process Mining in Emergencies
	Chapter 11: Interactive Process Mining in Surgery with Real Time Location Systems
	Chapter 12: Interactive Process Mining in Chronic Diseases: Diabetes
	Chapter 13: Interactive Process Mining in IoT and Human Behaviour Modelling
	Chapter 14: Interactive Process Mining in Medical Training
	Chapter 15: Interactive Process Mining for discovering Dynamic Risk Models
	Chapter 16: Interactive Process Mining-Informed Change Management Methodology for healthcare
Chapter 17:Interactive Process Mining Challenges	

Fig. 1 Book chapters

have focused on philosophical and organizational aspects. That means, the what and the how Interactive Process Mining Techniques can support professionals in the improvement of health processes.

Figure 1 shows the relation of chapters that are included in the book. The remainder of the book is the following:

The first chapter introduces the problem and explains the main concepts that will be revisited later in the book in more detail. Apart from this introduction, the book is organized into three parts and a final chapter discussing the challenges we are facing in the application of Interactive Process Mining in the medical domain.

The first part revisits the basic aspects and the current medical background. Chapter 2, analyze the effects that are producing the Health Digital Transformation in the medical domain and shows the aspects in the appearance of Value-Based Medicine Paradigm. Chapter 3 provides an introductory background to medical processes and what approaches exist for their design and automation. Chapter 4 introduces Process Mining focused on their application in the healthcare domain, highlighting the differences, singularities, and barriers in their application in real medical environments. Chapter 5 goes deeper into the problem of Data Quality, specifically in the case of Process Mining. To close this part Chap. 6 shows the use of semantics for a better way to define processes using Process Mining and Health Data Standards.

The second part of this book is focused on the presentation of the Interactive Process Mining Paradigm in the healthcare domain. Chapter 7 explains what is the Interactive Process Mining paradigm, presenting its singular advantages for application in the medical domain. Chapter 8 deepens the methodological aspects of Interactive Process Mining, revisiting the concept of Data Rodeos for supporting the deployment of Interactive Process Mining in health. Finally, Chap. 9 introduces the concept of Interactive Process Indicator (IPI) as a new way to provide information to the doctor to achieve better knowledge in medical processes and supporting them in taking better decisions.

The third part of the book is a selection of real cases for illustrating the application of Interactive Process Mining in the healthcare domain. Chapters 10, 11, 12, 13, 14, and 15 present real cases in real scenarios where Interactive Process Mining is being applied, highlighting specific aspects, advantages, and barriers of this methodology. The cases have been selected covering different fields inside the medical domain. Chapters are talking about applying this technology in hospitals with the existing information in medical databases, as well as enriched with Real-Time Location Systems, and supporting medical education. But we also have selected cases analyzing the patient process in chronic diseases, discovering its dynamical processes and analyzing the data that comes from the Internet of Things for discovering the patient's individual behavior.

Chapter 16 introduces the application of organizational techniques, like Change Management, proposing techniques for improving the success probability in the application of Interactive Process Mining in a singular case, like it is in healthcare domain. The last chapter summarizes new challenges that have to be addresses in the coming years in order to successfully apply this methodology in healthcare domains.

This book is the humble result of more than 15 years of research in the medical informatics field, looking for the best ways to support the decisions of health professionals, increase the quality of care, and achieve better patient experience via continuous improvement in medical processes.

A part of my life is in this book. I hope you enjoy reading.

Valencia, Spain   Carlos Fernandez-Llatas
May 2020

Acknowledgements

When one decides to start writing or editing a book, a clear motivation must be present. Every time, independent of the number of publications you have made in your life, the efforts that you finally devote to a book always achieve what you planned for. If a book is successful, it is never due to a single person's effort. Around each publication, there is a set of people who, being aware or not, are essential, and without them, a book such as this would never exist.

To Wil Van der Aalst, all that's written in this book is possible thanks to his work. Without Wil and his passion, all my research would have been conducted in other different directions. To Josep Carmona, for introducing and guiding me in the Process Mining community. To Andrea Buratin and Marco Montali for the interesting walks and talks around the world. Thanks to the IEEE Task Force on Process Mining and all their participants for pushing for the presence of Process Mining in the world.

To my colleagues of the Process-Oriented Data Science for Healthcare Alliance Steering Committee Jorge Munoz-Gama; Marcos Sepulveda for making me feel at home; Niels Martin, for his incredible *Niels-Level* capability to organize, work, and produce; and Owen Johnson and Emmanuel Helm for betting really big for our community. To Mar Marcos, Gustav Bellika, Roberto Gatta, Eric Rojas, Martin Wolf, Mario Vega, Onur Dogan, Emilio Sulis, Kassaye Yitbarek, Ilaria Amantea, Joyce Pebesma, and many others for believing in my work and devoting time to visit me at our lab. I thank them very much and the rest of the Process Oriented for Healthcare community, who were really pushing for the presence of Process Mining in healthcare domain.

To Fernando Seoane, for opening his life to me, for believing in my work even more than myself, and coaching and supporting me to grow up, and Ivan Pau, for his faith in me and my work.

To Farhad Abtani, Metin Akay, Maria Argente, Maria Teresa Arredondo, Panagiotis Bamidis, Jose Miguel Benedi, Ricardo Bellazzi, Ana Maria Bianchi, Cristina Bescos, Maria Fernanda Cabrera, Jose Manuel Catala, Paulo Carvalho, Angeles Celda, Inma Cervera, Arianna Dagliati, Javier Diez, Francisco Dolz, Choni Doñate, Luis Fernandez-Luque, Giuseppe Fico, Jorge Garcés, Elena Garcia, Juan Miguel

Garcia, Purificacion Garcia, Emilio Garijo, Maria Guillem, Sergio Guillen, Mercedes Gozalbo, Valeria Herskovic, Jorge Henriques, Blanca Jordan, Lenin Lemus, Jesus Mandingorra, Luis Marco, Jose Francisco Merino, Jose Millet, Sebastian Pantoja, Carlos Palau, Voro Peiro, Jorge Posada, Flavio Pileggi, Sofia Reppou, Elena Rocher, Luis Rodriguez, Jordi Rovira, Lucia Sacchi, Pilar Sala, Carlos Sanchez-Bocanegra, Shabbir Syed, Javier Urchueguia, Bernardo Valdivieso, Miguel Angel Valero, Salvador Vera, and many other technical and clinical partners that have interacted with me in more than 90 research projects during my personal career . Also to EIT Health, the European Commission, and the Spanish Government for their direct support to our Process Mining research via projects like VALUE (EIT-Health INNOVATION - 20328), LifeChamps (H2020-SC1 - 875329), PATHWAYS (EIT-Health CAMPUS - 19372), InAdvance (H2020-SC1 - 825750), CrowdHealth (H2020-SC1 - 727560), OR4.0 (H2020-EI-SMEInst - 812386), MOSAIC (FP7-ICT - 600914), FASyS (CDTI-CENIT-E 2009), eMOTIVA (MICyT- TSI-020110), VAALID (FP7 - 224309), PIPS(FP6-IST - 507019), and many others that indirectly feed the research which produced this book.

To all the contributors of the book and specially to David Novillo for his words and for accepting to write the Foreword in such less time.

To Vicente Traver, my boss, my friend since more than 20 years, nothing to say that hasn't been said. All that I have achieved or I will achieve in my professional and part of my personal life is thanks to him.

To my closest collaborators in constructing this book: Gema Ibanez-Sanchez and Zoe Valero-Ramon, who have supported me in the most complex and subtle parts of the book, offering me not only a helping hand in the worst moments but also their infinite friendship in all my life, and Juanjo Lull, who devotedly reviewed a huge part of this book. Their comments have improved significantly the content.

To the rest of members of SABIEN and the Process Mining 4 Healthcare Lab: Maria Jesus Arnal, Lucia Aparici, Jose Luis Bayo, Antonio Martinez-Millana, Alvaro Fides, Nacho Basagoiti, Maria Martinez, and Manuel Traver for keeping on believing in this adventure for more than 20 years and to those more than 100 people that have been working with us during these times in our lab.

To Marcos, my family, and friends and those special people, even those that I have known for a short time, that I have in my life and have suffered my absence during the gestation of this book. Yes, this is for you.

My last words go to all those who should have been reflected here, but who are not because of my damn memory. My most sincere and deepest apologies.

Valencia, Spain   Carlos Fernandez-Llatas
May 2020

Contents

Chapter 1
Interactive Process Mining in Healthcare: An Introduction

Carlos Fernandez-Llatas

1.1 A New Age in Health Care

In the last decades, in parallel to the industrial and social progress, several healthcare paradigms have appeared in the scientific medical community. These paradigms are proposing changes in the way in which healthcare is deployed in our society. The image of Traditional Medicine, were physicians are *artists* that are isolated and taking decisions based only on their knowledge and experience, arc changing to a new doctor always connected and with access to the last evidence existing in a globalized world.

With the development of Evidence-based Medicine in the 1990s [26] a new paradigm for standardizing the cares appears. Influenced by the fever of standardization of processes, Evidence-Based Medicine proposes the creation of protocols and guidelines using the best evidence existing in literature in combination with the running knowledge of the professionals taking into account the preferences of patients. However, in the implantation of Evidence-Based medicine in health centres have some barriers [16]. The collection of evidence was usually Knowledge-Driven by creating guidelines for disease cares as a result of consensus groups. However, these guidelines are usually written by professionals having the risk of incompleteness and ambiguity.

Other of the critics that are receiving the Evidence-Based Medicine is their impersonality. Excessively general protocols ignore the patients that have different responses to the treatment, that should be treated *out of the guideline*. This can sup-

C. Fernandez-Llatas (✉)
Process Mining 4 Health Lab – SABIEN – ITACA Institute, Universitat Politècnica de València, Valencia, Spain

CLINTEC – Karolinska Institutet, Sweden
e-mail: cfllatas@itaca.upv.es

C. Fernandez-Llatas (ed.), *Interactive Process Mining in Healthcare*, Health Informatics, https://doi.org/10.1007/978-3-030-53993-1_1

pose adverse effects in the treatments due to not taking into account the individuality of the patient before defining a treatment. In this line, other paradigms promote individualization of the cares. Personalized Medicine [15] or Precision Medicine [7] are examples of that. These paradigms are looking for new treatments that are taking the individual into account. This new concept is developing new strategies for analyzing individual variability for improving the cares by personalizing existing treatments. An example of that is human genomics, that takes into account the genetic information in humans for selecting the best treatments. However, Personal and Precision Medicine is not only genomics but also, use all data available of a single patient and build high computing systems that can support professionals in the selection of the best cares for each case. This is a new way to promote the creation of a new medical centre in patient's individualities.

This paradigm in combination with Integrated Care [2] one, looks for a complete view of the patient taking into account all the information available of the patient. This information can be collected from the data available in Electronic Health Records available on hospitals and primary care centres or Patient Health Records that store the information reported by the patient. Besides, other paradigms propose a more ambitious data collection and actuation protocols framework for providing an, even, richer data source that can offer a complete holistic view of the patient using, not only directly related medical information, that arse accessible in Electronic Health Records, but also personal, social and lifestyle information, that can support health professionals in the understanding of the behavioural models of the patients. Ambient Assisted Living and Internet of Things paradigms [9] propose the creation of always-connected smart environments, that not only provides a way to recover the information related to the daily routine of the patients but also build and smart environment to put in practice advanced Integrated Care treatments that can be deployed wherever the patient is.

In a world worried about the sustainability of health due to the increase of life expectancy and age-related commodities and chronic diseases, there is a need for a continuous evaluation of the health systems. The increase in the number of patients requires a more effective way to provide health to not collapse the system. In terms of defining health policies for next years, it is crucial to provide the best cares using the fewer resources a possible. Then, the deployment of new technologies and methodologies in medical domain for Health technology assessment is decisive in the supporting of the medical domain decisions.

When a new technology is deployed it necessary to evaluate variables as effectiveness, efficacy or the real cost. Sometimes, in complex environments like health, it is difficult to evaluate the cost-effectiveness of the actions performed. In this line, a new paradigm called Value-Based Healthcare [14] appeared in the field. Value-Based Healthcare promotes the assessment of the technologies based on the value chain that those technologies offer to the patient. In this line, Value-Based Healthcare, look for the analysis of technologies taking into account the information reported by the patient. In this way, there are defined two different kinds of measures reported by the patient; the Patient Reported Experience Measures (PREMs), that are referred to the experience perceived by the patient and the Patient-

Reported Outcomes Measures (PROMs) that are referent to the information about the effectiveness and safety of the treatment provided [3].

However, the value reported by the patient might be insufficient, to evaluate the cost-effectiveness of health technology. Other paradigms, like Quadruple Aim [4], offers others value perspectives. Quadruple Aim, define the value in four parts: The patient experience; that measures how the patient perceives their health. The population health, that evaluates the real health status of the patient in the most objective way as possible. The costs, that shows the resources (Economical, material, staff...) that should be used to provide the cares to the patient. And, finally, we should take into account the experience of the health professional. An adequate health technology assessment should be focused on the combination of those values, taking into account the different perspectives. This enables a better analysis of the value provided by the technology.

1.2   The Look for the Best Medical Evidence: Data Driven vs Knowledge Driven

Despite these large attempts to create an effective way of leading the digital health transformation, there are still problems to join in real practice all these research fields. In this scenario, it is clear the need for a way to provide technological tools to align all these paradigms and framework to daily practice.

The first attempt for developing an Artificial Intelligence system that supports medical doctors were the MYCIN system [27]. MYCIN was a Rule-based expert system that provides support in the daily practice decisions in a consultation. MYCIN was built using a simple inference engine that uses a knowledge base of around 500 rules. This expert system asked the doctor a predefined set of questions about the signs and symptoms of the patient, and according to the answers, the computer provides a set of possible causes. Posterior studies show that the accuracy of MYCIN was around 65%[30]. This percentage was better than non-specialist physicians (42.5% to 62.5%) but worst than a specialist (80%). In practice, the creation of this kind of expert systems can support the guidance of non-experts in their daily decisions. Currently, these systems are being successfully used for supporting doctors in their decisions through bots in specific diseases [19].

Rule-based systems are created based on the knowledge existing extracted from experts. These rules require the creation of consensus of experts that should formalize their knowledge in computer understandable statements. This requires a high exclusivity for expressing all the possible patterns in the medical knowledge, but with the adequate complexity to allow computerized automation. To approach this formalization, there are some tools and languages in literature [22]. Computer Interpretable Guidelines (CIG) ensures a correct and formal way for expressing Clinical Guidelines providing tools for automating them, avoiding ambiguities and inconsistencies.

However, the creation of those pathways has not acquired the expected penetration in healthcare domain to the difficulties in the manual creation of these formal models. The creation of these systems requires the consensus of experts groups that, usually have different opinion and approaches. The creation of this consensus is highly time-consuming. Besides, the high variability in healthcare increase the difficulty of model unambiguous and non-deterministic models to allow their automation. These barriers lead to simplified models that usually does not cover the reality of patients, inducing the frustration of professionals and, then, the rejection of the system.

In parallel, to the Knowledge-Driven paradigm, Data-Driven paradigms appear on scene. While Knowledge-Based systems are though to take decisions making deductions based on rules known from professionals, Data-Driven approaches want to learn the rules of the models based on the data existing in reality.

Leveraging current healthcare digital transformation era, Pattern Recognition [10], Machine Learning [1], and Deep Learning [23] paradigms can infer the real models from actual data existing in health databases.The use of big data technologies for inferring new evidence from patient information provides a great opportunity to support the diagnosis, treatments and healthcare holistically. Data-Driven Models can discover the reality inducing the relationship among the data available, even when these relations are not known from experts. This characteristic provides a significant advantage over Knowledge systems. The models are automatically inferred and show the statistical reality existing in the data, in an automated way without the necessity of the involvement of human experts in the loop reducing the time of creation, and offer a model able to represent new knowledge that is not known in the medical community.

However, behind this advantage, resides its main disadvantage. The new knowledge inferred in these models keeps hidden to health professionals. These systems are *Black Boxes* for Health professionals and should trust in their decisions, provoking an innumerable set of ethical issues [6]. Data-Driven systems are not infallible and an error can suppose the life of a patient.

1.3 To an Interactive Approach

At this point, although Data-Driven systems can create real scientific evidence to improve daily healthcare protocols, the lack of understandability is a huge barrier difficult to overcome. For that, the creation of mixed paradigms that allow the creation of models from data, but can be analyzed and understood by professionals to extract real scientific evidence can be the solution to this problem.

But, what means scientific evidence? Most studies in the medicine domain are based on descriptive statistics that are used classical methodologies used in classical studies like the well known Framingham study [20]. However, there is an increasing number of works that are demanding to evolve this way of producing evidence [13, 24, 28]. It is necessary to differentiate between Truth, Knowledge, and Certainty.

Truth, are the facts objectively correct; Knowledge is the information that we have due to our experience in our understanding, that means subjectively, and Certainty is a measure of confidence that we can apply to a fact that we are studying. In our problem, the Truth is the medical model that we are looking for; the Knowledge is what we *know* from the disease; and the Certainty is the tool that we have to evaluate the signs, symptoms and evolution that we see in the patients. So, Certainty is giving us the needed information for creating new Knowledge, in looking for the Truth.

Data-Driven models are giving to us *Black Box* Knowledge to take decisions. Cognitive Computing paradigm [21] promote to mimic the human brain in order to substitute the human in the knowledge phase and take the decisions based on the knowledge provided by the machine. But, that means to lose control over the information that we have. In that paradigm, our medical knowledge not only is not increasing but also we are giving our confidence to machines that are infinitely less powerful that our main computer system: The brain.

On the other hand, Interactive Models [12] promotes the interaction of the human with the machine using the human brain as another computation node in the learning system. While computers can provide the best memory and computation capabilities, Human brain can coordinate computation using heuristics, leading the experiments and isolating the atoms of evidence that are forming our medical knowledge. The Human-Computer interaction has been demonstrated its advantages in the learning domain decreasing the convergence time over classical cognitive models [12].

Interpreting Wisdom as the Decision we can show the differences between the paradigms based on the Pyramid of Wisdom [25]. Figure 1.1 shows this difference. Cognitive models provide computerized tools to provide models that provide the knowledge required for making the best decisions. Interactive Models advocate

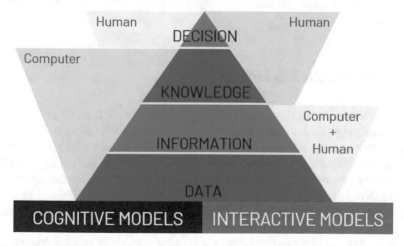

Fig. 1.1 Cognitive Models vs Interactive Models

producing the information in combination with computers letting the knowledge and the decision to the human.

However, the application of Interactive Methodology requires the involvement of human experts in the process of learning. This requires acceptance professionals. For achieving this aim, it is crucial to use adequate tools and methodologies to enable the interaction between the human and the learning systems. For that, the number of Data-Driven techniques that can be used in an interactive, are those that provide a way to communicate the results in a human-understandable way. Unfortunately, most used machine learning techniques, like Neural Networks, Hidden Markov Models, or Support Vector Machines are not thought to be humanly understandable. For that, to apply the Interactive Learning paradigm, it is necessary to select algorithms, methods and tools adapted for providing understandable information to discover new knowledge through new evidence.

As said, most of Machine Learning models are based on mathematical algorithms that produce accurate models, but not understandable. Currently, there are appearing works in literature demanding for an Explainable Artificial Intelligence in medical domain [17]. Explainable Artificial Intelligence is a research field that advocates for creating tools, methods and algorithms that translate the results of Machine Learning systems, to human-understandable information, providing not only the answer of a question, for example, a diagnosis, but also the reasons of the selection, the signs and symptoms that have pointed to the solution.

However, although the application of those techniques allows having the clues for a better understanding of the knowledge existing in the *Black Boxes*. The techniques are not designed to be understandable and there is not the needed fluid interaction between the expert and the machine. Also, Explainable models offer a unidirectional interaction, from the model to the expert. These systems can't be corrected and improved by experts reducing the capabilities of the interactive learning, that is based on the correction produced by experts to improve the system in the next iteration.

1.4   Why Process Mining?

Taking a look at the health paradigms analyzed in Sect. 1.1, in all of them there is an underlying process associated with the care protocols. Independently if the focus is based on the patient or the professional, clinical methodologies are based on processes. Clinical Guidelines created by health experts are usually described as processes, showing the behaviour of the disease and guiding the actions that should follow to correctly treat the disease. In this line, a process view can be a good interaction language. In this line, the Process Mining Paradigm can be an interesting suitable option for creating Interactive Learning systems.

Process Mining [29] is a relatively new paradigm that is increasing this presence in the medical domain by inferring the Processes based on data available from medical databases. Process Mining uses the events of the patients, that are the actions and its timestamp, for discovering the actual processes performed by patients, in a process view specially designed for being human understood. Also, Process Mining provides tools for enhancing the views highlighting the most interesting parts of the processes and techniques for comparing the processes, enabling the assessment of health protocols implemented [5].

Usually, Process Mining techniques are not the most accurate Data-Driven that you can apply to a machine learning problem, but its capability to be human-understandable supposes a new way to extract knowledge from the Data-Driven world. This allows mix Data and Knowledge-Driven worlds through the application of interactive models [12]. This not only increases the acceptability of the technology by the experts that can understand how its processes are deployed but also, the expert is enabled to correct the inferred model, the inference errors produced by the Data-Driven system, that are potentially zero in each stage [12].

1.5 Interactive Process Mining

The characteristics of Process Mining framework are perfect for applying Interactive paradigm in the optimization of process. The application of Interactive Process Mining techniques can support in the Data-Driven inference of the Protocols and guidelines that can be understood and adapted by healthcare professionals in an iterative way [12]. Evidence-Based Medicine paradigms can use these techniques for achieving a Data-Driven actual combination of human knowledge and best evidence in daily practice. This is because it allows the real interaction between the health professional running knowledge, and the best evidence existing that is accessible and understandable by the professional.

However, Interactive Process Mining technologies also can support health professionals for putting in practice these personalized paradigms. Process Mining is used for discovering individualized behaviours of patients [8, 11] using Ambient Assisted Living or Internet of Things information available in smart environments. This can provide new ways for helping health professionals not only in the individuals' processes discovery but also in the evaluation of the effects of new treatments in a holistic, integrated and personalized way. Besides, Process Mining can support in the value chain evaluation in the patient processes promoted in Value-Based Medicine according to Quadruple Aim aspects [18].

Interactive Process Mining supposes the application of machine learning algorithms that could offer an understandable view of processes. The purpose of that is taking advantage of human judgment in order to achieve the acquisition of real usable evidence from automatic data mining techniques. This allows not only answer research questions that physicians have in mind but also, produces new questions about the patients' patterns behaviour that, in another way, keep hidden into the data. This, on one hand, allow experts to use Interactive Process Mining looking for a first confirmation of the intuition evidence acquired from experience but, on the other hand, enable them to discover new evidence that is not expected and after that can be verified using clinical cases. These techniques allow a first step for selecting the best questions that can be stated for the development of clinical cases, with better guarantees, optimizing the process of obtaining evidence. Moreover, these techniques can support in the deployment of medical process resultant of the evidence acquisition, not only by helping in their traceability but also in the continuous adaption of the standardise process to the local reality in each medical centre in each moment in time, actions that are not sustainable using clinical cases.

The main aim of this book is to deepen in the aspects of this paradigm in the healthcare domain. In following chapters we analyze in more detail some aspects of the background, challenges and limitations, we propose a methodology, and we show a set of some real applications for showing how Process Mining can be used for interacting with medical experts to achieve evidence. Enjoy the reading!

References

1. Alpaydin E. Introduction to machine learning. MIT Press; 2020.
2. Amelung V, Stein V, Goodwin N, Balicer R, Nolte E, Suter E. Handbook integrated care. Springer; 2017
3. Black N, Varaganum M, Hutchings A. Relationship between patient reported experience (prems) and patient reported outcomes (proms) in elective surgery. BMJ Qual Saf. 2014;23(7):534–42.
4. Bodenheimer T, Sinsky C. From triple to quadruple aim: care of the patient requires care of the provider. Ann Fam Med. 2014;12(6):573–6.
5. Carmona J, van Dongen B, Solti A, Weidlich M. Conformance checking. Springer; 2018.
6. Char DS, Shah NH, Magnus D. Implementing machine learning in health care—addressing ethical challenges. N Engl J Med. 2018;378(11):981.
7. Collins FS, Varmus H. A new initiative on precision medicine. N Engl J Med. 2015;372(9):793–5.
8. Dogan O, Martinez-Millana A, Rojas E, Sepúlveda M, Munoz-Gama J, Traver V, Fernandez-Llatas C. Individual behavior modeling with sensors using process mining. Electronics. 2019;8(7):766.
9. Dohr A, Modre-Opsrian R, Drobics M, Hayn D, Schreier G. The internet of things for ambient assisted living. In: 2010 seventh international conference on information technology: new generations. IEEE, 2010. p. 804–9.
10. Duda RO, Hart PE, Stork DG. Pattern classification. Wiley; 2012.
11. Fernández-Llatas C, Benedi J-M, García-Gómez JM, Traver V. Process mining for individualized behavior modeling using wireless tracking in nursing homes. Sensors. 2013;13(11):15434–51.
12. Fernandez-Llatas C, Meneu T, Traver V, Benedi J-M. Applying evidence-based medicine in telehealth: an interactive pattern recognition approximation. Int J Environ Res Public Health. 2013;10(11):5671–82.
13. Goldberger JJ, Buxton AE. Personalized medicine vs guideline-based medicine. Jama. 2013;309(24):2559–60.
14. Gray M. Value based healthcare. BMJ. 2017;356:j437.
15. Hamburg MA, Collins FS. The path to personalized medicine. N Engl J Med. 2010;363(4):301–4.
16. Haynes B, Haines A. Barriers and bridges to evidence based clinical practice. BMJ. 1998;317(7153):273–6.
17. Holzinger A. From machine learning to explainable AI. In: 2018 world symposium on digital intelligence for systems and machines (DISA). IEEE; 2018. p. 55–66.

18. Ibanez-Sanchez G, Fernandez-Llatas C, Celda A, Mandingorra J, Aparici-Tortajada L, Martinez-Millana A, Munoz-Gama J, Sepúlveda M, Rojas E, Gálvez V, Capurro D, Traver V. Toward value-based healthcare through interactive process mining in emergency rooms: the stroke case. Int J Environ Res Public Health. 2019;16(10).
19. Lemaire J, Thouvenot VI, Toure C, Pons JS. Zero mothers die: a global project to reduce maternal and newborn mortality through the systematic application of mobile health and icts. J Int Soc Telemed eHealth. 2015;3:e8–1.
20. Mahmood SS, Levy D, Vasan RS, Wang TJ. The framingham heart study and the epidemiology of cardiovascular disease: a historical perspective. Lancet. 2014;383(9921):999–1008.
21. Modha DS, Ananthanarayanan R, Esser SK, Ndirango A, Sherbondy AJ, Singh R. Cognitive computing. Commun ACM. 2011;54(8):62–71.
22. Peleg M. Computer-interpretable clinical guidelines: a methodological review. J Biomed Inform. 2013;46(4):744–63.
23. Ravì D, Wong C, Deligianni F, Berthelot M, Andreu-Perez J, Lo B, Yang G-Z. Deep learning for health informatics. IEEE J Biomed Health Inform. 2016;21(1):4–21.
24. Romana H-W. Is evidence-based medicine patient-centered and is patient-centered care evidence-based? Health Serv Res. 2006;41(1):1.
25. Rowley J. The wisdom hierarchy: representations of the dikw hierarchy. J Inf Sci. 2007;33(2):163–80.
26. Sackett DL, Rosenberg WMC, Gray MJA, Haynes BR, Richardson SW. Evidence based medicine: what it is and what it isn't. BMJ. 1996;312(7023):71–2.
27. Shortliffe E. Computer-based medical consultations: MYCIN, vol. 2. Elsevier; 1976.
28. Sturmberg J, Topolski S. For every complex problem, there is an answer that is clear, simple and wrong: and other aphorisms about medical statistical fallacies. J Eval Clin Pract. 2014;20(6):1017–25.
29. van Der Aalst W. Process mining. Data science in action. Springer; 2016.
30. Yu VL, Fagan LM, Wraith SM, Clancey WJ, Scott AC, Hannigan J, Blum RL, Buchanan BG, Cohen SN. Antimicrobial selection by a computer. A blinded evaluation by infectious diseases experts. Jama. 1979;242(12):1279–82.

Part I
Basics

Chapter 2
Value-Driven Digital Transformation in Health and Medical Care

Fernando Seoane, Vicente Traver, and Jan Hazelzet

2.1 Evolution of Patient-Centric Medical Care

Since the beginning of modern medicine, medical care has been practiced with a strong focus on the patients needs beyond re-stating the patient's health. We can find in Hippocrates oath the origin for both patient safety stating the *nonmaleficence* principle and patient privacy. Therefore, we can state that medical care has been patient centric from the very beginning.

The development of public health between late 1700s and beginning of 1900s [44] first and the rising of Evidence-based medicine (EBM) [19] later where attempts to provide a standard of care of the highest quality to all. The remarked focus on population, seemed like medical care had shifted temporarily the focus away from the patient as individual. On the contrary, public health and EBM were actually incorporating more needs of the patient into the care process, needs of the patient not limited to the individual but as part of a society.

As response to such apparent focus shift at the end of the twentieth century, a renewed person-centric effort spread through care practitioners and medical care associations aiming to refocus care back into the patient [43] incorporating more patient needs beyond the medical interventions it-self, including patient values and

F. Seoane
Karolinska Institutet, Solna, Sweden
e-mail: fernando.seoane@ki.se

V. Traver (✉)
Process Mining 4 Health Lab – SABIEN – ITACA Institute, Universitat Politècnica de València, Valencia, Spain
e-mail: vtraver@itaca.upv.es

J. Hazelzet
Erasmus Medical Center, Rotterdam, Netherlands
e-mail: j.a.hazelzet@erasmusmc.nl

© Springer Nature Switzerland AG 2021
C. Fernandez-Llatas (ed.), *Interactive Process Mining in Healthcare*, Health Informatics, https://doi.org/10.1007/978-3-030-53993-1_2

Fig. 2.1 EBM triade inspired
on the original diagram in
[38] from 1996

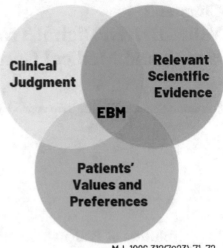

MJ. 1996;312(7023):71-72

preferences. As a result, the EBM concept developed into the EBM triad, including patient values, needs and preferences as one of its fundamental pillars [38] (See Fig. 2.1).

2.1.1 Holistic Approaches to Healthcare Improvement in a Patient-Centric Framework

While the patient centric movement [8] continued growing through the first decade of this century, new trends about healthcare delivery raised to meet the incipient challenge caused by the global demographic pressure of a larger, older and sicker population: Healthcare sustainability.

Concepts like value based health care (VBHC) introduced by Porter and Teisberg [33] or the triple aim of healthcare [4] promoted by the Institute of Healthcare Improvement (IHI) acknowledge the complexity of the healthcare ecosystem and presented a more holistic approach to provide care taking into consideration all significant factors influencing the future sustainability of healthcare (See Fig. 2.2).

2.1.2 VALUE Based HC Concept

While Value-based healthcare is a framework with a holistic approach integrating several dimensions, the initial given definition of value [34] "as the health outcomes achieved per dollar spent" was relatively limited, reducing the whole concept to a mere cost-efficiency question. Fortunately for the sake of future sustainability the

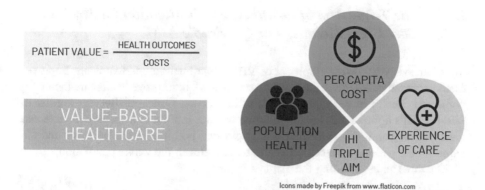

Fig. 2.2 Conceptual representation of Value-based Health care (left) and the triple aim of the Institute of Health Improvement

Table 2.1 Evolution of value definition in value-based health care. (**Source:** Modified from [10])

Narrow (price-based) utilisation of *Value* [13, 16, 29, 31]	Value defined as the ehealth outcomes by dollar spent
	$$Value = \frac{(Outcomes + Patient\ Experience)}{Cost(Direct + Indirect)of\ Care\ Intervention}$$
	$$Value = \frac{Healthcare\ that\ matters\ to\ the\ patient}{Cost\ along\ the\ entire\ cycle\ of\ care}$$
Comprehensive (normative) utilisation of "value"[17]	Allocative value: equitable distribution of resources across all patient groups
	Technical value: achievement of best possible outcomes with available resources
	Personal value: appropriate care to achieve patients' personal goals
	Societal value: contribution of healthcare to social participation and connectedness

definition of value has evolved in the last decade from a narrow, price-based, to a comprehensive, normative, definition, see Table 2.1 [10], not just preserving the wide holistic approach but making VBHC applicable to a wide range of healthcare systems.

2.1.3   The Triple Aim of Healthcare with Attention for Health Care Professionals: The Quadruple AIM

Simultaneously to the development of VBHC, the Institute of Healthcare Improvement proposed in 2007 a comprehensive framework to improve healthcare including population health in the triple aim [4] of healthcare. Conceptually very similar to VBHC, IHI's approach to health outcome was not limited to a specific disease and the care intervention provided. In the Triple aim, both the health outcome and the value for the patient were considered to a higher level: the whole population.

The three tenets building the Triple Aim are [4]:

- improving the individual experience of care,
- improving the health of populations and
- reducing the per capita costs of care for populations.

Probably, a wider framework that includes population health, i.e. incorporates the public health dimension with the patient centric approach and the financial aspect should be better useful to tackle the future sustainability challenge of healthcare.

Anyhow, it turned out that the triple aim was missing an essential component that is crucial for the other three tenets: The experience of the care team. As pointed out by Bodenheimer and Sinsky in 2014 [5] the triple aim cannot be achieved without including the wellbeing of the workforce. Any improvement achieved neglecting the experience of the health care staff will have a short-lasting effect, especially if it is achieved at their expenses. This way through the incorporation of the experience of the workforce, the triple aim evolved into the quadruple aim of healthcare [41] (See Fig. 2.3).

Fig. 2.3 Conceptual representation of the triple aim of the Institute of Health Improvement adding the perspective of the health care worker, known as the quadruple aim

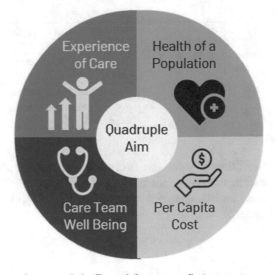

Icons made by Freepik from www.flaticon.com

2.2   Data-Driven Sustainable Healthcare Framework

2.2.1   *International Consortium for Health Outcome Measures*

The medical and healthcare community realized that the novel frameworks revolved around optimization concepts, targeting improvement, reducing cost and burden, increasing health outcome of intervention, and improving quality of life of patients. It was self-evident that the implementation of such holistic frameworks into practice required access to accurate information relevant to the different care processes. Not only such data should be condition specific but should be also standardized [12].

Health outcome measures have been collected and have been used for managing patients [36] for several decades. Accepting the claim by Porter in 2010 [30] that "Outcomes are the true measures of quality in health care" then measuring outcomes is indeed critical for assessing and maintaining the standard of quality of care provided to its prime.

Upon agreement that standardized health outcome measures were required to implement and maintain any healthcare improvement action [32] in any holistic manner, healthcare organizations collaborated and formed the International Consortium for Health Outcome Measures (ICHOM) in 2012. Since then, through a global collaboration effort ICHOM has developed more than 30 standardized sets of health outcomes measures with an evident patient-centric perspective.

ICHOM has identified and defined disease specific sets of clinical and Patient-Reported Outcomes Measures (PROMs), as well as Patient-Reported Experience Measures (PREMs) relevant for assessing value using outcomes that matter to patients and by doing so ICHOM has significantly contributed to spread the meaning of VALUE as the most comprehensive definition combining healthcare that matters to the patients with the cost along the entire cycle of care. This way unifying in a practical manner the conceptual frameworks proposed in VBHC and the multiple AIM of healthcare originally proposed by IHI.

2.2.2   *Digital Health Transformation*

Society as a whole and through specific branches has benefited from the application of advances in data storage, display technology, computing capacity and mobile data communications among others during more than a century, but specially in the two last decades. Despite that digital transformation is based on technological advances, it is not actually driven by technology but through the strategy of organizations aiming to meet certain needs or overcome specific challenges. The transformative power of novel technologies does not come from the enabling technologies but from the significance of the needs pulling for adopting given technological solutions, where disruptive innovation can multiply exponentially the value [22].

Table 2.2 Elements demanding a digital health transformation

Element	Constraints on Healthcare system		
	Patient	Cost	Quality
Population growth	Reduce access to care	Increase cost	Less time with patient
Increased patient demands	Demands better outcome	May lead to cost increase	Increase likelihood to perceive poor experience
Increased life expectancy	Increased likelihood to require care interventions	Increase cost	
Larger proportion of chronic patients	Patient required medical attention for life	Increase cost	Increase complexity of care delivery
Increased co-morbidities among chronic patient	Increased complexity of care	Increase cost per patient	
Care cost increase	Less budget available per patient		Less resources available
Inequity in care	Risk in drop in quality		Large variability

During the last 30 years a number of issues (see Table 2.2) have risen, demanding for changes in healthcare delivery of such magnitude that instead of changes it is actually a full transformation that is required, a transformation that can only be achieved through a paradigm shift (and thinking positively, the COVID-19 pandemic has pushed intensively towards such direction, forcing some of such expected changes).

As shown in Table 2.2, all changes, involve information: medical, clinical financial or patient-reported information and data. Basically, every single aspect of data is involved: collecting, storage, access, analysis, visualization, sharing, protecting etc. All the changes required to make future healthcare sustainable are data-related, consequently the seek transformation must be digital.

2.2.3 IT Infrastructure as Enabling Agent of Digital Transformation

The role of IT infrastructure and IT systems in health care has changed significantly in last decades. From originally heavily devoted to host the electronic patient record, basically just collecting the minimum necessary patient data and providing clinicians with limited access to patient data. IT systems at hospitals evolved to computer networks interconnecting the hospital databases, ensuring access to health-related data across the hospital and enabling information services to benefit all levels of the health care system [14].

Nowadays, IT systems at hospitals should focus mainly on data management, including data collection, data sharing, data presentation, preserving security and privacy while providing the data infrastructure required to leverage data analytics for both managerial, clinical and medical purposes. It is precisely the availability of high quality, relevant and shareable data, one of the factors digital healthcare transformation and consequently IT systems have become the core of the ongoing paradigm shift in healthcare.

2.2.4   Artificial Intelligence Widely Available for Contributing to the Transformation

Another enabling factor catalyzing digital transformation is Artificial Intelligence (AI). For over 40 years AI has been applied into medicine through the so-called Computer-Aided medical Diagnostics [1, 28] or Expert Systems [26, 40], but it has been during the last 10 years that AI has been incorporated into any future healthcare strategy. Such development has not been driven by only the strong pull of the market in need to meet increasing demands in number, expectations and complexity, but also by two very important facts:

- **Overwhelming number of success cases of AI analytics outside healthcare.** For over 40 years, enterprises have benefited from all sort of rule-based decision support [39] systems first, statistical descriptive analytics later and machine learning-based prediction analytics last. AI applications have showed their benefits through society from extremely application specific e.g. Identification of flicker disturbances in power quality [2], quality improvement in product manufacturing [23] to generic-daily life situations e.g. smartphone key typing [3], faceID unlocking tablets [6], best traffic route provided by google maps. Therefore, it is very well proven what AI-boosted analytics can do in basically any data-driven scenario.
- **The Birth of Big data.** The rapid expanding of big data through all branches of science, engineering [47] and business [25] fuelled by the emergence of the data scientist [11, 46] and the quick development of platforms for data management and cloud computing [20] like Hadoop prepared the runaway for AI predictive analytics to take off.

Through the years several different definitions have been given to AI, currently the official definition given by the EU parliament is the following "AI is the capability of a computer program to perform tasks or reasoning processes that we usually associate with intelligence in a human being." In the right conditions, that is with accurate and trustable data available, AI solutions can have a significant impact in several areas of healthcare [21], see Table 2.3. AI enabling (1) improvement of

Table 2.3 Mapping AI potential impact areas with current constraint dimensions in Healthcare

Healthcare area	Cost	Quality	Patient
Self-care, prevention and wellness	x	x	x
Triage and diagnosis		x	
Diagnostics	x	x	
Chronic care management	x	x	x
Care delivery		x	
Clinical decision support		x	x

population-health management, (2) improvement of operations and (3) strengthening innovation would most likely will contribute to the revolution required to ensure future sustainability of the healthcare systems.

When mapping these potential areas where AI can make a difference with the constraints in healthcare imposed by the elements demanding a digital health transformation listed in Table 2.2, it is possible to identify a large overlap that indicates the true transformative power of AI in Healthcare.

2.3 Challenges and Adoption Barriers to Digital Healthcare Transformation

Despite the strong pull from the healthcare systems with needs specifically demanding solutions with the transformative power of digital technologies, there are all sort of implementation challenges, organizational hurdles and acceptance barriers stopping to fully embrace digital healthcare transformation just yet.

Many of those challenges and hurdles [24] are generally related to incorporating digital technologies and implementation novel data management approaches within hospital operation and clinical practice but others are specifically related to aspects of AI.

2.3.1 Data Management Clash

Availability of all sort of data, patient, operational, financial, medical, is one of the catalyzers behind digital transformation, but patient privacy from one side and data interoperability [18, 27] issues from another are slowing down adoption of digital healthcare.

Legislation to enforce patient privacy should be in place, and in Europe, the GDPR has precisely defined it to preserve the privacy of everyone in the current information era. Unfortunately for Big Data Analytics in healthcare, GDPR is limiting heavily potential applications at the moment due to uncertainties from legal stand points of what can be done or not with certain data and how and in which way it should be interpreted to preserve the legal framework defined by GDPR [9]. This caution has resorted in many healthcare organizations through Europe to complete standstill, awaiting for other first adopters to present viable solutions, or specific guidelines from European or national authorities about how AI and big data analytics should be implemented under the umbrella of GDPR.

The true potential of big data AI-driven analytics requires that all sort of data is collected, stored, computed and visualized in completely different IT systems, that implies that data is shareable through the IT systems. Unfortunately, that is not the case in most of practical scenarios. Despite important initiatives to define interoperability frameworks for data sharing, currently, old legacy systems remain being active and used among hospitals all over the world slowing down the path to the digital healthcare transformation journey.

2.3.2   Organizational Self-awareness for Digital Adoption Readiness

The journey towards digital health transformation requires to interconnect many different dimensions within a care organization and requires certain level of readiness across the whole organization to implement any data analytics strategy, otherwise the implementation will fail and the potential benefits will not be achieved. The depth of such interrelation required to successfully implement any given data analytics solution is commonly underestimated, between the manual collection of a given parameter during daily routine to the availability of such value in a database of a hospital information system may pass days even weeks. Moreover, just because the parameters are digitalized, further data manipulation might be required due to incompatibility issues and lack of interoperability.

2.3.3   Inherent Risks of AI

Data analytics boosted by AI is certainly very useful but even when used to analyze what happens it is not infallible and is subjected to external factors, human error often. When AI is boosting predictive data analytics, the source of error might not be only external but inherent to the core fundamentals of AI.

One of the fundamental pillars of AI is a strong statistical core, the more solid the statistics available for an application the more accurate the analysis will be done and the more certain the predictions. It happens that when the number of cases are low the supporting statistics will be poor and the produced prediction will not be reliable. Inconveniently, in medical care when a practitioner is unsure and requires support this is often not with common everyday cases, where AI-support potentially will perform at its best, but with odd and complex cases, for which AI predictions will fail most often. Such kind of performance issue when AI is needed the most, creates a bad reputation and produces mistrust among practitioners that will impact their acceptance.

Limited traceability is also a common and significant downfall when dealing with machine learning based algorithms. In medical care patient safety and quality of care in general are critical factors driving clinical operations. Therefore, when there is a failure, sources must be identified, and measures should be taken to prevent the same failure to occur again. While the learning capacity of AI systems will potentially and eventually deal after several failures, preventing the miss-judgement, the opacity of [35] black-box model at the core of the most of AI algorithms will make it impossible to trace back the stage within the algorithm that failed and led to a wrong prediction. Nowadays in normal circumstance in clinical practice it is not acceptable to work with a tool that if it fails, the source for the failure cannot be located.

The inherent probability of an error in certain circumstances, and the lack of the true understanding of the underlying process at the core of the AI process, will impact heavily the acceptance of most clinicians to adopt the use of these tools into clinical practice.

Even in organizations with high data analytics maturity and strong user pull to incorporate already-proven innovative technologies, and even when considering the current landscape of AI solutions provided by trust-worthy vendors of established reputation, the task of selecting the most appropriate technological solution is tedious and complex, and requires a careful planning incorporating a holistic approach.

2.3.4   Actions to Reduce Challenges, Hurdles and Barriers

The shadow casted by the relatively novelty of the GDPR over healthcare organization requires certain guidelines with clear examples from the responsible authorities or the development of best practice guidelines to enlighten up the journey.

A well-thought strategy to implement digital health transformation accounting for all aspects intertwined with the future implementation steps required to take would definitely facilitate the digitalization journey. Such a strategy should be designed according to the maturity level of the organization for adopting data analytics and the implementation should be paced accordingly to the progression of the maturity level for adopting data analytics of the healthcare organization.

For nearly a decade ago, HIMSS, the Healthcare Information and Management Systems Society, developed the adoption model for analytics maturity (AMAM) and has been using it to support healthcare organizations to evaluate and advance their own analytics capabilities. HIMSS in a new effort to support healthcare organizations to eliminate organizational challenges and technology readiness barriers has just launched the HIMSS Digital Health Framework [42] and the Digital Health Indicator.

A framework based on the seven maturity levels developed by HIMSS and an indicator to measure progress towards a digital health ecosystem by measuring both operational features of digital health systems, as well as transformation of digital care delivery.

The trust of clinicians and medical managers is critical to increase the acceptance of AI solutions within healthcare. Education actions targeted to improve the understanding of the black-box engine driving the AI algorithms would increase the technology readiness of users and decision makers but the true impact on improving understandability among clinical stakeholders would come from using understandable AI methods with an inclusive methodology engaging the clinician in the whole AI modelling process.

Under the umbrella of Artificial Intelligence and information theory, Process Mining [45] is a research discipline that uses existing information to create human-understandable views that support healthcare stakeholders in enhancing their insight in the clinical process. One of the distinct features of process mining is that it focuses on the analysis of logs of activities from process creating visual models. The direct visualization of the modeling output and direct connection of the model elements with the source provides the method with a transparency that allows to identify causality and enhance traceability. Such transparency is the opposite of a black box model and it is an incentive for users in the health care field, demanding to be able to inspect the inside of analytical and predictive core.

A novel interactive process mining methodology [15] has been developed that specifically requires the engagement of the clinicians in the extraction of the operational model. Such engagement provides the clinician with insights about the internal functioning of the analysis phase that preserve their trust, wondering the reasons and engaging them in the continuous improvement loop, following a question-based methodology [37].

Another initial advantage intrinsic to process mining analysis methods is that the object of study are processes from events logs not patient data per se, therefore reducing constraints imposed by preserving privacy.

Availability of evidence is critical to reach an acceptance across the health and medical care community, therefore a well-documented catalogue of success cases of improving healthcare through assessing value for patients using digital health solutions is required.

Giving the need for healthcare improvement with a holistic perspective and the target pursued by process mining, improvement of output based on the key performance processes, seems like a match difficult to overlook.

2.4   Summary

Medical care has been patient centered from the origin and has evolved closely along the evolution of patient needs from the patient as individual to the patient as population, pursuing to provide the medical care of the highest quality standard.

The holistic unification of patient individual health and patient population approaches through health and patient outcomes as predicted by Cairns back in 1996 [7] and has been catalysed first by the availability of information technologies and then the rising and development of VBHC.

Considering value in VBHC as achieving the best outcomes from the perspective of the patient versus executing the care process needed to achieve these outcomes in the most optimal way. It is of paramount importance to identify and understand the processes to be improved in order to be able to improve the outcomes.

Digital health tools enable deployment of information services and data analysis technologies like process mining precisely adequate for discovery, analysis and optimizing of the operational models underlying the actual care processes.

Despite that the undergoing transformational change is pulled by global needs and driven by information technologies, data availability and data science, the journey ahead for digital health transformation is full of all sort of barriers: regulatory, clinical adoption, medical trust, and patient acceptance.

References

1. Adams JB. A probability model of medical reasoning and themycin model. Math Biosci. 1976;32(1–2):177–86.
2. Axelberg PGV, Bollen MHJ, Yu-Hua Gu I. Trace of flicker sources by using the quantity of flicker power. IEEE Trans Power Delivery. 2007;23(1):465–71.
3. Balakrishnan A. How the first iphone blew the blackberry away with an amazingly accurate on-screen keyboard, 26 June 2017; 2017.
4. Berwick DM, Nolan TW, Whittington J. The triple aim: care, health, and cost. Health Aff. 2008;27(3):759–69.
5. Bodenheimer T, Sinsky C. From triple to quadruple aim: care of the patient requires care of the provider. Ann Fam Med. 2014;12(6):573–6.
6. Bud A. Facing the future: the impact of apple faceid. Biom Technol Today. 2018;2018(1):5–7.
7. Cairns J. Measuring health outcomes, 1996.
8. Capko J. The patient-centered movement. J Med Pract Manage. 2014;29(4):238.
9. Cole A, Towse A, et al. Legal barriers to the better use of health data to deliver pharmaceutical innovation. London: Office of Health Economics; 2018.
10. European Commission. Expert panel on effective ways of investing in health. opinion on defining value in "value-based healthcare", 2019.
11. Davenport TH, Patil DJ. Data scientist. Harv Bus Rev. 2012;90(5):70–6.
12. Deerberg-Wittram J, Guth C, Porter ME. Value-based competition: the role of outcome measurement. In: Public health forum, vol. 21. De Gruyter; 2013, p. 12–3.
13. EFPIA. Value-based healthcare – an industry perspective. 24 June 2019, 2019.
14. Egan GF, Liu Z-Q. Computers and networks in medical and healthcare systems. Comput Biol Med. 1995;25(3):355–65.
15. Fernandez-Llatas C, Bayo JL, Martinez-Romero A, Benedí JM, Traver V. Interactive pattern recognition in cardiovascular disease management. a process mining approach. In: 2016 IEEE-EMBS international conference on biomedical and health informatics (BHI). IEEE, 2016, p. 348–51.
16. Gerecke G, Clawson J, Verboven Y. Procurement: the unexpected driver of value-based health care. Boston: Boston Consulting Group; 2015.
17. Gray JM, Abbasi K. How to get better value healthcare. J R Soc Med. 2007;100(10):480.

18. Greenlaw R, Scholl S. Interaction design patterns for using emergent in social apps. Hum Factors. 2014;37(1):65–84.
19. Evidence-Based Medicine Working Group et al. Evidence-based medicine. a new approach to teaching the practice of medicine. Jama. 1992;268(17):2420.
20. Abaker Targio Hashem I, Yaqoob I, Anuar NB, Mokhtar S, Gani A, Khan SU. The rise of "big data" on cloud computing: review and open research issues. Inf Syst. 2015;47:98–115.
21. EIT HEALTH. Transforming healthcare with ai. March 2020, 2020.
22. Hwang J, Christensen CM. Disruptive innovation in health care delivery: a framework for business-model innovation. Health Aff. 2008;27(5):1329–35.
23. Köksal G, Batmaz İ, Testik MC. A review of data mining applications for quality improvement in manufacturing industry. Expert Syst Appl. 2011;38(10):13448–67.
24. Kruse CS, Goswamy R, Raval YJ, Marawi S. Challenges and opportunities of big data in health care: a systematic review. JMIR Med Inform. 2016;4(4):e38.
25. McAfee A, Brynjolfsson E, Davenport TH, Patil DJ, Barton D. Big data: the management revolution. Harv Bus Rev. 2012;90(10):60–8.
26. Miller RA, Pople Jr HE, Myers JD. Internist-i, an experimental computer-based diagnostic consultant for general internal medicine. N Engl J Med. 1982;307(8):468–76.
27. Nohl-Deryk P, Brinkmann JK, Gerlach FM, Schreyögg J, Achelrod D. Barriers to digitalisation of healthcare in germany: a survey of experts. Gesundheitswesen (Bundesverband Der Arzte Des Offentlichen Gesundheitsdienstes (Germany)) 2018;80(11):939–45.
28. Pauker SG, Gorry GA, Kassirer JP, Schwartz WB. Towards the simulation of clinical cognition: taking a present illness by computer. Am J Med. 1976;60(7):981–96.
29. Porter ME. Defining and introducing value in health care. In: Evidence-based medicine and the changing nature of health care: 2007 IOM annual meeting summary. Institute of Medicine Washington, DC, 2008, p. 161–72.
30. Porter ME. Measuring health outcomes: the outcomes hierarchy. N Engl J Med. 2010;363:2477–81.
31. Porter ME, et al. What is value in health care. N Engl J Med. 2010;363(26):2477–81.
32. Porter ME, Lee TH. The strategy that will fix health care. Harv Bus Rev. 2013;91(10):1–19.
33. Porter ME, Teisberg EO. Redefining competition in health care. Harv Bus Rev. 2004;82:64–77.
34. Porter ME, Teisberg EO. Redefining health care: creating value-based competition on results. Harvard Business Press; 2006.
35. Nicholson Price II W. Black-box medicine. Harv J Law Technol. 2014;28:419.
36. Roach KE. Measurement of health outcomes: reliability, validity and responsiveness. JPO J Prosthet Orthot. 2006;18(6):P8–12.
37. Rojas E, Sepúlveda M, Munoz-Gama J, Capurro D, Traver V, Fernandez-Llatas C. Question-driven methodology for analyzing emergency room processes using process mining. Appl Sci. 2017;7(3):302.
38. Sackett DL, Rosenberg WMC, Muir Gray JA, Brian Haynes R, Scott Richardson W. Evidence based medicine. Br Med J. 1996;313(7050):170.
39. Scott-Morton MS, Keen PGW. Decision support systems: an organizational perspective. Reading: Addison-Wesley; 1978.
40. Shortliffe EH. Medical expert systems—knowledge tools for physicians. West J Med. 1986;145(6):830.
41. Sikka R, Morath JM, Leape L. The quadruple aim: care, health, cost and meaning in work. BMJ Qual Saf. 2015;24:608–10.
42. Snowdon A. White paper 2020. digital health: a framework for healthcare transformation, 2020.
43. Stewart M, Brown JB, Weston WW, McWhinney IR, McWilliam CL, Freeman TR. Patient-centered medicine: transforming the clinical method. 1995. Sage Publications: Thousands Oaks. Amin Z Ambulatory care education. Singap Med J. 1999;12:760–3.
44. Tulchinsky TH, Varavikova EA. The new public health. Academic; 2014.
45. Van Der Aalst W. Data science in action. In: Process mining. Springer; 2016, p. 3–23.

46. Van der Aalst WMP. Data scientist: the engineer of the future. In: Enterprise interoperability VI. Springer, 2014, p. 13–26.
47. Wu X, Zhu X, Gong-Qing Wu, Ding W. Data mining with big data. IEEE Trans Knowl Data Eng. 2013;26(1):97–107.

Chapter 3
Towards a Knowledge and Data-Driven Perspective in Medical Processes

Carlos Fernandez-Llatas and Mar Marcos

3.1 Introduction

Healthcare is one of the most challenging problems that our society is facing currently. The population of the world is growing around 1% per year [33]. In addition, the expectancy of life is increasing thanks to the new advances and the better quality of health solutions. For this reason, people are reaching older ages, which entails more chronic illnesses, with more co-morbidities. This supposes a great increase in the complexity of the illnesses. In addition, thanks to the new age of internet patients are more aware of their illnesses, having higher expectations of the health system. Altogether, this causes a great impact in the sustainability of healthcare, which should cover this scenario with the same budget. This juncture is demanding a new paradigm that will be able to deal with the complexity and continuous changes in the health domain in the coming years, in order to guarantee the sustainability of the system.

From the 1990s, when the Evidence-Based Medicine paradigm emerged [35], there has been an increasing interest in providing tools for empowering health professionals in the application of new methodologies and paradigms that could solve this problem. Sacket defined Evidence-Based Medicine as the *"conscientious, explicit, and judicious use of current best evidence in making decisions about*

C. Fernandez-Llatas (✉)
Process Mining 4 Health Lab – SABIEN – ITACA Institute, Universitat Politècnica de València, Valencia, Spain

CLINTEC – Karolinska Institutet, Sweden
e-mail: cfllatas@itaca.upv.es

M. Marcos
Department of Computer Engineering and Science, Universitat Jaume I, Castelló de la Plana, Castelló, Spain
e-mail: mar.marcos@uji.es

the care of individual patients" [35]. This paradigm tried to unify knowledge gathered from the best research evidence (what the literature says), with the clinical experience (what the clinician knows), centered in providing the best experience to the patient (what the patient wants). In this scenario, the idea of creating formalized processes that support the daily clinical practice with the best evidence available arises. In this scenario, the idea of creating formalized processes (or protocols) that support the daily clinical practice with the best evidence available arises. It promotes the formalization of clinical research results so that they can be applied in daily practice by clinical professionals. This is done through the specification of protocols that are thought to be well-defined standards of care. In this line, these protocols can serve to improve the clinical effectiveness, provide solutions for risk management, and trace the actual care process to reduce the variability of the treatments in healthcare.

In the literature there are different approaches for the definition of such formalized processes. The aim of this chapter is to analyse the most prominent approaches for supporting clinical experts in the representation of medical processes. First, the two process-related perspectives in healthcare (which we have named as patient & process centered and clinician & knowledge centered, respectively) are presented and compared. Moreover, the different instruments developed by the medical profession related to this concept are described. After that, the two main approaches available in the literature for building medical processes are reviewed: on one hand, knowledge-driven Clinical Decision-Making technologies, and, on the other hand, Clinical Process Management technologies, which rely on a data-driven approach. Finally, the concluding section discusses new challenges towards the formalization of medical processes leveraging the advantages of these two technologies.

3.2   Process-Related Perspectives in Healthcare

Health systems are struggling to meet the growing demand for healthcare services from ageing population while maintaining consistent quality standards. As Peleg and González-Ferrer point out, two strategies are being used for this purpose, both sharing a process-based perspective [30]. One strategy focuses on improving the management of the processes (e.g. interventions, interactions) that the patient goes through in relation to a clinical encounter. The other strategy concentrates on supporting decision making by the clinician at the point of care using specific-purpose tools (i.e. dedicated to a specific medical condition) that incorporate knowledge about clinical processes. This knowledge is mostly based on the best evidence available that can be found in documents such as clinical practice guidelines, but can also refer to medical background knowledge contained in textbooks and manuals. The former strategy takes the perspective of the patient journey and considers organizational issues of healthcare processes, including the coordination of multidisciplinary teams and the allocation of resources, and thus can be described as *patient & process centered*. In contrast, the latter strategy focuses on the perspective of the clinician when managing an individual patient, with an

Table 3.1 Summary of the features of the *clinician & knowledge centered* (CKC) and *patient & process centered* (PPC) strategies in healthcare

Strategies / Features	CKC	PPC
Main subject	Health professional	Patient
Main process	Health professional's actions and decisions	Patient journey
Patients	Individual patient	Multiple patients
Health professionals	Individual health professional	Multidisciplinary health team
Diseases	Single disease	Single or multi-disease
Main usage	Prescriptive	Analytical
Orientation	Knowledge-driven	Knowledge or data-driven

emphasis on knowledge-intensive decision tasks, therefore it might be considered as *clinician & knowledge centered*.

There exist significant differences in how the previous strategies can be exploited in the healthcare context. Most notably, the clinician & knowledge centered (CKC) strategy, relying on the recommendations issued by medical experts, can be used to determine *what should be performed* (or *what is prescribed*) given the specific clinical circumstances of a patient, typically in the context of a single disease. On the other hand, the patient & process centered (PPC) strategy can be applied to inspect *what has been performed* and makes it possible e.g. to monitor the itinerary (or itineraries) actually followed by patients with a particular clinical profile, possibly involving multiple diseases. In other words, the usage of the CKC strategy would be primarily prescriptive, whereas that of the PPC one would be analytical. Lastly, the two strategies may differ in their positioning with respect to knowledge and data. Although a knowledge-driven orientation can be taken in both cases, in the case of the PPC strategy the use of process models obtained from clinical data in the Electronic Health Record, i.e. a data-driven orientation, is a common practice. Table 3.1 summarises the main characteristics (and differences) of these strategies.

The instruments developed by the medical profession to support the concept of consistent and high-quality healthcare are very much related to what has been exposed. *Clinical Practice Guidelines (CPGs)* are the core instrument. According to the most recent definition, CPGs are defined as *"statements that include recommendations intended to optimize patient care that are informed by a systematic review of evidence and an assessment of the benefits and harms of alternative care options"* [15]. In line with the view of Evidence-Based Medicine, the development of CPGs is usually commissioned to a group of experts who are responsible for collecting and analysing the best and most up-to-date evidence about a particular clinical condition, and for agreeing a set of general recommendations regarding the main management aspects thereof.

Clinical Protocols are related yet distinct from CPGs. A clinical protocol is a locally agreed statement about a specific clinical issue with steps based on CPGs and/or organizational consensus [2]. Usually, clinical protocols are specific to a

health organization. *Care Pathways* likewise adapt CPG recommendations to the
needs and particularities of a health organization. Thus, both clinical protocols and
care pathways can be regarded as instruments for the implementation at local level
of the evidence base from CPGs. However, care pathways differ in that they describe
many more aspects (and in more detail), including: an explicit statement of the goals
and key elements of care when solving one or several clinical issues, the description
of the communication among the care team members and with patients and their
families, and the specification of the coordination aspects of the care process (with
roles, sequencing of decisions and actions, etc.) [36]. Care pathways also define
the information to be recorded so that it is possible to monitor deviations of the
actual care with respect to the recommended procedure. *Clinical Pathways (CPs)*
in turn differ from care pathways in that they are confined to the paths within a
hospital, i.e. excluding outpatient clinic and follow-up activities. Common to most
of the concepts, it is possible to distinguish the general instrument (template) from
the versions adapted to the values and preferences of the patient, giving rise e.g.
to "personalised care pathways". Figure 3.1 depicts the relationships among these
concepts.

As explained before, the CKC strategy strongly relies on knowledge about
clinical processes and decisions. Most typically, CPGs are used as source for such
knowledge. For their part, CPs (and pathways in general) are very well suited for the
purposes of the PPC strategy, due to their focus on the monitoring of care processes.
Naturally, CPGs have a knowledge-driven orientation, whereas either a knowledge-
driven or a data-driven orientation can be adopted for CPs.

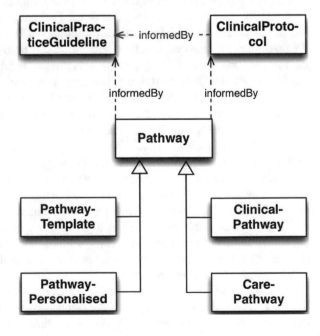

Fig. 3.1 Relationships between clinical practice guidelines, clinical protocols, and pathways, including pathway variations. (Adapted from Figure 1 in Benson's article [2])

3.3   Technologies for Clinical Decision-Making

3.3.1   Computer-Interpretable Guidelines

CPGs have shown the potential to foster the translation of clinical research results into practice, and to improve the quality and outcomes of healthcare. However, the practical utility of CPGs is often hindered by the text-based format in which they are predominantly disseminated. Another problem is their emphasis on the general principles of care, rather than on the actual processes along the patient journey [30]. In this context, *Computer-Interpretable Guidelines (CIGs)* emerge as a tool to make patient-customized CPG recommendations available to clinicians in an easier and more immediate way, compared to text-based CPGs. Thus, CIGs can be defined as formalized versions of CPG contents intended to be used as decision-support systems. The beneficial effects of the use of CIGs in the clinical setting have been documented in the literature, and include improved CPG adherence and increased efficiency of the healthcare processes (e.g. thanks to the reduction of unnecessary test requests) [20].

Several CIG representation languages have been proposed in the fields of Artificial Intelligence in Medicine and Medical Informatics, the most prominent of which are Arden Syntax, PROforma, Asbru, EON, GLIF, and GUIDE [5, 31]. CPGs contain a wealth of knowledge of diverse types. To accommodate this variety, CIG languages provide a wide range of modelling constructs. Peleg et al. recognize two main representational categories, namely structuring in plans of decisions and actions, and linking to patient data and medical concepts, and identify a total of eight dimensions within them [31]. These dimensions are: (1) organization of plans, (2) goals, (3) action model, (4) decision model, (5) expression language, (6) data interpretation/abstraction, (7) medical concept model, and (8) patient model.

Many of the CIG languages take an approach to the description of plans (above dimensions (1) through (4)) which has been named *Task-Network Model (TNM)*. The TNM approach consists in describing guidelines in terms of a hierarchical decomposition of networks of component tasks. The task types, as well as the types of control-flow constructs (sequence, in parallel, etc.), vary in the different TNM approaches. Still, all of them provide support for actions, decisions and nested tasks. A highly distinctive feature of CIG languages lies in the decision model. In this regard, PROforma's decision model, which was subsequently adopted by other CIG languages, deserves a special mention. In PROforma, decisions are described in terms of the alternative options (or candidates) considered, each one with an associated set of arguments. These arguments are logical conditions that, when they are met, provide different kinds of support for the candidate, namely for, against, confirming or excluding the candidate.

As an illustration, Fig. 3.2 shows a PROforma excerpt corresponding to the algorithm for the diagnosis of heart failure in the non-acute setting [23], based on the 2016 guidelines of the European Society of Cardiology. It comes as no surprise that, although CIG languages were specifically geared for CPGs, they have also

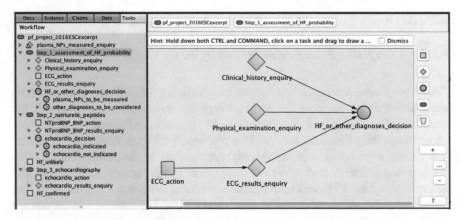

Fig. 3.2 PROforma model for the diagnosis of heart failure in the non-acute setting [23]. To the left, task tree representing the hierarchical decomposition of tasks; to the right, task network corresponding to the plan `Step_1_assessment_of_HF_probability` (first step of diagnosis), including action, enquiry and decision tasks

proven to be useful for modelling and supporting complex clinical processes from a broad spectrum. This includes care pathways for different purposes, e.g. for the management of triple assessment in breast cancer [28] or for the monitoring of patients with multiple comorbidities [21].

3.3.2 Development and Maintenance Issues with Computer-Interpretable Guidelines

The representational richness of CIG languages makes them difficult to use (not to mention mastering them) for non-technical users like clinicians. Furthermore, it is well recognized that CPG knowledge is intrinsically complex and hence difficult to comprehend and formalize [19]. As a consequence of these factors, the encoding of CPG knowledge in a CIG language is a difficult and labour-intensive task which requires the joint collaboration of both clinical and IT professionals. On the one hand, clinical expertise is essential for a complete and adequate understanding of CPG recommendations. On the other hand, IT skills are required to analyse the clinical processes they include, as well as to shape them in terms of the constructs of the CIG language chosen [25]. This explains why the topic of CIG knowledge acquisition and specification has been the focus of a large number of research works in the literature. Concretely, in relation with the life-cycle of CIG development, knowledge acquisition and specification is the topic to which more efforts have been devoted, after CIG languages [29]. Noteworthy among these approaches are the application of cognitive methodologies to guide the encoding of CPGs into CIGs, and the use of pattern-based information extraction methods to support the translation of CPG texts into a semi-structured format. Despite these efforts, CIG development tasks remain largely manual. This may lead to a significant delay between the time when a CPG is issued and the time when a fully functional and validated CIG is ready for its implementation, which could be unacceptable from a clinical perspective.

Once implemented, CIGs necessitate some kind of quality control to determine whether the impact they have on the healthcare processes is as expected. The aim of clinical decision support systems in general, and of CIGs in particular, is to improve the quality, safety and cost-effectiveness of care processes. A monitoring of evidence-grounded quality metrics, together with an appropriate feedback to the health organization, can serve as a stimulus for process improvement [8]. Quality metrics provide a framework for comparison, e.g. to detect outlier cases in which CPG recommendations have not been followed. Such cases may point to procedure parts where modifications should be considered. CIG compliance analysis has been the topic of a number of works in the literature [29]. There are two types of approaches for evaluating compliance with CIGs: approaches directly comparing the concrete actions performed by the physician, and those comparing the actual processes discovered from clinical activity logs using Process Mining methods. The former range from informal (manual) methods to more formal methods based e.g. on model checking. The approaches based on Process Mining methods have recently attracted growing interest because of their potential to recognize variations with respect to the prescriptive process embodied in CIGs.

3.4 Technologies for Clinical Process Management

3.4.1 Process Discovery and Continuous Improvement

Due to the difficulties of the manual development process of CPGs, data-driven approaches have emerged in the literature for supporting health experts in the definition of guidelines. Data-driven models use the data available in healthcare databases to infer the underlying processes and thereby provide Decision Support Systems without the need for a purely manual development by clinical experts. The idea is to develop algorithms that discover automatically such underlying processes.

Data-driven solutions have been used successfully for the automatic learning of models that can support experts in different fields. With this aim, different approaches within this paradigm have been applied to the medicine domain. One of the most common approach is the creation of classifiers for supporting in the daily decisions [40]. However, these tools do not provide a process view. These systems only provide a statistical probability of the current status of the patient at a certain moment in time. Other options, like Temporal Abstractions [4], offer a vision about the trends in the biomedical signals that enable a dynamic measure of the patient status. However, although these techniques can be incorporated in the CKC or PPC strategies, they do not allow to discover the rules behind the progression of the disease in the patient.

Other works have tried to discover the behaviour of the medical processes by inferring their inherent rules using information routinely collected in healthcare databases [6]. However, from a process management perspective, these rules do not provide the natural view of the process as it is provided by workflows. This fact has a negative impact on the understandability of these systems, which as a consequence usually appear as *black boxes* in the eyes of medical practitioners.

Process Mining appears in the middle of this juncture [38]. This paradigm uses time-stamped events existing in healthcare databases to offer a workflow-based view. Using these techniques, there are works providing tools to infer the underlying medical process, offering partial patterns [18], general patterns avoiding infrequent behavior [17], or complete views of CP [11, 39]. But Process Mining is not only about the discovery of processes. Process Mining aims to provide a complete set of technologies for supporting medical professionals not only in the process design phase but also in the traceability, analysis and optimization of the process deployed. Health systems produce continuous data flow that can be used for analyzing how the processes behave in actual scenarios [9]. With that, it is possible not only to show a snapshot of the pathway, but also to make a comparison over time to discover any variation of the medical procedures, e.g. due to the application of new protocols [3, 32].

Figure 3.3 shows an example of how Process Mining can represent the processes inferred from data available in medical databases. This process represents the flow of patients in a surgery area, and was automatically inferred from real data in existing databases [9]. The model not only represents the flow of the process but, also, colours represent the performance in their execution. This information can be crucial for a better understanding of how processes are deployed in a real scenario.

These technologies can be applied in a iterative way allowing for a continuous optimization of the process [12]. This allows the user not only an easier design of the process, but also an iterative adaption of the process that converges to the best optimized solution.

3.4.2 Workflow Inference Models

For achieving an adequate process standardization, algorithms should provide formal models that can be used for standardize the care. In this line, The Business Process Management (BPM) field [7] aims to offer solutions for supporting the creation of those processes in a general-purpose way. In this way, the concept of *Workflow* is proposed. The Workflow Management Coalition defines it as *"the computerised facilitation or automation of a business process, in whole or part"* [16]. In other words, a Workflow is a formal specification designed to automate a process. Process Mining provides tools for building Workflows from events existing in medical databases.

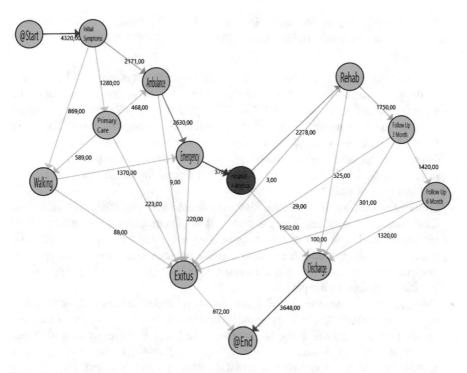

Fig. 3.3 Process inferred using a Process Mining Discovery algorithm. The colours of the nodes represent the average Length of Stay in each one of the stages, and the colours in the arcs represent the percentage of patients that follows each path

Workflows are designed to deal with process standardization via the definition of graphical structures, without ambiguities and focused on their automation, with a view towards automatic guidance by computer systems or replication by human experts. Workflows are devised for supporting the design of a process that: (1) needs high-level legibility, intended to be understood by human experts, not only for its creation but also for its optimization; (2) requires traceability, to make possible a continuous analysis of the current status of the process flow; and (3) guides users over a set of steps, allowing them to know the trace of the process flow to the current status and showing the possibilities after it.

BPM techniques have been tested in the medical field for representing clinical workflows. In this line, there are some works in the literature dealing with different Workflow models. Some works use well known mathematical representation languages like: Petri Nets [22, 32]; Deterministic Finite Automatons (DFA) or graphs [26]; other more specific formal mathematical models like Timed Parallel Automatons (TPA) [10]; and other models specifically created for increasing the understandability like the Business Process Management Notation (BPMN) [27].

To select an adequate Workflow Language for each problem it is necessary to analyze its characteristics. In healthcare, three characteristics should be taken into account [10]:

- **Expressivity**. It is the capability for representing all the dynamic flow behaviours of the processes in the field. This characteristic can be measured thanks to the so-called *Workflow Patterns* [34]. Workflow patterns are different situations that are possible in a process (sequences, parallelism, milestones, etc.). The more workflow patterns a language can express, the best expressivity it has. The objective is to have the best language able to express all the possible patterns in each medical field. Otherwise, the lack of expressivity can result in inaccurate and ambiguous models.
- **Understandability**. It represents how easy to read and understand is a language. Clinicians are not IT engineers and not all the languages are suitable for them to comprehend. The lack of understandability increases the risk of rejection by the clinician. Even worst, it can result in inaccuracies and errors in the models' design that could not only make the system to fail but also lead to an inappropriate recommendation for the patient.
- **Complexity**. The complexity of a language is related to the quantity of information that it conveys and how computers can process it. This complexity depends on the grammar on which the language is based. The complexity of a grammar has an influence on its interaction with computers. It is well known in compilation theory that the more complex a language of a specific grammar is, the more difficult it is to process and interpret it [1]. A complex language is harder to execute and to infer using data-driven techniques. So, the more complex a language is, the more difficult it is to create applications to understand it and to create data-driven accurate models without the use of heuristics.

Selecting the best language for a specific field requires a trade-off between having the desired expressivity, while maximizing the understandability and keeping the least possible complexity. For example, Petri Nets are probably the most expressive language for representing any kind of process, but the difficulty for clinicians to understand it and its complexity makes it necessary to use heuristics for the inference algorithm. On the other hand, DFA has a very low complexity and this allows an easy interpretation and very powerful techniques for inference. It is also easy to understand, however its expressivity is very limited. There are mixed solutions like TPAs, which are expressive as Safe Petri Nets and low complexity as DFAs. Other specific languages, like BPMN, have been specifically created so that the users can understand them, using graphical metaphors for adding semantics to workflows in a human-understandable way. However, BPMN has a higher complexity to be executed. In this line, all the characteristics of the problem to be solved should be evaluated, for selecting an adequate solution in each case.

3.5 Challenges of Clinical Decision-Making and Process Management Technologies

Despite the hard work in research to leverage the advantages of clinical decision-making and process management technologies in the medical domain, there is still a big gap between the possibilities of these technologies and their joint application in real scenarios.

On one hand, from the perspective of clinicians, there is a need for creating safe, non-intrusive, adaptive and trusted tools that offer the confidence required for their implementation in real scenarios. CPGs and CIGs can offer solutions in this direction, but the problems associated to their development process, requiring a high consensus of experts and the need for a continuous revision, make the judicious and successful use of these instruments a challenge. On the other hand, from a cognitive and perceptual computing perspective [37], there is a need for more data as well as for better self-adaptive algorithms to provide a holistic approach from a data-driven point of view [39]. However, this would imply reducing to a minimum human intervention during the process of model creation and adaption. But, is there a real need for completely self-adaptive tools? Why exclude the human in the process of automatic learning? In the Interactive Pattern Recognition paradigm, it has been demonstrated that the involvement of the expert in the loop not only provides better and quicker results than classical Data-Driven approaches, but also ensures a better understanding and improved confidence in each iteration [12].

The research community of the fields of CIGs and process mining for health is claiming for the combination of these technologies, taking advantage of the best of two worlds [14]. The importance of combining clinical decision-support and workflow technologies to provide realistic support for complex processes, like extended care pathways and multidisciplinary care, was identified more than a decade ago [13]. Beyond that, the need for human expert participation is key for ensuring the adequacy of the models inferred by data-driven approaches. With this assistance experts could incorporate their background knowledge in the model, e.g. to correct possible inference errors. This would allow the creation of models, Workflow or CIG ones, of a better quality and error-free. Furthermore, in process mining, the implementation of solutions to the problem of data denoising would be more effective in an interactive way [24].

The involvement of the expert in the loop using an interactive paradigm mixing data and knowledge-driven solutions opens a set of new perspectives with huge potential. On one hand, process mining approaches could greatly benefit from knowledge intensive models such as CIGs, e.g. using them as a layer for the purpose of improving the explainability of their models to clinicians. On the other hand, the application of interactive process mining methods could play a role of paramount importance in the development and continuous adaption of CPGs (and CIGs), e.g. enabling the integration of tried-and-tested procedures inferred from healthcare data as a complementary source of knowledge in addition to evidence-based and expert knowledge. The main challenge will be how to articulate the design of tools so that a perfect integration of these two technologies can be achieved and, at the same time, their respective benefits can be leveraged to improve both the quality standards and the management aspects of healthcare processes.

References

1. Aho AV, Sethi R, Ullman JD. Compilers, principles, techniques. Addison Wesley. 1986;7(8):9.
2. Benson T. Care pathways. Technical report, NHS National Programme for Information Technology (NPfIT), 2005.
3. Conca T, Saint-Pierre C, Herskovic V, Sepúlveda M, Capurro D, Prieto F, Fernandez-Llatas C. Multidisciplinary collaboration in the treatment of patients with type 2 diabetes in primary care: analysis using process mining. J Med Internet Res. 2018;20(4).
4. Concaro S, Sacchi L, Cerra C, Fratino P, Bellazzi R. Mining healthcare data with temporal association rules: improvements and assessment for a practical use. In: Conference on artificial intelligence in medicine in Europe. Springer; 2009. p. 16–25.
5. de Clercq PA, Blom JA, Korsten HHM, Hasman A. Approaches for creating computer-interpretable guidelines that facilitate decision support. Artif Intell Med. 2004;31(1):1–27.
6. Du G, Jiang Z, Diao X, Yao Y. Knowledge extraction algorithm for variances handling of cp using integrated hybrid genetic double multi-group cooperative pso and dpso. J Med Syst. 2012;36(2):979–94.
7. Dumas M, La Rosa M, Mendling J, Reijers HA, et al. Fundamentals of business process management, vol. 1. Springer; 2013.
8. Eisenberg F. Chapter 4 – the role of quality measurement and reporting feedback as a driver for care improvement. In: Greenes RA, editor. Clinical decision support. The road to broad adoption. 2nd ed. Oxford: Academic; 2014. p. 145–64.
9. Fernandez-Llatas C, Lizondo A, Monton E, Benedi J-M, Traver V. Process mining methodology for health process tracking using real-time indoor location systems. Sensors. 2015;15(12):29821–40.
10. Fernandez-Llatas C, Pileggi SF, Traver V, Benedi JM. Timed parallel automaton: a mathematical tool for defining highly expressive formal workflows. In: 2011 Fifth Asia modelling symposium. IEEE; 2011. p. 56–61.
11. Fernandez-Llatas C, Valdivieso B, Traver V, Benedi JM. Using process mining for automatic support of clinical pathways design. In: Data mining in clinical medicine. Springer; 2015. p. 79–88.
12. Fernández-Llatas C, Meneu T, Traver V, Benedi J-M. Applying evidence-based medicine in telehealth: an interactive pattern recognition approximation. Int J Environ Res Public Health. 2013;10(11):5671–82.
13. Fox J, Black E, Chronakis I, Dunlop R, Patkar V, South M, Thomson R. From guidelines to careflows: modelling and supporting complex clinical processes. Stud Health Technol Inform. 2008;139:44–62.
14. Gatta R, Vallati M, Fernandez-Llatas C, Martinez-Millana A, Orini S, Sacchi L, Lenkowicz J, Marcos M, Munoz-Gama J, Cuendet M, et al. Clinical guidelines: a crossroad of many research areas. Challenges and opportunities in process mining for healthcare. In: International conference on business process management. Springer; 2019. p. 545–56.
15. Graham R, Mancher M, Miller Wolman D, Greenfield S, Steinberg E. Clinical practice guidelines we can trust. Washington, DC: The National Academies Press; 2011.
16. Hollingsworth D, Hampshire UK. Workflow management coalition: the workflow reference model. Workflow Management Coalition. Document Number TC00-1003. 1995;19:16.
17. Huang Z, Lu X, Duan H. On mining clinical pathway patterns from medical behaviors. Artif Intell Med. 2012;56(1):35–50.

18. Huang Z, Lu X, Duan H, Fan W. Summarizing clinical pathways from event logs. J Biomed Inform. 2013;46(1):111–27.
19. Kaiser K, Marcos M. Leveraging workflow control patterns in the domain of clinical practice guidelines. BMC Med Inform Decis Mak. 2016;16:20.
20. Latoszek-Berendsen A, Tange H, van den Herik HJ, Hasman A. From clinical practice guidelines to computer-interpretable guidelines. A literature overview. Methods Inf Med. 2010;49(6):550–70.
21. Lozano E, Marcos M, Martínez-Salvador B, Alonso A, Alonso JR. Experiences in the development of electronic care plans for the management of comorbidities. In: Riaño D, Teije A, Miksch S, Peleg M, editors. Knowledge representation for health-care. Data, processes and guidelines. Berlin/Heidelberg: Springer; 2010. p. 113–23.
22. Mahulea C, Mahulea L, García-Soriano J-M, Colom J-M. Petri nets with resources for modeling primary healthcare systems. In: 2014 18th International conference on system theory, control and computing (ICSTCC). IEEE; 2014. p. 639–44.
23. Marcos M, Campos C, Martínez-Salvador B. A practical exercise on re-engineering clinical guideline models using different representation languages. In: Marcos M, Juarez JM, Lenz R, Nalepa GJ, Nowaczyk S, Peleg M, Stefanowski J, Stiglic G, editors. Artificial intelligence in medicine: knowledge representation and transparent and explainable systems. Springer International Publishing; 2019.
24. Martin N, Martinez-Millana A, Valdivieso B, Fernández-Llatas C. Interactive data cleaning for process mining: a case study of an outpatient clinic's appointment system. In: International conference on business process management. Springer; 2019. p. 532–44.
25. Martínez-Salvador B, Marcos M. Supporting the refinement of clinical process models to computer-interpretable guideline models. Bus Inform Syst Eng. 2016;58(5):355–66.
26. Mesner O, Davis A, Casman E, Simhan H, Shalizi C, Keenan-Devlin L, Borders A, Krishnamurti T. Using graph learning to understand adverse pregnancy outcomes and stress pathways. PloS One. 2019;14(9):e0223319.
27. Müller R, Rogge-Solti A. Bpmn for healthcare processes. In: Proceedings of the 3rd central-European workshop on services and their composition (ZEUS 2011), Karlsruhe, vol. 1, 2011.
28. Patkar V, Fox J. Clinical guidelines and care pathways: a case study applying proforma decision support technology to the breast cancer care pathway. Stud Health Technol Inform. 2008;139:233–42.
29. Peleg M. Computer-interpretable clinical guidelines: a methodological review. J Biomed Inform. 2013;46(4):744–63.
30. Peleg M, González-Ferrer A. Chapter 16 – guidelines and workflow models. In: Greenes RA, editor. Clinical decision support. The road to broad adoption. 2nd ed. Oxford: Academic; 2014. p. 435–64.
31. Peleg M, Tu S, Bury J, Ciccarese P, Fox J, Greenes RA, Hall R, Johnson PD, Jones N, Kumar A, Silvia Miksch, Quaglini S, Seyfang A, Shortliffe EH, Stefanelli M. Comparing computer-interpretable guideline models: a case-study approach. J Am Med Inform Assoc. 2003;10(1):52–68.
32. Rebuge Á, Ferreira DR. Business process analysis in healthcare environments: a methodology based on process mining. Inf Syst. 2012;37(2):99–116.
33. Roser M, Ritchie H, Ortiz-Ospina E. World population growth. Our world in data, 2013.
34. Russell N, Van Der Aalst W, Ter Hofstede A. Workflow patterns: the definitive guide. MIT Press, 2016. https://ieeexplore.ieee.org/book/7453725.
35. Sackett DL, Rosenberg WMC, Gray MJA, Haynes BR, Richardson SW. Evidence based medicine: what it is and what it isn't. BMJ. 1996;312(7023):71–2.
36. Schrijvers G, van Hoorn A, Huiskes N. The care pathway: concepts and theories: an introduction. Int J Integr Care. 2012;12(Spec Ed Integrated Care Pathways):e192.
37. Sheth A. Internet of things to smart iot through semantic, cognitive, and perceptual computing. IEEE Intell Syst. 2016;31(2):108–12.
38. Van Der Aalst W. Process mining. Data science in action. Springer; 2016.

39. Yang W, Su Q. Process mining for clinical pathway: literature review and future directions. In: 2014 11th international conference on service systems and service management (ICSSSM). IEEE; 2014. p. 1–5.
40. Yoo I, Alafaireet P, Marinov M, Pena-Hernandez K, Gopidi R, Chang J-F, Hua L. Data mining in healthcare and biomedicine: a survey of the literature. J Med Syst. 2012;36(4):2431–48.

Chapter 4
Process Mining in Healthcare

Carlos Fernandez-Llatas, Jorge Munoz-Gama, Niels Martin, Owen Johnson, Marcos Sepulveda, and Emmanuel Helm

4.1 Process Mining

Since medical processes are hard to be designed by consensus of experts, the use of data available for creating medical processes is a recurrent idea in literature [3, 7, 8]. Data-driven paradigms are named to be a feasible solution in this field that can support medical experts in their daily decisions [20]. Behind this paradigm, there are frameworks specifically designed for dealing with process-oriented problems. This is the case of process mining.

Process Mining [32] is a relatively new framework that is thought to provide useful human-understandable information about the processes that are being executed in reality. The process mining paradigm provides tools, algorithms and visualization

C. Fernandez-Llatas (✉)
Process Mining 4 Health Lab – SABIEN – ITACA Institute, Universitat Politècnica de València, Valencia, Spain

CLINTEC – Karolinska Institutet, Sweden
e-mail: cfllatas@itaca.upv.es

J. Munoz-Gama · M. Sepulveda
Pontificia Universitat Católica de Chile, Santiago, Chile
e-mail: jmun@uc.cl; marcos@ing.puc.cl

N. Martin
Research Foundation Flanders (FWO), Hasselt University, Hasselt, Belgium
e-mail: niels.martin@uhasselt.be

O. Johnson
Leeds University, Leeds, UK
e-mail: O.A.Johnson@leeds.ac.uk

E. Helm
University of Applied Sciences Upper Austria, Wels, Austria
e-mail: emmanuel.helm@fh-hagenberg.at

© Springer Nature Switzerland AG 2021
C. Fernandez-Llatas (ed.), *Interactive Process Mining in Healthcare*, Health Informatics, https://doi.org/10.1007/978-3-030-53993-1_4

instruments to allow human experts to obtain information about the characteristics of execution processes, by analyzing the trace of events and activities that occurs in a determinate procedure, from a process-oriented perspective.

Process mining has a close relationship with workflow technologies. Usually, process mining algorithms represent their findings as workflows. Workflows are the most commonly used representation framework for processes. Workflows are not only used in enterprises to automate processes but also clinical guidelines represent some decision algorithms using workflows due to their simplicity and ease of understanding [14]. Besides, the use of formal workflows allows the creation of engines that can automate flows in computer systems. Figure 4.1 shows a possible use of process mining technology. Process mining algorithms use the events recorded in each process and represent it as a workflow. This workflow represents the real flow in an understandable and enriched way, for supporting experts in the actual knowledge of what is occurring in reality. For that, this paradigm can offer a high-level view to professionals, allowing a better understanding of the full process.

Process Mining algorithms are usually divided in three groups [32]

- Process Mining Discovery Algorithms [31]: these are systems that can create graphically described workflows from the events recorded in the process. Different process discovery algorithms are used in several healthcare scenarios [5]. The selection of an adequate discovery algorithm depends on the quantity of data available, and the kind of representation workflow desired. Figure 4.1 shows the inference of a discovery algorithm. This algorithm graphically represents the flow of the patient process from raw data coming from events and activities.

- Process Mining Conformance Algorithms: Process Mining Conformance Algorithms [2] can detect if the flow followed by a patient conforms to a defined process. This can be used to measure the patient's adherence to a specific treatment but allows also the graphical representation of the moments the patient is not fulfilling the treatment flow, supporting the physicians in the improvement process of patients' adherence. These techniques can be also used to compare processes to detect the differences in their executions. Conformance algorithms can compare workflows and show the differences graphically, allowing experts to quickly detect changes in different processes. For example, this technique has been used to detect behavioural changes over time in humans [12].

- Process Mining Enhancement Algorithms: Process Mining Enhancement Algorithms extend the information value of a process model using colour gradients, shapes, or animations to highlight specific information in the workflow, providing an *augmented reality* for a better understanding of the process. For example, Fig. 4.1 shows an example of the enhancement of a workflow. In this case, the workflow is representing the common flow of patients in the surgical area of a hospital [9]. A workflow with colour gradients in nodes is shown, representing the duration of the stay in each stage of the surgical process, and in arrows, representing the change frequency among phases. With this information, experts can have a better idea of the dynamic behaviour of the process and can perform changes to improve the process and evaluate the effectiveness of actions by comparing the current flow with past inferences.

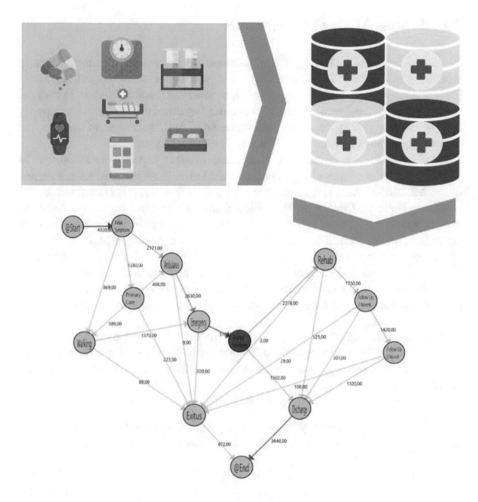

Icons made by Smashicons, Monkik, Itim2101, Pixel Buddha and Freepik from www.flaticon.com

Fig. 4.1 Process mining discovery

The main issue to solve when applying an interactive pattern recognition problem is that the experts should understand the model inferred to provide corrections and infer knowledge from the models [11]. Process mining technology is data-driven but with a focus on understandability. In this line, we can define process mining as *a Syntactic Data Mining technique that supports the domain experts in the proper understanding of complex processes in a Comprehensive, Objective way.* This characteristic makes process mining one of the most suitable technologies for applying interactive models.

4.2   Process Mining in Healthcare

Recent reviews are analyzing the application of process mining techniques in healthcare in detail [5, 27]. Some works analyze the change of hospital processes [27], and management of emergencies [1], support the medical training in surgical procedures [21], the flow of patients in specifically critical departments, like surgery [9], or oncology [26], or even, this framework has been used to analyze the behavioural change in humans to detect early dementia signs [12].

In [5], 447 Process Mining for Healthcare relevant papers were identified. 24 of these papers are indexed on PubMed. PubMed is the most used search engine of the MEDLINE database, containing biomedical research articles offered for the Medicine National Library of the United States. That means that only 5% of the papers that are considered relevant in the Process Mining for Healthcare literature are indexed in the clinical domain. That points to clear difficulties in the application of process mining techniques in real domains. Figure 4.2 shows the trends in publishing in PubMed Library since 2005. This histogram shows that, although there are works about process mining technologies since the start of the century [31], the penetration of these technologies are now starting to be applied in the medical domain.

The difficulties to apply process mining in the healthcare domain are due to distinguishing characteristics of the clinical domain. In this way, it is crucial to take these particularities into account to create a successful process mining system in the health domain:

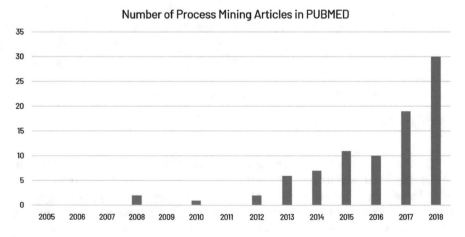

Fig. 4.2 Number of Process Mining articles in PubMed library 2005–2018

4.2.1 Variability in the Medical Processes

Medical processes are intended to holistically cover clinical treatments. Medical processes do not only cover diagnosis, treatments, and clinical decisions but also care prevention, patient preferences and medical expertise. That implies that medical processes inherit the complexity of the treatments and diagnosis, as well as the intangible know-how of healthcare professionals [25]. Moreover, patients are usually involved in several health episodes at the same time which causes the co-existence of a different set of pluripathologies and co-morbidities associated to the same patient that can be related, or not, among themselves. This scenario requires close collaboration where many different health professionals interact to define, usually offline, a multi-disciplinary strategy for each patient.

Besides, medical paradigms, like evidence-based medicine [29], value-based healthcare [15], or personalized medicine [16] put the patient in the centre of the medical process. In these paradigms, the attitudes and beliefs of patients are taken into account. This provokes different responses to the treatments, due to the psychology and personal behaviour that take part in the decisions of the patient in terms of the acceptation, or not, of the treatment proposed by the doctor. The adherence of the patient regarding the treatment is one of the most important problems when applying a new treatment to patients [23]. The adherence is key dealing with a disease. The selection of the treatment not only depends on the best option available according to medical evidence, but also on the beliefs, family condition, fears, ambitions, and quality of life of the patient. We should not forget that the real decision-maker in the medical treatment of the patient. In this way, it is crucial to understand their psychological and physical situation before making a clinical decision.

This variability in the medical processes increases the size of the model in terms of arcs and nodes. This provokes one of the most well-known problems in process mining literature, the *Spaghetti Effect*. The application of process discovery algorithms on highly variable systems results in unreadable models. In this way, it is important to select adequate tools for each problem that support the highlighting of the interesting process structures and abstracting or splitting the model in simpler protocols that show the relevant information for the doctors [10]. Process mining researchers should be aware of this problem and provide solutions, tools and frameworks to characterize and extract information about this variability, to extract better and more understandable knowledge of real patients.

4.2.2 Infrequent Behaviour Could be the Interesting One

One of the most common solutions that process mining and other data mining practitioners use to infer models is to discard *outliers* in the data. These outliers are considered as noise and are removed from the data. This decreases the variability, which creates cleaner models that can provide better understandable solutions. However, infrequent behaviour should not always be discarded from the system like, for example, for the detection of adverse effects [30].

Outlier-free logs will produce clean models that produce views representing the most common paths that are followed by the most common patients occurring in most common cases. This implies that the inferred model should be close to the standard clinical processes that are, generally, followed by the patient, and should match with the perception of the medical experts which are providing care. That means that these logs, formed by standard patients, will allow discovering the standard process. However, the standard process is not always the most interesting one. Health professionals usually are familiar with the standard case. The standard patient is covered by the standard treatment. As a consequence, showing the standard model inferred to the doctor does not provide any knowledge to him.

Infrequent cases are cases that do not follow the standard process properly. That means that these cases are the patients that are usually out of the guideline and require special treatment. In those cases, the medical doctor needs help, not as in the standard case. Infrequent behaviour patients processes do not only provide a view about the flow of non-standard cases, but can also provide help to understand the different patient circuits, or even find non-standard similar patients that have followed the same path [22]. This can be a real support to health professionals in daily practice that can't be offered by standard noise reduction techniques.

4.2.3 Medical Processes Should be Personalized

Since the appearance of the evidence-based medicine paradigm, there have been attempts to automate the care provided to patients [29]. The idea of this paradigm is to discover the best medical protocols that can be applied to take care of the disease not only in terms of treatment but also in terms of diagnosis and prevention. However, evidence-based medicine detractors criticize the lack of flexibility in the definition of these protocols [13, 28]. Standard protocols produced by evidence-based medicine has been perceived as incompatible with patient-centred care [28]. Patient-centred care pleads for a more personal application of health where individual's health beliefs, values and behaviours are taken into account when deciding on the best treatments.

All of this criticism on evidence-based medicine originates from the difficulties in the application of clinical pathways due to different health deployment cultures existing in health systems [6, 24]. That means that the application of health care protocols to tackle the same illness can differ significantly from one centre to another, depending not only on the culture of the local population but also on time constraints, the level of staff involvement, the costs associated, among a huge quantity of different factors [6]. Consequently, to replicate the best practices based on medical evidence, it is crucial to iteratively adapt medical processes based on continuous analysis and refinement of the deployed protocols, taking into account the cultural differences of the target population. Process mining techniques should provide tools and paradigms that allow evolving iteratively the clinical protocols using with the real information collected from target scenarios and led by health professionals. This should be done not only for discovering the standard processes but also supporting health experts in the understanding of the personal characteristics of individual patients.

4.2.4   Medical Processes Are Not Deterministic

Differences in personal preferences of patients, their beliefs and attitudes affect the effectiveness and efficacy of the treatments. That means that in healthcare, cause-effect relationships are often fuzzy. Medical evidence is based on estimations extracted from clinical trials that usually works in most of the cases. However, The same treatment, provided to two different patients with the same illness and, even, the same co-morbidities can result in totally different processes due to many additional factors that cannot be observed or taken into account in the model. This is because there is a gap between each patient and the medical model that represent the clinical knowledge. Formal medical processes are supposed to be automatable and unambiguous, but this is incoherent with the intrinsic nature of patients flow.

This uncertainty is critical in data-driven models. While knowledge systems can offer semantic explanations and rules for describing the ambiguities. Data-driven models can only offer statistical approaches that can inform about the probabilities. The incorporation of process mining techniques, that allow dealing with in-determinism in medical models, like the inference of semantics [4] or the incorporation of information that can point to the ambiguity reasons should be taken into account for better support of the medical decision.

4.2.5   Medical Decisions Are Not Only Based on Medical Evidence, But Also on Medical Expertise

Although one of the most key features of evidence-based medicine is to extract medical evidence, the final decision in medical treatments is always taken by the health professional. Evidence-based medicine looks for the fusion of the best medical evidence with the personal knowledge of medical professionals. This means that medical processes are, in fact, guidelines, that might be followed by the physician. Clinical guidelines aim to offer support to healthcare professionals, based on insights from accumulated clinical evidence.

Data driven systems should focus on providing the most relevant information in the most understandable way to support the practitioner in their daily practice. The decisions taken by health professionals are determined by medical knowledge, represented by guidelines proposed in the medical models, and their personal feelings obtained from the communication with the patient, which can be verbal or not. The validation of these decisions should aim to provide a holistic value-based healthcare analysis in order to provide medical indicators (like P-Value [18]) that allow professionals to trust the tools provided. These decisions, which can be different from the ones recommended by the models, are registered in the logs and can, consequently, be used in next iterations to improve the models through interactive models [11].

4.2.6 Understandability Is Key

Given the difficulties of the manual definition of medical protocols, pathways and guidelines, data-driven technologies are being called to support medical professionals in their formalization. Traditional machine learning techniques are thought to provide the best accuracy in the models, but the interaction with professionals is not available due to the lack of readability of these techniques. Consequently, the resulting models are *black boxes* for health professionals. Machine learning inferred models are based on statistical mathematical models. In this line, the more patients we have in the dataset, the more precise models we can infer [19]. On the contrary, the fewer patients we have the more probable is that the system fails in their prediction. For that, machine learning models are accurate in the prediction of standard cases, but, have a higher probability to fail in infrequent cases. The standard case is usually covered by standard treatment and, in those cases, the expert does not need support. The expert needs support for infrequent cases, where the machine learning models have more problems. This creates suspicion amongst the experts whether to trust a system that has a higher probability of failure for the cases when they are more needed. This is pushing to a new way of explainable machine learning for creating understandable models for health professionals [17].

In the healthcare domain, process mining algorithms should be thought to maximize the understandability of the models inferred. While classical data mining solutions are intended to provide accurate models, process mining enables health professionals a better understanding of the processes and the correction of the models based on their knowledge. Understandable data-driven systems, like process mining, allow the expert to understand the reasons behind the system's recommendation, providing clues for better decisions in daily practice. Besides, it is key to select the correct graphical models that allow the understanding of the processes. Highly expressive models, like Petri nets, can be too complex for the understanding of non-process experts like clinicians, that are used to define their models with more graphically oriented systems as was explained in the previous chapter.

4.2.7 Must Involve Real World Data

Due to the necessity to preserve the privacy of individuals, current laws impose a high barrier for the creation of adequate data-driven models. One potential solution is the use of simulated data for the creation of algorithms to create healthcare solutions. However, the complexity of simulation models is bounded by their model representation capability, which is always much lower than complexity in the real world. Great algorithms and tools that have demonstrated impressive efficacy in other application contexts, can be pointless in healthcare due to unexpected aspects due to unknown variability in the health domain that cannot be simulated. Simulated data cannot offer medical evidence, so, we cannot assume that techniques are adequate for health if we have not tested them with real data.

4.2.8 Solving the Real Problem

The medical expert is the only one able to notice if discovered evidence is relevant or not. Data scientists can find impressive results by creating algorithms to highlight specific aspects of a process. However, if these results do not tackle a real medical problem, or the discovered evidence is well known in the medical community, it makes no sense to use these algorithms. The involvement of medical professionals in the definition of problems and the interpretation of results is key in the creation of useful tools and the discovery of new medical evidence.

4.2.9 Different Solutions for Different Medical Disciplines

Medicine is a huge field formed by several disciplines and specialities having very different variables to measure. Health managers should have different views of the process than clinicians, but even in a single clinical domain, different specialities should have different views. For example, the key biomedical variables for an endocrinologist can be different than the information relevant for a cardiologist. The information available in the medical domain is so huge that it is mandatory to provide the adequate tools and views for each problem to solve, taking into account the real needs of the health professional at any moment. The information overload provokes a paradox effect: the more information is accessible, the more difficult it is to find the relevant one.

For that, the application of process mining technologies in the healthcare domain should be completely adapted to the medical field, creating customized methods and tools for supporting physicians in their daily practice, avoiding one-fits-all solutions and creating adaptive and customizable frameworks for facilitating their real use and highlighting the relevant information in each case.

4.2.10 Medical Processes Evolve in Time

Medical processes are being improved every day due to the continuous appearance of new clinical evidence in the literature. Also, as patients are humans, their personality, beliefs and general behaviour evolve in time. That means that the treatment response of a patient changes depending on several factors that can or cannot be observable. A change in a medical process might suppose an indeterminate change in the behaviour of the process in the next iteration. This is because the effects of change in medical protocols are dependent on an unknown number of variables that makes the result indeterministic.

In this way, process mining technologies should be not only focused on discovering better processes for taking care of the patients but also to be constantly aware of their continuous evolution. This requires tools to trace, measure and analyze how patients adapt their life to the proposed treatments in each stage of their disease. Within a process mining approach, the process can be continuously tracked iteratively. In each one of the iterations of creating optimized and adapted medical protocols, the experts can understand and correct the processes, allowing to be resilient to the concept drift problem produced by the evolution in time of medical processes via the utilization of interactive methods. This is because the interactive paradigm ensures the convergence in the limit of the learning process by involving the expert in the loop [11].

4.3 Conclusion

In the domain of data-driven technologies, process mining has acquired a certain prominence in case of process oriented problems. Its capability to discover, analyze and enhance graphical processes in an easy to understand way supposes a new way to provide information to professionals by involving them in the process of generating knowledge. This characteristic is especially valuable in healthcare, were the expert usually has no engineering knowledge and no data science skills. Unlike other data science paradigms, process mining can provide information to the expert about what is actually occurring with their patients, allowing them in a better understanding of the effectiveness of the treatments selected. This facilitates close collaboration between the computer and the experts that might enable the imbrication between the clinical evidence and the professional knowledge that is required in the evidence-based medicine paradigm.

However, to ensure the applicability of process mining technologies to the clinical domain, it is necessary to take into account their special characteristics. Selected process mining algorithms, methods and tools should be specifically designed to deal with this highly demanding field. In this chapter, we have analyzed and stated the most important of these specificities. The selection of the best process mining technologies for each specific case is crucial for creating successful deployments of intelligent systems in health centres.

References

1. Andrews R, Wynn MT, Vallmuur K, Ter Hofstede AHM, Bosley E, Elcock M, Rashford S. Leveraging data quality to better prepare for process mining: an approach illustrated through analysing road trauma pre-hospital retrieval and transport processes in queensland. Int J Environ Res Public Health. 2019;16(7):1138.
2. Carmona J, van Dongen B, Solti A, Weidlich M. Conformance checking. Springer; 2018.
3. Chowriappa P, Dua S, Todorov Y. Introduction to machine learning in healthcare informatics. In: Machine learning in healthcare informatics. Springer; 2014. p. 1–23.
4. De Medeiros AKA, van der Aalst WMP. Process mining towards semantics. In: Advances in web semantics I. Springer; 2008. p. 35–80.
5. Erdogan TG, Tarhan A. Systematic mapping of process mining studies in healthcare. IEEE Access. 2018;6:24543–67.
6. Evans-Lacko S, Jarrett M, McCrone P, Thornicroft G. Facilitators and barriers to implementing clinical care pathways. BMC Health Serv Res. 2010;10(1):182.
7. Fatima M, Pasha M, et al. Survey of machine learning algorithms for disease diagnostic. J Intell Learn Syst Appl. 2017;9(01):1.
8. Fernández-Llatas C, García-Gómez JM. Data mining in clinical medicine. Springer; 2015.
9. Fernandez-Llatas C, Lizondo A, Monton E, Benedi J-M, Traver V. Process mining methodology for health process tracking using real-time indoor location systems. Sensors (Basel, Switzerland). 2015;15(12):29821–40.
10. Fernandez-Llatas C, Martinez-Millana A, Martinez-Romero A, Benedi JM, Traver V. Diabetes care related process modelling using process mining techniques. Lessons learned in the application of interactivepattern recognition: coping with the Spaghetti Effect. In: 2015 37th annual international conference of the IEEE engineering in medicine and biology society (EMBC), 2015. p. 2127–30.
11. Fernandez-Llatas C, Meneu T, Traver V, Benedi J-M. Applying evidence-based medicine in telehealth: an interactive pattern recognition approximation. Int J Environ Res Public Health. 2013;10(11):5671–82.
12. Fernández-Llatas C, Benedi J-M, García-Gómez JM, Traver V. Process mining for individualized behavior modeling using wireless tracking in nursing homes. Sensors. 2013;13(11):15434–51.
13. Goldberger JJ, Buxton AE. Personalized medicine vs guideline-based medicine. Jama. 2013;309(24):2559–60.
14. Gooch P, Roudsari A. Computerization of workflows, guidelines, and care pathways: a review of implementation challenges for process-oriented health information systems. J Am Med Inform Assoc. 2011;18(6):738–48.
15. Gray M. Value based healthcare. BMJ. 2017;356:j437.
16. Hamburg MA, Collins FS. The path to personalized medicine. N Engl J Med. 2010;363(4):301–4.
17. Holzinger A. From machine learning to explainable AI. In: 2018 world symposium on digital intelligence for systems and machines (DISA). IEEE; 2018. p. 55–66.
18. Ibanez-Sanchez G, Fernandez-Llatas C, Celda A, Mandingorra J, Aparici-Tortajada L, Martinez-Millana A, Munoz-Gama J, Sepúlveda M, Rojas E, Gálvez V, Capurro D, Traver V. Toward value-based healthcare through interactive process mining in emergency rooms: the stroke case. Int J Environ Res Public Health. 2019; 16(10). https://www.mdpi.com/1660-4601/16/10/1783.

19. Jain AK, Chandrasekaran B. 39 dimensionality and sample size considerations in pattern recognition practice. Handb Stat. 1982;2:835–55.
20. Kononenko I. Machine learning for medical diagnosis: history, state of the art and perspective. Artif Intell Med. 2001;23(1):89–109.
21. Lira R, Salas-Morales J, Leiva L, Fuentes R, Delfino A, Nazal CH, Sepúlveda M, Arias M, Herskovic V, Munoz-Gama J et al. Process-oriented feedback through process mining for surgical procedures in medical training: the ultrasound-guided central venous catheter placement case. Int J Environ Res Public Health. 2019;16(11):1877.
22. Mansour A, Ying H, Dews P, Ji Y, Yen J, Miller RE, Massanari RM. Finding similar patients in a multi-agent environment. In: 2011 annual meeting of the North American fuzzy information processing society. IEEE; 2011. p. 1–6.
23. Osterberg L, Blaschke T. Adherence to medication. N Engl J Med. 2005;353(5):487–97.
24. Pace KB, Sakulkoo S, Hoffart N, Cobb AK. Barriers to successful implementation of a clinical pathway for chf. J Healthcare Qual Off Publ Natl Assoc Healthcare Qual 2002;24(5):32–8.
25. Rebuge Á, Ferreira DR. Business process analysis in healthcare environments: a methodology based on process mining. Inf Syst. 2012;37(2):99–116.
26. Rinner C, Helm E, Dunkl R, Kittler H, Rinderle-Ma S. Process mining and conformance checking of long running processes in the context of melanoma surveillance. Int J Environ Res Public Health. 2018;15(12):2809.
27. Rojas E, Munoz-Gama J, Sepúlveda M, Capurro D. Process mining in healthcare: a literature review. J Biomed Inform. 2016;61:224–36.
28. Romana H-W. Is evidence-based medicine patient-centered and is patient-centered care evidence-based? Health Serv Res. 2006;41(1):1.
29. Straus SE, Richardson WS, Glasziou P, Haynes RB. Evidence-based medicine: how to practice and teach EBM. 3 ed. Churchill Livingstone; 2005.
30. Stricker BHCh, Psaty BM. Detection, verification, and quantification of adverse drug reactions. BMJ. 2004;329(7456):44–7.
31. Van der Aalst W, Weijters T, Maruster L. Workflow mining: discovering process models from event logs. IEEE Trans Knowl Data Eng. 2004;16(9):1128–42.
32. van der Aalst WMP. Process mining: data science in action. Springer; 2016.

Chapter 5
Data Quality in Process Mining

Niels Martin

5.1 Introduction

Healthcare organizations such as hospitals are confronted with multiple challenges such as tightening budgets combined with increased care needs due to an aging population [19, 21]. To cope with these challenges, hospitals need to understand their processes in order to improve their effectiveness and efficiency. In this respect, the previous chapter has discussed the potential of process mining. Process mining will enable healthcare organizations to gain profound insights in, amongst others, the order of activities prevailing in reality, the relationship between the involved resources, and the real-life performance of the process. To obtain such a real-life view on the process, event logs originating from process-aware information systems such as a Hospital Information System (HIS) are used.

In the last decade, a multitude of algorithms have been developed to retrieve valuable process-related information from event logs [2]. Despite the great potential of these algorithms to analyze healthcare processes, the reliability of process mining outcomes ultimately depends on the quality of the input data used by the algorithm [21]. Consistent with the notion "Garbage In, Garbage Out", applying process mining algorithms to low quality data can lead to counter-intuitive or even misleading results [5]. Using such results for decision-making purposes entails the risk of taking ineffective actions, which could cause adverse effects in healthcare processes such as inefficient resource allocations, leading to increased waiting times and patient dissatisfaction.

N. Martin (✉)
Research Foundation Flanders (FWO), Brussels, Belgium

Hasselt University, Diepenbeek, Belgium ·

Vrije Universiteit Brussel, Brussels, Belgium
e-mail: niels.martin@uhasselt.be

© Springer Nature Switzerland AG 2021
C. Fernandez-Llatas (ed.), *Interactive Process Mining in Healthcare*, Health Informatics, https://doi.org/10.1007/978-3-030-53993-1_5

Fig. 5.1 Chapter overview

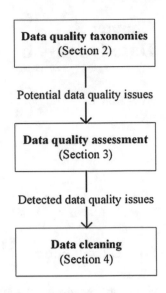

Real-life event logs typically suffer from several data quality issues [3, 9, 21, 31]. This especially holds in flexible and dynamic environments with extensive manual recording, such as healthcare [9, 28]. For instance: suppose that a nurse performs several activities for different patients and only records these activities in the system at a later point in time. When the insertion time in the system is automatically recorded as the timestamp of an activity, this can constitute a data quality issue from a process mining perspective as there is a discrepancy between the moment at which the activity is actually executed and its trail in the HIS. This could, for instance, lead to misleading process performance information and could even change the order of activities, depending on the order in which activities are entered into the system.

This chapter provides an introduction to data quality in the process mining field. As shown in Fig. 5.1, three main topics are discussed. Firstly, Sect. 5.2 discusses the key data quality taxonomies defined in literature, which describe potential data quality issues. A distinction is made between generic taxonomies and taxonomies from the process mining field, where the latter focus on the specific input data format that process mining uses. Secondly, Sect. 5.3 focuses on data quality assessment, which reflects the identification of data quality issues in a dataset. Besides some examples of assessment results of real-life healthcare logs, three data quality assessment frameworks from process mining literature are discussed. Moreover, the available tool support is briefly introduced. Finally, Sect. 5.4 centers around data cleaning, which involves the use of heuristics to tackle specific data quality issues present in the event log.

5.2   Data Quality Taxonomies

Given the potential impact of data quality issues on process mining outcomes, a profound insight in the variety of issues that can be present in real-life data is required. In literature, several authors have conceptualized the data quality notion and proposed taxonomies to categorize them. This section discusses a selection of these taxonomies. While Sect. 5.2.1 focuses on general taxonomies, i.e. classifications without a specific process mining focus, Sect. 5.2.2 discusses the key data quality taxonomies in the process mining field.

5.2.1   General Data Quality Taxonomies

Before proceeding to the key data quality taxonomies in the process mining field, some general taxonomies are outlined first. While a full outline of these taxonomies is beyond the scope of this chapter, some concepts are highly relevant for the process mining context. These will be briefly discussed in the remainder of this section.

When identifying data quality issues, the 'fitness for use' notion is often highlighted. This implies that data is of sufficient quality when it is fit for use for the question at hand [35]. This suggests that data quality is a relative notion, in the sense that it depends upon the goal(s) of the analysis. For instance: when resource information is missing in the event log, this only constitutes a relevant data quality issue when the analysis would require the use of this information.

Building upon the 'fitness of use' perspective and based on surveys amongst professionals and MBA students, Wang and Strong [35] distinguish four types of data quality: intrinsic, contextual, representational and accessibility data quality. Firstly, intrinsic data quality refers to characteristics such as the data's believability, accuracy, objectivity, and the reputation of the data source. Secondly, contextual data quality, amongst others, refers to the relevance of the data, its completeness, the adequacy of the volume of available data, and how recent the available data is. Thirdly, representational data quality relates to the interpretability of the data, its ease of understanding, the consistency of its format, and the conciseness of its representation. Finally, accessibility data quality includes characteristics such as the ease with which the data can be accessed, and which security measures are in place to avoid access by unauthorised individuals or organizations [35]. While the taxonomy of Wang and Strong [35] is widely applicable, a simplified version is converted to a clinical research setting by Kahn et al. [17].

Besides 'fitness for use', other common dimensions to classify data quality issues are included in the taxonomy of Rahm and Do [27]. These authors firstly distinguish between single-source and multi-source quality issues, referring to the number of data sources from which the dataset originates. When the dataset is composed based on multiple data sources, i.e. in a multi-source setting, issues related to differences in data representation and the presence of contradicting data values can occur. Within both single-source and multi-source problems, a further distinction is made between schema level and instance level errors. Issues at the schema level originate from problems with the data model design or a poor enforcement of data entry rules. For instance: if two nurses share the same unique staff identifier, a schema level issue is present. Instance level issues, such as typos or contradicting values, are related to the specific values of a data field and, hence, cannot be avoided at the schema level [15, 27].

Gschwandtner et al. [15] use the distinction between single-source and multi-source problems with a particular focus on time-oriented data. In a single-source setting, different categories of data quality issues are specified: missing data, duplicate data (e.g. the same patient occurs twice in the dataset with slightly different timestamps), implausible values (e.g. a nurse with a 20-hour shift), outdated values (e.g. only very old data is included in the dataset), wrong data, and ambiguous data (e.g. unknown abbreviations). When multiple data sources are involved in the composition of the dataset, other data quality issues can occur: heterogeneous syntax (e.g. different date formats in distinct data sources), heterogeneous semantics (e.g. timestamps are recorded at different levels of granularity), and reference-related issues (e.g. incorrect references across different data sources). It should be noted that the single-source quality issues can also be present in the individual components of a dataset in a multi-source setting.

While the aforementioned taxonomies tend to have a high-level nature and refrain from identifying specific data quality issues, others define issues at a lower level of granularity. Consider, for example, the taxonomy of Kim et al. [18], where data quality issues such as wrong data entries, duplicated data and different word orderings are identified. These issues are categorised, starting from a general distinction between missing data and non-missing data. While the former relates to data values which should be present, but are absent, the latter category refers to data values which are present, regardless of whether or not they are correct. The category non-missing data is further subdivided in wrong data on the one hand and not wrong, but unusable data on the other hand. Wrong data are all data entries that do not correspond to the true data value when the data is consulted. Not wrong, but unusable data is data which is not wrong in itself, but which can lead to misleading results when used for analysis purposes. The inconsistent use of abbreviations is an example of the latter [18].

5.2.2   Data Quality Taxonomies in Process Mining

Section 5.2.1 presented some general data quality classifications. While these taxonomies highlight some relevant concepts for process mining, they are not geared towards the specific data structure used as an input for process mining. This specific data structure, i.e. an event log, can give rise to specific data quality issues, e.g. related to the relationship between events within a case [31]. Several process mining researchers have conceptualised the notion of event log quality. This section outlines the key data quality taxonomies in the process mining field.

5.2.2.1   Process Mining Manifesto

A high-level taxonomy of event log data quality is provided in the Process Mining Manifesto [3], a document compiled by the IEEE Task Force on Process Mining.[1] Even though no detailed data quality issues are defined, the event log maturity levels which are introduced provide a preliminary view on event log data quality. In total, five maturity levels are specified, where the first level represents a poor quality event log, while the fifth level reflects an event log of excellent quality. In general, the maturity levels can be described as follows:

- **Maturity level 1.** Event log in which events are typically not recorded automatically. In such a log, events might not correspond to reality or can be missing.
- **Maturity level 2.** Event log in which events are recorded automatically, but where a systematic approach for logging is absent. Moreover, the system can be circumvented. As a consequence, events can be missing or might not correspond to reality.
- **Maturity level 3.** Event log in which events are recorded automatically, but no systematic approach is followed for logging. Even though events might be missing, there is reasonable confidence that the events which are recorded match reality.
- **Maturity level 4.** Event log in which events are recorded automatically and systematically, i.e. the log's content is both reliable and complete. Moreover, explicit case and activity notions are present.
- **Maturity level 5.** Event log in which events are recorded automatically and systematically. These high-quality event logs also assign clear semantics to all events and attributes. This implies that ontologies exist to which events and attributes are explicitly related. Moreover, privacy and security concerns are tackled [3].

Even though it is technically possible to apply process mining techniques to an event log of maturity level 1 or 2, the outcomes tend to be highly unreliable. Hence, as a general recommendation, event logs at maturity level 3 or higher are required to perform process mining [3].

Within a healthcare context, an example of an event log at maturity level 1 would be a log composed using input from a paper-based file system. When moving towards higher levels of maturity, event logs will originate from a HIS. The maturity level of these logs will depend, amongst others, upon the type of HIS, the usage patterns of the system, and the extent to which the recorded events have clear semantics. Inevitably, some events will be recorded manually by medical staff,

---

[1] https://www.tf-pm.org

Table 5.1 Data quality taxonomy by Bose et al. [9]

	Case	Event	Belongs to	Case attribute	Position	Activity name	Timestamp	Resource	Event attribute
Missing data	I1	I2	I3	I4	I5	I6	I7	I8	I9
Incorrect data	I10	I11	I12	I13	I14	I15	I16	I17	I18
Imprecise data			I19	I20	I21	I22	I23	I24	I25
Irrelevant data	I26	I27							

asynchronously from the execution of an activity. A prime example of the latter are patient-related activities. This stresses that data quality should always be a key concern when performing process mining in healthcare.

5.2.2.2 Taxonomy by Bose et al. [9]

While the Process Mining Manifesto [3] conveys some high-level ideas on event log quality, Bose et al. [9] define more specific data quality issues. Based on their experience with process mining projects within a variety of organisations, Bose et al. [9] define 27 distinct classes of event log quality issues, which are summarized in Table 5.1. These issues are subdivided in four classes:

- **Missing data.** Pieces of data which are missing, even though they should be present in the event log. The absence of data typically indicates issues with the logging process.
- **Incorrect data.** Data entries which are present, but for which the recorded values do not reflect reality.
- **Imprecise data.** Pieces of data are imprecise when they are recorded at an insufficiently detailed level.
- **Irrelevant data.** A data entry is considered irrelevant when it cannot be used in its current format. Filtering or transformation might be required to retrieve useful information from this data entry [9].

When combining these four classes with key event log components (e.g. activity label, timestamp) and characteristics (e.g. position of an event within a trace), the set of 27 event log quality issues is obtained. These include missing events (i.e. events which occurred in reality, but were not recorded in the event log), incorrect timestamps (i.e. timestamps which do not correspond to the moment at which an event took place in reality), imprecise resources (i.e. resource information recorded at a coarse-grained level) and irrelevant cases (i.e. cases which are not relevant for the question at hand). A brief description of all event log quality issues is included in Table 5.2.

Table 5.2 Description of the event log quality issues according to Bose et al. [9]

Class	Code	Quality issue	Description
Missing data	I1	Missing cases	Cases which have been processed in reality are not included in the event log. In this way, process mining outcomes might not reflect reality
	I2	Missing events	Events which are not recorded within a trace, causing the retrieval of relationships which might not hold in reality
	I3	Missing relationships	The absence of an explicit link between an event and a case, causing difficulties to retrieve the correct relationships between events
	I4	Missing case attributes	Case attribute values which are not recorded, requiring algorithms using these values to leave out the case
	I5	Missing position	In the absence of timestamps, missing position implies that the position of an event within the trace is unknown
	I6	Missing activity names	Events for which the activity name is not present, making the origin of this event unclear
	I7	Missing timestamps	Events for which the timestamp is not recorded in the log. Besides making process performance analysis a complex task, control-flow discovery might also become unreliable (unless the position within the trace is guaranteed to be correct)
	I8	Missing resources	The resource associated to an event is not registered, impacting all process mining algorithms using resource information
	I9	Missing event attributes	Event attribute values which are absent, causing difficulties for algorithms using these values
Incorrect data	I10	Incorrect cases	Cases in the event log which, in reality, relate to a different process. These cases will behave as outliers in process mining analyses
	I11	Incorrect events	Events which are recorded incorrectly, e.g. events that did not occur in reality are present in the log
	I12	Incorrect relationships	An incorrect link between a case and an event is recorded, causing events to be associated to the wrong case
	I13	Incorrect case attributes	Case attribute values which are logged incorrectly, causing difficulties for algorithms using these values
	I14	Incorrect position	When timestamps are absent, this issue occurs when an event is incorrectly positioned within the trace
	I15	Incorrect activity names	Events for which the activity name is incorrectly recorded
	I16	Incorrect timestamps	Events for which the timestamp does not correspond to the time that the event took place in reality

(continued)

Table 5.2 (continued)

Class	Code	Quality issue	Description
	I17	Incorrect resources	The resource associated to an event is incorrect, leading to issues with algorithms using resource data
	I18	Incorrect event attributes	Event attribute values which are logged incorrectly, causing problems when applying algorithms which leverage these values
Imprecise data	I19	Imprecise relationships	Events which cannot be linked to a particular case specification because of the case specification that is chosen for log construction purposes. For instance, it is no longer possible to connect an event to a patient consult because the log is constructed with a patient as a case
	I20	Imprecise case attributes	Case attribute values which cannot be used because they are recorded in a coarse-grained wat
	I21	Imprecise position	In the absence of timestamps, an imprecise position implies that events that occur in parallel are recorded sequentially in a systematic way
	I22	Imprecise activity names	Events for which the activity name is recorded in a coarse-grained way, leading to multiple events having the same activity name, even though they refer to different activities
	I23	Imprecise timestamps	Events having a timestamp which is recorded at a coarse level of granularity. Consider, for instance, that timestamps are recorded at the day level, even though a large number of events occurs for a particular case on a single day
	I24	Imprecise resources	The resource information available in the event log is of a more coarse-grained nature than the resource information that is actually known. This limits the potential of resource-related algorithms
	I25	Imprecise event attributes	Event attribute values which cannot be used because they are recorded at a coarse level
Irrelevant data	I26	Irrelevant cases	Cases which are not relevant for the analysis question at hand. Including such cases can have a negative impact on the understandability of the process mining outcomes
	I27	Irrelevant events	Events which are not relevant for the analysis in their current form, implying that filtering and aggregation are required

5.2.2.3 Taxonomy by Verhulst [33]

Another event log quality taxonomy has been proposed by Verhulst [33]. It is a literature-based framework, drawing upon both general data quality literature, the taxonomy of Bose et al. [9] and the guidelines for event log creation defined by van der Aalst [1]. Based on an analysis of this literature, 12 event log

Table 5.3 Description of the event log quality dimensions according to Verhulst [33]

Quality dimension	Description
Completeness	Dimension capturing how complete the data is, e.g. whether missing values are present, whether transactional information is present
Uniqueness/duplicates	Dimension expressing the attribute values which only occur once, which also relates to the presence of duplicate events
Timeliness	Quality dimension demonstrating whether the event log fits the expected timeframe
Validity	Dimension highlighting whether the data conform to the syntactical requirements in its definitions, e.g. related to data types
Accuracy/correctness	Dimension capturing whether the available values closely match the (unknown) real values
Consistency	Dimension related to the consistency of data entries, e.g., expressed in terms of the length of data entries
Believability/credibility	Dimension expressing whether users have confidence in the objectivity of the data entries
Relevancy	Dimension measuring the importance of data entries
Security/confidentiality	Dimension capturing the ability to safeguard the data
Complexity	Dimension outlining the complexity of the process generating the data
Coherence	Quality dimension focusing on the logical interconnection between data entries
Representation/format	Dimension capturing whether data is presented in a compact way and in the same format

data quality dimensions are specified. These dimensions, which are summarized in Table 5.3, include completeness (expressing how complete the data is) and accuracy/correctness (expressing whether values closely match reality). While these examples constitute dimensions which are closely related to the specific data entries in the event log, Verhulst [33] also incorporate dimensions such as the timeliness of the log (i.e. whether it fits the expected timeframe) and the security of the data (i.e. the ability to safeguard the data).

For most dimensions, Verhulst [33] provide a measuring method to quantify a dimension. Quantification is performed by either assigning a score to the log (e.g. for completeness, a score between 0 and 10 is required), or by adding a boolean true/false judgment (e.g. for timeliness). For some dimensions, such as believability/credibility, it is stated that no measurement is possible [33].

5.2.2.4 Event Log Imperfection Patterns by Suriadi et al. [31]

Another important contribution to event log quality research are the event log imperfection patterns defined by Suriadi et al. [31]. Based on their experience with real-life case studies in a variety of domains, they define 11 imperfection patterns. These patterns highlight data quality issues which are specific to event logs. While Bose et al. [9] and Verhulst [33] categorise event log quality and provide a taxonomy, Suriadi et al. [31] focus on providing an elaborate description on the 11 fine-grained patterns they distinguish. These patterns are:

- **Form-based event capture.** This imperfection occurs when event data is captured using electronic forms in an information system. Working with forms typically causes multiple events to be recorded when the form is submitted in the system. These events will share the same timestamp, even though the underlying actions might have taken place at different points in time.
- **Inadvertent time travel.** Inadvertent time travel occurs when events carry incorrect timestamps because the real timestamp is 'close' to the wrong value. Consider, for instance, a setting in which timestamps are manually recorded and events occur just after midnight. Under these conditions, staff members recording the date of the day before, together with the correct time, would cause inadvertent time travel in the event log.
- **Unanchored event.** This issue takes place when timestamps are recorded in a different format from the format expected by the tooling.
- **Scattered event.** This imperfection patters refers to the presence of information in the attribute values which highlights the presence of additional events. However, these events are not explicitly recorded, but are hidden in the attribute values which are recorded in the log. For example: the attribute values of an event in an operating theatre log conveys information on the phases of the surgery, which could be used to enrich the log with additional events.
- **Elusive case.** This issue occurs when events are not linked to a case, as is often observed when data originates from information systems which are not process-aware.
- **Scattered case.** A scattered case refers to a case for which key activities are not recorded in the event log under consideration. However, events related to these activities are present in a different system. To obtain insights in the full process flow for this case, the log needs to be composed using the content of several information systems.
- **Collateral events.** Collateral events are several events which refer to the same process action.
- **Polluted label.** This imperfection pattern occurs when several event attribute values have the same structure, but differ in terms of their specific values. Consider, for instance, that each activity label includes a reference to a specific patient and staff member (e.g. 'Clinical examination – patient 51545 – physician 4'). When such a log would be used for control-flow discovery purposes, it would suffer from the large number of unique activity labels.
- **Distorted label.** Distorted labels are multiple event attribute values which are not identical, but demonstrate very strong syntactic and semantic similarities. When, the diagnosis attribute contains values 'neurological condition' and 'neurologcal condition' (with an 'i' missing in the latter specification), this constitutes an example of a distorted label.

- **Synonymous labels.** This issue occurs when several values differ at the syntactic level, but are similar at the semantic level. For instance: in two distinct information systems, the same activity is referred to with two different labels.
- **Homonymous labels.** This imperfection pattern manifests itself when an activity is repeated for a particular case, but the semantics of this activity is not the same across these instances. For instance: when the activity 'Initial assessment' occurs for the first time, it implies that an ED physician has seen the patient. However, when this same activity takes place a second time, it implies that a medical specialist from an inpatient unit has been called to see a patient [31].

5.2.2.5   Taxonomy by Vanbrabant et al. [32]

In contrast to the prior taxonomies and the imperfection patterns of Suriadi et al. [31], Vanbrabant et al. [32] developed a taxonomy starting from a healthcare use case, i.e. the development of a simulation model for an emergency department. A simulation model is a computer model used to evaluate *'what if?'*-scenarios in order to reason about potential process changes [4]. As process mining techniques can be used during the development of such a simulation model [24, 30], event log data quality is also a prime concern within this context.

To provide a structured insight in the variety of event log quality issues, Vanbrabant et al. [32] propose a taxonomy based on a thorough analysis of both general and healthcare-specific taxonomies in literature. From this analysis, the authors conclude that, while their categorisation tends to differ, most taxonomies demonstrate strong similarities regarding the specific data problems that are specified. In their synthesized taxonomy, Vanbrabant et al. [32] distinguish between missing data and non-missing data, where the latter category is further subdivided in wrong data on the one hand and not wrong but not directly usable data on the other hand. These generic categories, which are consistent with Kim et al. [18], are translated into 14 specific event log quality issues.

Missing Data

Missing data relates to data entries which are absent in the log, even though they should be recorded. Within this category, three quality issues are identified:

- **Missing values.** Missing values are data values which should be present, but which are not recorded. In this respect, a distinction needs to be made between genuinely missing values and data entries for which it makes sense that no value is recorded. For instance: for patients who did not undergo a blood test, it makes sense that an attribute related to blood results has no value.
- **Missing attributes.** Missing attributes refer to attributes which are needed for the analysis, but which are not present in the event log. This can be either because it has not been exported to the provided dataset, or because it is not recorded in the

system altogether. While missing values reflect specific data entries which are missing for particular patients, missing attributes imply that an attribute value is missing for all patients.

- **Missing cases.** Missing cases implies that cases, which were handled in reality, do not appear in the event log. In healthcare, this could, for instance, imply that data of particular patients is not included in the log [32].

Non-missing Data

The category non-missing data contains event log quality issues which are related to data values which are recorded in the log. Within this category, a distinction is made between wrong data on the one hand and not wrong, but not directly usable data on the other hand.

The first subcategory, *wrong data*, consists of the following data quality issues:

- **Violation of logical order.** A violation of logical order implies that the order of particular activities is incorrect due to issues with the recorded timestamps. This could, for instance, lead to data entries making it seem as if a patient is discharged before receiving treatment.
- **Violation of mutual dependency.** A violation of mutual dependency occurs when two mutually dependent attributes have contradicting values. For example: when an infant patient is not assigned to a paediatrician, this could be considered as a violation of mutual dependency.
- **Inexactness of timestamps.** Inexact timestamps are timestamps which do not reflect the actual time at which an event took place. This is a common data quality issue in healthcare as many timestamps are recorded following a manual action by healthcare staff (e.g. sending a request or saving a file). When there is a discrepancy between the moment at which an action is executed and the moment at which it is recorded in the system, this data quality issue occurs.
- **Typing mistakes.** Typing mistakes in textual fields can also cause errors in attribute values, leading to issues for algorithms which use these attributes.
- **Outside domain range.** Domain range violations refer to timestamps, numerical and categorical data values which are outside the range of possible values. For instance: triage codes at the emergency department are often expressed as a number between, and including, 1 and 5. Within that context, a value of 7 would be outside the domain range, indicating that an entry error took place.
- **Other implausible values.** This issue is a residual category of wrong data values which do not correspond to one of the earlier specifications [32].

As shown in Fig. 5.2, the aforementioned wrong data issues are combined in two groups. A violation of logical order and a violation of mutual dependency are grouped as 'violated attribute dependencies', while the remaining issues are categorized as 'incorrect attribute values'.

Next to wrong data, the second subcategory of non-missing data consists of *not wrong, but not directly usable data*. This subcategory reflects data which is

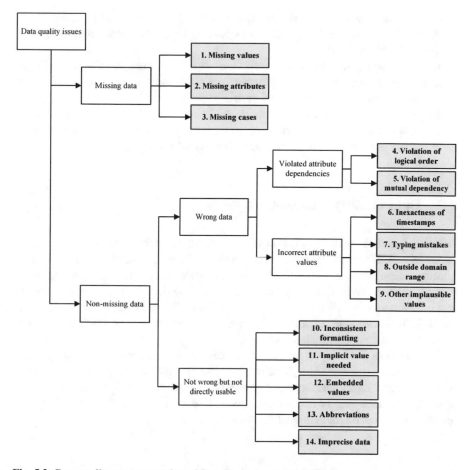

Fig. 5.2 Data quality taxonomy adapted from Vanbrabant et al. [32]

not wrong, but for which preprocessing is required in order to use it for analysis purposes. The following event log quality issues are specified:

- **Inconsistent formatting.** Inconsistent formatting implies that the format of data values of a particular attribute, or different attributes of the same type, is not consistent within a case or across cases. For instance: the timestamp format might differ when data originates from different systems.
- **Implicit value needed.** This quality issue refers to attribute values which are not available explicitly, but which can be derived from available data. Suppose, for instance, that the height and weight of a patient is available. In that case, the Body Mass Index is implicitly available as it can be calculated based on the recorded data.
- **Embedded values.** Embedded values are attribute values which are an aggregation of several usable pieces of information. Consider, for example, that gender

and age are codified in the dataset as F28 for a 28 year old female patient. When
the format is consistent, a gender and age attribute can be obtained by separating
this codified data entry.

- **Abbreviations.** Abbreviations are often used to shorten specific domain terminology. From an analysis perspective, abbreviations can be problematic,
  especially when they are not used consistently.
- **Imprecise data.** Imprecise data refers to data entries which are not specified at
  the required level of granularity. An example are timestamps which are recorded
  at the day level instead of at the minute or second level [32].

5.3 Data Quality Assessment

From the previous section, it follows that a multitude quality issues can potentially
occur in real-life event logs. This observation stresses the need for thorough data
quality assessment, i.e. determining whether data quality issues are present in the
event log. When an analyst is aware of the prevailing data quality issues, initiatives
can be taken to alleviate them (e.g. by collecting additional data) or, in case it is not
possible to tackle an issue, knowledge about its presence can be taken along when
conducting process mining analyses.

This section focuses on the topic of data quality assessment. Section 5.3.1
discusses some case studies to illustrate data quality issues prevailing in real-
life healthcare logs. Section 5.3.2 presents frameworks having the ambition to
structure the data quality assessment process. Section 5.3.3 discusses tools which
are available to conduct data quality assessment.

5.3.1 Data Quality Issues in Real-Life Healthcare Logs

Taking the taxonomies presented in Sect. 5.2.2 as a starting point, this subsection
illustrates data quality issues actually detected in real-life healthcare event logs.

While the taxonomy of Bose et al. [9] does not focus on a particular application
domain, three healthcare-related logs are used to illustrate the presence of event
log quality issues. Firstly, the logs from X-ray machines of Philips healthcare are
evaluated. These machines record high volumes of fine-grained data on a wide
variety of examinations. An additional source of variation are the personal habits
of physicians when executing a particular examination. Three data quality issues
are observed: incorrect timestamps (due to synchronisation issues with the clocks in
the system), irrelevant cases (depending on the analysis goals) and irrelevant events
(also depending on the analysis goals) [9].

Secondly, the public BPI challenge 2011 log is assessed, which relates to the
treatment procedures of cancer patients at a large Dutch academic hospital. Besides
the high control-flow complexity due to the variety of procedures included in the log,

several data quality issues are detected: missing resources, missing event attributes (e.g. diagnosis codes), imprecise activity names (mixed granularity of activity names and duplicate activity names), imprecise timestamps (several timestamps are recorded at the day level) and irrelevant events (i.e. each case contains events linked to a variety of departments and patient visits, which can be irrelevant for the question at hand) [9]. The same BPI challenge 2011 log is also assessed by Verhulst [33]. They detected that the granularity level of timestamps is inconsistent: while some timestamps are recorded at the level of seconds, others are recorded at the hour or even at the day level. Moreover, 2% traces contain duplicate events and multiple data types are detected for a single attribute (*Activity Code*) as this attribute contains integer, double and string values.

Finally, Bose et al. [9] study an event log originating from the systems of the intensive care unit at the Catharina Hospital in the Netherlands. The log mainly consists of events on the characteristics of patients, examinations which are conducted and clinical measurements which are performed. The identified data quality issues in this log are missing events (due to manual recording of some activities), missing case attributes (such as the main diagnosis at discharge), missing event attributes (e.g. related to blood results), incorrect timestamps (batch registration due to manual recording), imprecise activity names (duplicate activity names), imprecise timestamps (several timestamps are recorded at the day level) and irrelevant cases (due to the presence of patients with a variety of diagnoses in the same log) [9].

The taxonomy of Bose et al. [9] is also used by Mans et al. [21] to evaluate the data quality of the hospital information system at the Maastricht University Medical Centre. This evaluation is conducted by interviewing domain experts familiar with the raw data, and the assessment of the database tables by the authors. Based on this input, the prevalence of each data quality issue from the taxonomy of Bose et al. [9] is estimated. As shown in Table 5.4, three prevalence levels are considered: *N* refers to event log quality issues which do not occur, *L* indicates a low prevalence and *H* reflects a higher prevalence. Cells which are empty reflect event log quality issues

Table 5.4 Data quality assessment of the HIS at the Maastricht University Medical Centre [21]

	Case	Event	Belongs to	Case attribute	Position	Activity name	Timestamp	Resource	Event attribute
Missing data	N	H	L	L	N	L	N	N	L
Incorrect data	N	L	L	L	N	L	L	N	L
Imprecise data			N	N	N	N	H	H	N
Irrelevant data									

Empty cells reflect a event log quality issue which is not applicable. For the other issues, *N* indicates that the issue does not occur, *L* indicates a low prevalence and *H* indicates a higher prevalence which are not applicable. For instance: irrelevant cases and events are not applicable as each HIS data point is considered to be relevant for a particular patient.

From their case study at Maastricht University Medical Centre, Mans et al. [21] conclude that the three data quality issues which occur the most frequently are:

- **Missing events.** Missing events, i.e. events which took place in reality, but were not recorded in the system, are one of the most frequent event log quality issues. This can be attributed to the fact that many events require manual recording on behalf of caregivers, entailing the risk that they forget to record some actions that were executed.

- **Imprecise timestamps.** Several departments within the hospital use dedicated systems alongside the HIS. For instance, the radiology department uses a specific system for the creation, processing and management of medical images. For billing purposes, all departments transfer data to the HIS at a later stage. During this export, detailed timestamps are not always transferred and times might be defined at the day level in the HIS. More fine-grained timestamps are typically retrievable from the dedicated systems of a department.

- **Imprecise resources.** Imprecise resource data is the third frequently occurring event log quality issue. While the HIS records information about the resource entering an event, this resource does not always link to a specific staff member. For instance: the resource associated to an event might relate to a physical location within the hospital instead of to a staff member [21].

While the case of Mans et al. [21] aims to assess the data quality of a HIS as a whole, Suriadi et al. [31], Vanbrabant et al. [32] focus on one specific department: the emergency department. In the Belgian emergency department considered by Vanbrabant et al. [32], the largest data quality issue is batch recording of statuses as for 91.68% of all patients, several statuses are recorded within the same minute. This implies that, for many of these statuses, the recorded timestamp does not correspond to the moment in time at which an action was actually performed. Besides batch recording, several other data quality issues are detected. An example relates to the absence of required activities in the event log. Domain experts indicate that, for each patient, registration, triage, clinical examination, medical completion by a physician, and departure need to be recorded. However, for all patients, at least one of these actions is missing. For instance, for 88.53% of the patients, the clinical examination was missing. The absence of required actions can be problematic for control-flow discovery purposes [32].

In contrast to Vanbrabant et al. [32], Suriadi et al. [31] do not study the entire patient population at the emergency department, but focus on patients with chest pain. The raw data used to analyze the process flows of this patient population was provided in four distinct tables. Several data quality issues are detected, including form-based event capture as many medical parameters are recorded in a single form, leading to several events sharing the same timestamp. Moreover, Suriadi et al. [31] want to follow patients throughout their entire stay at the emergency department and, when relevant, during their admission to an inpatient unit. However, when a patient is admitted to the hospital, a different identifier is used for this patient, which constitutes a data quality issue. Other event log imperfection patterns, such as unanchored and scattered events, are also detected.

With the aforementioned BPI Challenge 2011 log as an exception, all event logs discussed until this point consist of private data. Open source healthcare data can, amongst others, be retrieved from the Medical Information Mart for Intensive Care III, or MIMIC-III in short, composed by the MIT Lab for Computational Physiology.[2] Kurniati et al. [20] evaluate the data quality of MIMIC-III for process mining purposes. An important data quality issue, which is purposefully introduced for anonymization purposes, is date shifting. This implies that all timestamps, which are recorded at the date level of granularity, are shifted by a random offset. As this offset is not consistent for all actions related to a specific patient, this causes issues for process mining purposes as the order of activities in the data might be changed. A multitude of other issues were detected, including missing events, missing timestamps, incorrect timestamps and duplicated events. Moreover, the system capturing the data has changed during the data collection period, which causes data format changes within the dataset. Despite the multitude of data quality problems, Kurniati et al. [20] still consider MIMIC-III a valuable data source for process mining purposes given the richness of the data in terms of attributes.

5.3.2   Data Quality Assessment Frameworks

The presence of a wide range of data quality issues in real-life healthcare event logs demonstrates the importance of thorough data quality assessment when applying process mining techniques. Existing frameworks which aim to structure process mining projects, such as the L*-methodology [2], the Process Diagnostics Method [10] and the PM^2-methodology [13], have limited attention for data quality assessment. However, recent literature provides some frameworks which have a more predominant focus on data quality assessment. These will be discussed in the remainder of his subsection.

5.3.2.1   Framework by Fox et al. [14]

The framework by Fox et al. [14] aims to mark electronic health records data with quality labels bad, compromised, or good. While bad data is of unacceptable quality, compromised data has issues but can still be used for some purposes. To add these quality markings, the Care Pathway Data Quality Framework (CP-DQF) is proposed, consisting of three key steps.

In the first step, a data quality register for the research question(s) (called experiments in Fox et al. [14]) at hand is created. This involves adding known data

---

[2]https://mimic.physionet.org/

quality issues to the register and linking each research question to these issues. At a later stage, these links will be used to determine which data cannot be used to answer particular questions due to the presence of data quality problems.

The second step, the application of CP-DQF on the available data, consists of several substeps:

- Metadata fields are added to the available data, which will be used to add quality labels. Fox et al. [14] suggest the addition of a Boolean *BadRow* and a vector string *BadRowCodes*, where the latter can hold several data quality issue codes.
- For each data quality issue, it is determined whether they can be handled by means of preprocessing, or whether they should be outlined in the discussion section of the report of the results.
- It is decided whether the presence of a particular quality issue would make the data unusable for a particular research question. When this is the case, the research question is marked and the data should be excluded for this research question.
- Following the conclusions from the previous step, the effect of excluding the data is determined. Marking some data as bad data might cause particular data integrity constraints to be violated.
- Marking code is written or executed to populate the metadata fields related to data quality, which were added in the first substep.
- In case mitigation code is available or can be developed to tackle a data quality issue, this is written or executed.
- Information about the scope of data quality issues and the mitigation actions that have been implemented are recorded in the data quality register for documentation purposes.
- To obtain a dataset to answer a research question, dataset collection code is written. This code takes into account the values of the metadata fields that have been added [14].

The final step of the framework entails reporting about the outcomes of the prior two steps. This involves a discussion of topics such as the general data quality of the available data, and the impact that data quality issues can have on the results [14].

5.3.2.2 Framework by Andrews et al. [6]

Andrews et al. [6] propose a framework which is inspired on the Cross Industry Standard Process for Data Mining (CRISP-DM). They specify steps that should take place before the final data extraction, i.e. in the early stages of a process mining project. This cyclical framework, visualized in Fig. 5.3, consists of seven steps:

- **Step 1: Process understanding.** In this step, the analyst should get acquainted with the process. To this end, potential information sources include existing process models and consultations with stakeholders.

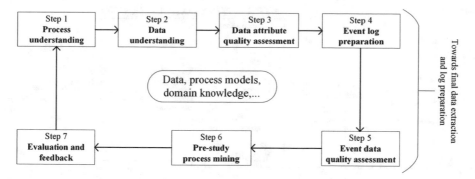

Fig. 5.3 Data quality assessment framework adapted from Andrews et al. [6]

- **Step 2: Data understanding.** Data understanding involves understanding the data, using instruments such as data dictionaries.
- **Step 3: Data attribute quality.** This step involves investigating the quality of the data at the level of individual attributes, e.g. by determining their completeness.
- **Step 4: Event log preparation.** While steps 2 and 3 consider the raw data, this step requires that the raw data is transformed into an initial event log. This log can be used for pre-study process mining purposes (step 6).
- **Step 5: Event quality.** In this step, the data quality is checked at the level of events. To this end, taxonomies such as the ones proposed in Sect. 5.2.2 can be used.
- **Step 6: Pre-study process mining.** Pre-study process mining implies that some initial process mining algorithms are applied to the event log to highlight data quality issues, e.g. by applying control-flow discovery algorithms.
- **Step 7: Evaluation and feedback.** Based on the input of the prior steps, this step involves communicating the identified issues to process owners, checking and potentially revising the questions at hand, and shaping the final event log that will be used to perform the study [6].

5.3.2.3   Framework by Martin et al. [25]

Martin et al. [25] propose an interactive data cleaning framework, which is shown in Fig. 5.4. Within this framework, a distinction is made between two types of data quality assessment: data-based and discovery-based assessment. Data-based assessment focuses on the identification of problematic patterns in the event log, i.e. by solely looking at the available data. However, even when data quality tests are thoroughly applied to the event log, there still exists a real risk that some issues are overlooked. To this end, Martin et al. [25] suggest to add discovery-based data quality assessment. A discovery-based approach implies that data quality problems are retrieved by discovering process models. For instance, the discovery of a control-flow model might visualize incorrect relationships between activities. From these

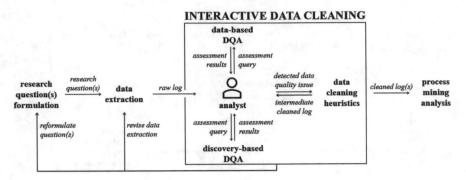

Fig. 5.4 Data quality assessment framework of Martin et al. [25]

erroneous relationships, such as a patient being discharged before being registered, incorrect timestamps for some cases can be discovered [25]. The discovery-based component in the framework of Martin et al. [25] conveys a similar idea than step 6 in the framework of Andrews et al. [6]. Both frameworks highlight the potential of applying, for instance, control-flow discovery algorithms to detect data quality issues.

When the data quality assessment results highlight the presence of quality issues, which will often be the case in real-life healthcare data, three main courses of actions are available to the analyst. Firstly, it might be possible to solve the problem by applying a particular data cleaning heuristic. Such a heuristic implements a particular data cleaning action, which will be the topic of Sect. 5.4. Secondly, data quality issues such as missing events might be rectified by collecting additional data, i.e. by returning to the data extraction phase. After additional data has been retrieved from the information systems, new assessment queries can be specified to verify whether the quality issues are resolved. Finally, quality assessment results might make it impossible to answer a particular research question. Consider, for instance, questions regarding resource involvement in case no resource information is available in the event log. Under these circumstances, the detected data quality issues require a reformulation of the research questions [25].

As shown in Fig. 5.4, the analyst is positioned at the center of the data quality assessment and data cleaning process. This stresses the interactive character of the framework, in which the analyst is in full control during the specification of data quality assessment queries and data cleaning heuristics.

5.3.3 Tools for Data Quality Assessment

Within the process mining field, data quality assessment often occurs on an ad-hoc basis [5, 22]. This implies that some tests are being performed, often based on an analyst's experience within the healthcare organization. Given the key importance of data quality to ensure reliable process mining outcomes, more elaborate data quality assessment is warranted. This would be facilitated when it is supported by adequate tooling. Such tooling should move beyond showing error messages when data inputs are inconsistent with the expected data format, as this only constitutes one potential data quality issue.

In an effort to support systematic event log quality assessment, the open source R-package DaQAPO[3], Data Quality Assessment for Process-Oriented data, has been developed [23]. R[4] is a programming language providing extensive functionalities for data manipulation and statistical analysis. Additional functionalities can be obtained by installing packages with a specific purpose, of which DaQAPO focuses on supporting data quality assessment of process execution data. The package is part of bupaR,[5]which is an integrated suite consisting of R-packages targeted towards handling and analyzing process execution data [16].

The key functionalities of DaQAPO can be grouped in three categories: (1) functions to read in data, (2) functions to identify data quality issues, and (3) a function to remove anomalies from the data. Within the second category, DaQAPO provides a wide range of functions which detect commonly occurring data quality issues in healthcare data. These include missing values, incomplete cases, batch registration of events by a staff member (e.g. a physician who records his/her findings after having seen several patients), and the absence of related activities (e.g. a bed at an inpatient unit being assigned without being requested). Every function can be fine-tuned to the context of a specific hospital by entering the appropriate parameter values. The function-based architecture enables users of DaQAPO to iteratively and interactively dig deeper to gain a thorough insight in the prevailing data quality issues.

Within the same line of thought, i.e. enabling efficient and effective data quality assessment, the recent work of Andrews et al. [5] is promising. They introduce the foundations of a new log query language QUELI, Querying Event Log for Imperfections. In the long run, QUELI should evolve into a query language which can be used to detect the event log imperfection patterns discussed in Sect. 5.2.2.4. At the time of writing, detection algorithms had been developed for the following five imperfection patterns: form-based event capture, inadvertent time travel, collateral events, synonymous labels and homonymous labels.

5.4   Data Cleaning

Based on the data quality assessment results, healthcare organizations gain insight in the data quality issues which are prevailing. These insights should be taken into account when performing process mining analyses as the identified issues might

---

[3]https://github.com/nielsmartin/daqapo/
[4]https://www.r-project.org/
[5]https://bupar.net/

impact the credibility of the results. For some specific data quality issues, heuristics have been developed in an effort to rectify them. While some researchers proposed alternative solutions to data quality issues in HIS-data, such as its integration with alternative sources of process execution information [22], this section focuses on data cleaning heuristics using the event log as the only source of process execution data. In particular, Sect. 5.4.1 describes exemplary data cleaning heuristics and Sect. 5.4.2 contains a reflection on such heuristics.

5.4.1 Data Cleaning Heuristics

Several data cleaning heuristics have been proposed in literature. These typically target one particular data quality issue and build upon several assumptions about the event log or the way in which the event log quality issue manifests itself. This subsection describes data cleaning heuristics regarding the following event log quality issues: incorrect timestamps (Sect. 5.4.1.1), missing case identifiers (Sect. 5.4.1.2), missing events (Sect. 5.4.1.3), and incorrect/missing attribute values at a more generic level (Sect. 5.4.1.4).

5.4.1.1 Incorrect Timestamps

From Sect. 5.3.1, it follows that many event log quality issues originate from timestamp-related problems. These might, for instance, be incorrect or might be recorded at different granularity levels because they originate from different systems [9, 32]. Such timestamp-related data quality issues are problematic for control-flow discovery purposes as they distort the order of events. Within this context, Dixit et al. [12] propose an interactive approach to rectify such event ordering issues. Their approach consists of the following four steps:

- **Step 1: Automated detection.** The first step automatically generates a list of potential timestamp-related data quality problems. To this end, three indicators for such issues are considered: (1) the level of granularity of timestamps, (2) potential order anomalies based on the algorithm's guess about the correct order, and (3) statistical anomalies, e.g., based on the temporal position of an event compared to other events.
- **Step 2: User-driven repair.** Based on the list of potential data quality issues from step 1, the user can start to interactively repair these issues. To this end, the user can model relationships between events in an interactive Petri Net editor and highlight the way in which the timestamps should be repaired. Besides changing a timestamp, repair actions can also involve the addition of removal of events. To actually repair the event log, alignment techniques from the conformance checking field are used.

- **Step 3: Impact analysis.** Besides the repaired event log, a copy of the log before the repair action is also saved. In the third step of the approach, impact analysis, the impact of the repair on the event log is made explicit. Several metrics are used, including the Levenshtein distance between both logs, the number of removed events, and the number of events for which the timestamp has been changed.
- **Step 4: Log update.** Based on the impact analysis results, the user should decide whether or not the repair is confirmed. When the change to the log is confirmed, the repaired log will replace its predecessor before the repair action was taken.

5.4.1.2   Missing Case Identifiers

Bayomie et al. [7] propose an approach to handle missing case identifiers. However, in contrast to a situation in which case identifiers are missing for some events, they consider a setting in which all case identifiers are missing. The developed method, which is built around the concept of decision trees, requires the event log and a correct control-flow model as input, together with the mean and standard deviation of the duration of each activity. This latter information can be provided by domain experts, or retrieved from the event log. The generated output is a series of event logs with case identifiers, together with a measure expressing the level of confidence in the imputed case identifiers [7].

In order to apply the method of Bayomie et al. [7], the following assumptions must hold: (1) an event's timestamp should mark the completion of the current activity and the start of the next activity, (2) the process control-flow does not contain loops, and (3) the process has a single start activity which makes it possible to recognize a new case.

5.4.1.3   Missing Events

Another common data quality issue are missing events, i.e. events which took place in reality, but were not recorded in the event log. In this respect, Rogge-Solti et al. [29] propose a method to add missing events and impute an appropriate timestamp value. To this end, the most likely missing events are determined based on path probabilities of process models developed by domain experts (modeled using Stochastic Petri Nets). Afterwards, Bayesian networks are leveraged to determine the most likely timestamp for the imputed events. The approach of Rogge-Solti et al. [29] builds on several assumptions, including the fact that all non-missing timestamps are correct, that events are missing at random, and that activity durations follow a normal distribution.

Regarding the same data quality issue, i.e. missing events, Di Francescomarino et al. [11] highlight that, e.g., manual activities are often not recorded in the information system and, hence, not present in the event log. Such non-observable activities are considered problematic from a process mining perspective as they will not appear in process mining outcomes such as a control-flow model. To this end,

Di Francescomarino et al. [11] propose a technique to add non-observable activities to traces in the event log using action languages. Focusing on event logs without timestamps, the proposed algorithm uses a control-flow model and data attributes to complete traces. This control-flow model, delivered by domain experts and assumed to be correct and complete, is encoded as a planning problem. Besides the constraints that the control-flow model imposes, additional constraints can originate from data attributes. For instance: a particular activity might only be executed when the patient has a particular characteristic. To formulate the planning problem, the action language K is used [11].

Besides Rogge-Solti et al. [29] and Di Francescomarino et al. [11], other heuristics have also been developed to add missing events. These include Wang et al. [34], where a method is developed to add missing events to an event log without timestamps using a branching framework, and Bertoli et al. [8], where the notion of a satisfiability problem is leveraged. Both Wang and Strong [35] and Bertoli et al. [8] assume the availability of a control-flow model, the former in the form of a Petri net and the latter as a BPMN-model.

5.4.1.4 Incorrect/Missing Attribute Values

The heuristics outlined in Sects. 5.4.1.1, 5.4.1.2 and 5.4.1.3 all require domain knowledge to perform data cleaning. Domain expertise can, for instance, be conveyed by means of a process model, which is a commonly required input for existing data cleaning algorithms. Recently, Nguyen et al. [26] proposed a data cleaning approach which does not require any form of domain expertise. Their approach focuses on two data quality issues, i.e. the correction of incorrect attribute values and the imputation of missing attribute values. To tackle these issues without the need for any domain expertise, they use autoencoders, which are a specific type of neural network which is trained using unlabelled data.

Even though preliminary results on structured artificial data are promising, their approach still experiences difficulties to manage the complexity of real-life data. Especially the correction of timestamps in real-life event logs proves to be a daunting task for autoencoders. The authors attribute the algorithm's underperformance to correct these timestamps to the significant variability of case and activity durations in real-life data. In contrast, the generated artificial data used normal distributions for timestamp specification, which facilitates the training of the autoencoder [26]. Moreover, the approach of Nguyen et al. [26] assumes randomly introduced anomalies and missing values, while in practice some patterns might exist. Given such limitations, future refinements of this type of algorithms would benefit from incorporating domain knowledge in the data cleaning process.

5.4.2 A Reflection on Data Cleaning Heuristics

From the previous, it follows that data cleaning heuristics have been developed to tackle some specific event log quality issues. However, these heuristics tend to be based on strong assumptions, which can hamper their application in a real-life context. When certain assumptions do not hold in reality, the application of data cleaning heuristics might lead to unwarranted manipulations of the data. This can, in its turn, lead to incorrect and misleading conclusions when used for process mining purposes. Besides the need to check the validity of the assumptions, domain expertise will also be required to determine whether the corrections proposed by the algorithm make sense in practice. This stresses the potential of interactive data cleaning approaches (e.g., the one proposed in Sect. 5.3.2.3) in which the healthcare professional is in full control of the data cleaning efforts.

Regardless of the data cleaning approach that has been used, it is important to take into consideration the fact that the original data has been changed in the remainder of the process mining analysis. Some conclusions might immediately follow from changes that have been made to the event log. Such conclusions need to be handled with care and have to be interpreted against the background of the performed data cleaning actions.

5.5 Conclusion

Given its impact on the reliability of process mining outcomes, data quality should be a prime concern to all researchers and practitioners in the field. This especially holds in healthcare, where real-life data typically suffers from a multitude of data quality issues, amongst others because many events are recorded following a manual action by healthcare staff.

Against this background, this chapter provided an introduction to data quality in the process mining field. Firstly, data quality taxonomies were discussed in which potential data quality issues are described. A distinction is made between generic taxonomies and dedicated taxonomies from the process mining domain. The issues identified in this latter category of taxonomies show that process mining is confronted with specific data quality problems due to the specific characteristics of an event log. Secondly, attention was attributed to data quality assessment, i.e. the identification of data quality issues prevailing in an event log. As insights in the existing data quality issues are indispensable for the remainder of the process mining project, data quality assessment should be an integral part in each process mining project. Finally, this chapter outlined some data cleaning heuristics which aim to alleviate specific event log quality issues. However, such methods often build upon strong assumptions which might not hold for a real-life healthcare process. This highlights the need to closely involve domain experts during the data cleaning process.

Even though literature provides data cleaning heuristics to cope with some specific event log problems, it needs to be recognized that improved data collection at the source is always desirable. In that respect, healthcare organizations are encouraged to take measures to improve the accuracy of data registration. Management can emphasize the importance of accurate data registration to nurses and physicians by making its potential explicit. Moreover, investments can be done in systems which enable swift data registration as healthcare staff tends to already experience a high work pressure. Efforts to promote better data registration at the source are worthwhile as they would enable process mining to reach its full potential in helping healthcare organizations to understand their processes. These process insights can be leveraged to instigate process improvement initiatives.

References

1. van der Aalst WMP. Extracting event data from databases to unleash process mining. In: vom Brocke J, Schmiedel T. editors. BPM – driving innovation in a digital world. Cham: Springer; 2015. p. 105–28.
2. van der Aalst WMP. Process mining: data science in action. Heidelberg: Springer; 2016.
3. van der Aalst WMP, Adriansyah A, Wynn M. Process mining manifesto. Lect Notes Bus Inf Process. 2012;99:169–94.
4. Altiok T, Melamed B. Simulation modeling and analysis with Arena. San Diego: Elsevier; 2010.
5. Andrews R, Suriadi S, Ouyang C, Poppe E. Towards event log querying for data quality. Lect Notes Comput Sci. 2018;11229:116–34.
6. Andrews R, Wynn MT, Vallmuur K, Ter Hofstede AH, Bosley E, Elcock M, Rashford S. Leveraging data quality to better prepare for process mining: an approach illustrated through analysing road trauma pre-hospital retrieval and transport processes in Queensland. Int J Environ Res Public Health. 2019;16(7):1138.
7. Bayomie D, Awad A, Ezat E. Correlating unlabeled events from cyclic business processes execution. Lect Notes Comput Sci. 2016;9694:274–89.
8. Bertoli P, Di Francescomarino C, Dragoni M, Ghidini C. Reasoning-based techniques for dealing with incomplete business process execution traces. In: Proceedings of the congress of the italian association for artificial intelligence. Springer; 2013. p. 469–80.
9. Bose RJCP, Mans RS, van der Aalst WMP. Wanna improve process mining results? It's high time we consider data quality issues seriously. Tech. Rep. BPM Center Report BPM-13-02, Eindhoven University of Technology, 2013.
10. Bozkaya M, Gabriels J, van der Werf JM. Process diagnostics: a method based on process mining. In: Proceedings of the 2009 international conference on information, process, and knowledge management. IEEE; 2009. p. 22–7.
11. Di Francescomarino C, Ghidini C, Tessaris S, Sandoval IV. Completing workflow traces using action languages. Lect Notes Comput Sci. 2015;9097:314–30.
12. Dixit PM, Suriadi S, Andrews R, Wynn MT, ter Hofstede AH, Buijs JC, van der Aalst WMP. Detection and interactive repair of event ordering imperfection in process logs. Lect Notes Comput Sci. 2018;10816:274–90.
13. van Eck ML, Lu X, Leemans SJJ, van der Aalst WMP. PM^2: a process mining project methodology. Lect Notes Comput Sci. 2015;9097:297–313.
14. Fox F, Aggarwal VR, Whelton H, Johnson O. A data quality framework for process mining of electronic health record data. In: Proceedings of the 2018 IEEE international conference on healthcare informatics. IEEE; 2018. p. 12–21.

15. Gschwandtner T, Gärtner J, Aigner W, Miksch S. A taxonomy of dirty time-oriented data. Lect Notes Comput Sci. 2012;7465:58–72.
16. Janssenswillen G, Depaire B, Swennen M, Jans M, Vanhoof K. Bupar: enabling reproducible business process analysis. Knowl Based Syst. 2019;163:927–30.
17. Kahn MG, Raebel MA, Glanz JM, Riedlinger K, Steiner JF. A pragmatic framework for single-site and multisite data quality assessment in electronic health record-based clinical research. Medical Care 2012;50:S21–9.
18. Kim W, Choi BJ, Hong EK, Kim SK, Lee D. A taxonomy of dirty data. Data Min Knowl Disc. 2003;7(1):81–99.
19. Kirchner K, Herzberg N, Rogge-Solti A, Weske M. Embedding conformance checking in a process intelligence system in hospital environments. Lect Notes Comput Sci. 2013;7738: 126–39.
20. Kurniati AP, Rojas E, Hogg D, Hall G, Johnson OA. The assessment of data quality issues for process mining in healthcare using medical information mart for intensive care III, a freely available e-health record database. Health Inf J. 2019;25(4):1878–93.
21. Mans RS, van der Aalst WMP, Vanwersch RJB. Process mining in healthcare: evaluating and exploiting operational healthcare processes. Heidelberg: Springer; 2015.
22. Martin N. Using indoor location system data to enhance the quality of healthcare event logs: opportunitics and challenges. Lect Notes Bus Inf Process. 2018;342:226–38.
23. Martin N, Van Houdt G. DaQAPO – data quality assessment for process-oriented data. Https://github.com/nielsmartin/daqapo, 2019.
24. Martin N, Depaire B, Caris A. The use of process mining in business process simulation model construction. Bus Inf Syst Eng. 2016;58(1):73–87.
25. Martin N, Martinez-Millana A, Valdivieso B, Fernández-Llatas C. Interactive data cleaning for process mining: a case study of an outpatient clinic's appointment system. Lect Notes Bus Inf Process. 2019;362:532–44.
26. Nguyen HTC, Lee S, Kim J, Ko J, Comuzzi M. Autoencoders for improving quality of process event logs. Expert Syst Appl. 2019;131:132–47.
27. Rahm E, Do HH. Data cleaning: problems and current approaches. IEEE Data Eng Bull. 2000;23(4):3–13.
28. Rebuge Á, Ferreira DR. Business process analysis in healthcare environments: a methodology based on process mining. Inf Syst. 2012;37(2):99–116.
29. Rogge-Solti A, Mans RS, van der Aalst WMP, Weske M. Repairing event logs using timed process models. Lect Notes Comput Sci. 2013;8186:705–8.
30. Rozinat A, Mans RS, Song M, van der Aalst WM. Discovering simulation models. Inf Syst. 2009;34(3):305–27.
31. Suriadi S, Andrews R, ter Hofstede AH, Wynn MT. Event log imperfection patterns for process mining: towards a systematic approach to cleaning event logs. Inf Syst. 2017;64:132–50.
32. Vanbrabant L, Martin N, Ramaekers K, Braekers K. Quality of input data in emergency department simulations: framework and assessment techniques. Simul Model Pract Theory. 2019;91:83–101.
33. Verhulst R. Evaluating quality of event data within event logs: an extensible framework. Master's thesis, Eindhoven University of Technology, 2016.
34. Wang J, Song S, Zhu X, Lin X, Sun J. Efficient recovery of missing events. IEEE Trans Knowl Data Eng. 2016;28(11):2943–57.
35. Wang RY, Strong DM. Beyond accuracy: what data quality means to data consumers. J Manag Inf Syst. 1996;12(4):5–33.

Chapter 6
Towards Open Process Models in Healthcare: Open Standards and Legal Considerations

Luis Marco-Ruiz, Thomas Beale, Juan José Lull, Silje Ljosland Bakke, Ian McNicoll, and Birger Haarbrandt

6.1 Introduction

6.1.1 Pathways, Guidelines and Computerized Clinical Decision Support

Previous chapters have explained the relationship between clinical process workflows and process mining. In order to discuss further topics related to interoperability and specification of workflows, a more thorough description becomes handy.

L. Marco-Ruiz (✉)
Peter L. Reichertz Institut für Medizinische Informatik, TU Braunschweig and Hannover Medical School, Hannover, Germany

Norwegian Centre for E-Health Research, University Hospital North Norway, Tromsø, Norway
e-mail: Luis.Marco-Ruiz@plri.de

T. Beale
Ars Semantica Ltd., London, UK

openEHR International, London, UK

J. José Lull
Process Mining 4 Health Lab – SABIEN – ITACA Institute, Universitat Politècnica de València, Valencia, Spain

S. Ljosland Bakke
openEHR International, London, UK

Helse Vest IKT AS, Bergen, Norway

I. McNicoll
openEHR International, London, UK

B. Haarbrandt
Peter L. Reichertz Institut für Medizinische Informatik, TU Braunschweig and Hannover Medical School, Hannover, Germany

© Springer Nature Switzerland AG 2021
C. Fernandez-Llatas (ed.), *Interactive Process Mining in Healthcare*, Health
Informatics, https://doi.org/10.1007/978-3-030-53993-1_6

In the following, we leverage the definitions provided by Field and Lorr [28], Fox [19], Kinsman et al. [32], and the openEHR specifications [5] to define the types of workflow models in the clinical domain as:

- Clinical guidelines are *"systematically developed statements designed to assist practitioner and patient on decisions about appropriate health care for specific clinical circumstances"* [28].
- A care pathway is a structured multidisciplinary description of a set of time-framed activities focused on a specific condition that provide guidance on how to deal with the situations that may arise during the treatment of the condition [5, 19, 32]. Care pathways aim to reduce variability and are developed considering clinical guidelines adapting their content to local contexts [5, 32].
- A care plan is a concrete set of activities to be performed for the treatment of a specific patient in order to achieve a pre-defined goal leveraging patient's specific features (preferences, co-morbidities, etc.) [5, 19].
- A task plan is the term we will use to refer to the computable specification of the tasks and goals that formally define a care plan [5].

The medical informatics community has traditionally approached the support of clinical processes as part of Computerized Clinical Decision Support (CCDS). Particularly, the CCDS community has focused on providing support for the interoperability of workflows by implementing computer interpretable clinical guidelines (CIGs) [47, 48]. In a nutshell, CIGs attempt to formally specify the ideal clinical process and interact with the EHR to recommend appropriate actions to clinicians with the objective of increasing the adherence to clinical guidelines [47]. Various standards have been developed to specify clinical guidelines (published as free text documents) as CIGs and defining the architecture to allow their interoperation with the EHR [35]. However, several challenges have imposed strong barriers for their general adoption and, nowadays, the real use of (EHR-embedded) CIGs is scarce [47]. Examples of these challenges are the complexities inherent to the description of processes that need to be agreed at national level, the lack of good options to deal with ambiguity, and the local adaption needed to deal with the specificities inherent to each clinical organization [35, 47].

Several studies have pointed out the complexities in the clinical knowledge elicitation process [31, 35, 52]. An example are national infrastructures for CCDS [31, 36] and the conceptual CREDO framework proposed by Fox [18]. Those frameworks are interesting for understanding the decision making process and its connection with CIGs development. However, there is a challenge in being able to measure the effect and observing the full care process that may not be directly observable by clinicians due to its complexity. Currently, this problem is one of the main barriers for CIGs adoption since local adaptation to specific contexts where the particularities of the local workflow need to be leveraged has proved to be one of the main barriers affecting CIGs adoption and interoperability [41, 47].

Interestingly, the information for describing the real process is available in EHRs. But it is represented in a format that does not easily allow for understanding the full process details. The format that EHRs use is oriented towards providing one specific patient care rather than representing pathways common to a specific cohort of patients. In order to observe clinical processes, it is necessary to filter noise and present events in a human-comprehensible way so the clinical expert can make sense of them [45]. This requirement is also related to the perceptual computing paradigm, the concept of computing for the human experience [53, 54] and the co-pilot paradigm [4]. In perceptual computing, Artificial Intelligence (AI) serves as a mechanism for balancing the human perception enabling better decisions and perceiving aspects crucial for treating complex cases that, otherwise, would remain hidden in health information systems´ logs. When combined with clinical knowledge, Process Mining has the potential to act as a perceptual mechanism that allows the clinical expert to explore, understand, and identify areas of improvement of the clinical process [57]. Its main difference with respect to the CIGs and BPM approaches is that, instead of defining an ideal workflow that must be mapped to a particular organization, it analyzes the logs of the information system to infer the actual events and traces present in each system. Therefore, the workflow described is based on events from the real one, rather than an ideal workflow from a guideline. In medical organizations, this means that Process Mining has the potential to let us observe the real operation of different actors by connecting the events recorded in the EHR. This has the potential to determine in a quantitative manner which parts of a clinical workflow deviate significantly from the ideal path described by a clinical guideline and understand why a deviation is caused. In most cases, these deviations have a clear reason with a specific clinical interest since they are related to cases that do not comply with the ideal patient that a specific guideline focuses on, but on complex cases that require the interaction of various medical experts in order to determine the optimal treatment for one patient. That is the case of patients suffering from multimorbidities. Process Mining can help clinicians to better understand those cases and facilitate the decision on how to deal with those patients by, for example, developing computable phenotypes for detecting those uncommon cases so their optimal treatment can be rapidly determined using previous experiences with similar cases.

This vision complements frameworks like CREDO [18] in two ways. First, it allows for visualizing and understanding the real process before designing new care plans, thus determining what stages of the new care plan require interventions for approaching the ideal care pathway. Second, it allows for observing the effect after adopting the new care plan. This sets the foundations for working iteratively performing DMAIC cycles implementing continuous improvement in complex areas that require constant monitoring, thus, helping to realize the concept of Learning Healthcare System (LHS) [21, 44].

6.2 The Need of Semantics for Clinical Processes

The ability to observe real processes in operation and, furthermore, the results of a specific CCDS intervention is needed for the implementation of the LHS [20, 44].

In this sense, the results of Process Mining techniques should not only be delivered to a process manager in a report; but they should be delivered as tailored advice back to clinicians embedded in their clinical workflow [2]. This would enable the implementation of cognitive health information systems capable of learning and improving from their own experience. For this, Process Mining would need to be combined with EHR information representation formats so daily EHR operation can be analyzed by Process Mining algorithms, and the results of these analyses can be delivered back to clinicians as tailored CCDS. However, nowadays, the automatic generation of workflow models is mostly limited to formalisms that do not allow for embedding clinical semantics. One of these formats are Petri nets and their derivatives [58]. While Petri Nets, YAWL, and other process specification formalisms, are very powerful in terms of expressing complex workflows with branching, conditional executions, etc. they are mathematical abstractions that lack clear semantics and context. In addition, they are designed to define systems where the actor is a passive agent, while in the healthcare domain actors are active agents who make choices, react to drugs etc. [5].

Noteworthy, clinical processes are extremely sensitive to context semantics. This is depicted in Fig. 6.1 where the left side shows how traditional enterprise Data Warehousing (DW) methods require effectiveness to deal with massive amounts of data and few contextual data to make sense of these large data sets [34, 39]. However, as shown on the right of Fig. 6.1, clinical DW traditionally operates with lower amounts of data, but it requires complex data structures and semantic enrichment to be able to interpret clinical data sets [34, 39]. For example, spine surgery to relieve back pain is a concept which requires many contextual attributes to correctly specify the exact process: the surgical approach (laminectomy, fusion surgery, etc.), the access devices used (bone flap elevator, microscope, immobilization frame, spinal decompression cutter), the access approach to the spine (anterior or posterior), the programmed date for the procedure, the parties that will carry out the procedure, and so on. In fact, this example only refers to situational context, more contextual properties are commonly linked to EHR data such as protocols, order workflows, episodes of care, etc. [7]. Therefore, there is a need for representing processes that are discovered and linked to the context where their traces originated. This requires the specification of different types of semantics in order to ensure the adequate interpretation of clinical information. Otherwise, the

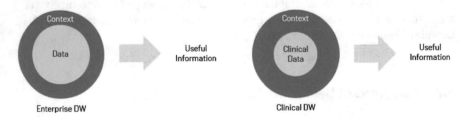

Fig. 6.1 Amount of contextual semantics needed in Enterprise Data Warehouses and Clinical Data Warehouses

complexity inherent to the clinical domain can easily become ambiguous in the definition of clinical terms. Processes and actions are not an exception to this since clinical processes often involve various professionals that are placed in different organizations. Examples include: the treatment of COPD patients which usually involves lung specialists, GPs, and physiotherapists; the follow-up and treatment of pre-birth cardiac pathologies which are carried out by the collaboration of the gynecologist and a team usually situated in a reference hospital consisting of pediatric cardiologists; the performance of genetic analyses which are often undertaken by a molecular biologist in a specialist laboratory and reported to the requester physician, etc. Furthermore, enabling continuous improvement requires understanding how the same type of complex patient was managed by various health organizations. However, this is problematic when the semantics of the clinical concepts involved in the process are not precise since they cannot be traced across different health organizations [11, 34].

The Process Mining community has approached this challenge in a general way by defining the cXtensible Event Stream (XES) standard [59]. As shown in the figure, XES defines logs as the wrapper element of process information, which in turn contain traces formed by several events. Attributes of various data types can be bound to these entities for describing information about them. XES provides an important contribution since it establishes a way for defining events and traces in XML format. An excerpt of the XES class diagram is provided in Fig. 6.2. As shown in the diagram, an event log can declare the so-called extensions for defining more granular attributes to define the semantics of processes.

However, at the time of writing, these extensions have not been further developed and it is up to the specialists of each domain to define them for allowing the definition of their processes. If one considers the complexity of the clinical domain, the semantic extensions using XES would take an enormous amount of effort to be developed. For example, the core of 100 archetypes approved and published by the Norwegian Clinical Knowledge Manager (CKM) have taken 6 years to be developed and clinically approved since the CKM began its operation in 2014 as a collaboration among Norwegian health regions that provided clinical reviewers [26]. In addition, the archetypes that conform the openEHR EHR structure in Norway have not been developed in isolation, but they have been developed and approved in collaboration with the International openEHR CKM that receives feedback from various countries, thus increasing their robustness as generic information models [26]. Furthermore, the amount of experts to develop them would be unaffordable and the models developed may, in the best case, be iso-semantic (e.g. structurally different but semantically equivalent) to those defined as archetypes or FHIR profiles [29]. A more sensible approach is to directly reuse the existing methods in the healthcare domain for specifying clinical data and process features. However, this requires to carefully assess the different types of semantics involved in the specification of a process to make it clinically relevant and precise enough to drive conclusions from its analysis.

When it comes to healthcare, the semantic extension of processes involves the definition of different types of semantics. Different classifications of semantics exist

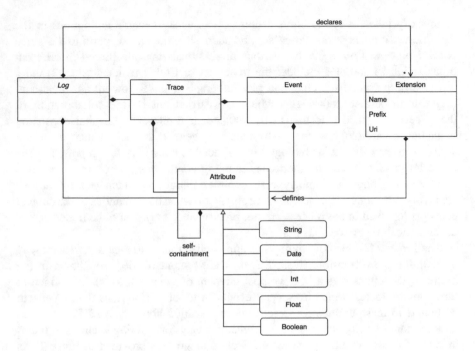

Fig. 6.2 Extract of XES model class diagram

depending on the point of view [39, 46, 50]. For convenience, in this chapter, we will classify the semantics involved in three main types:

- The first type is **data semantics** that capture the information recorded with regards to a process in one particular stage of this process. For example, in a blood pressure measurement, data semantics specify the values observed as systolic = 110, and diastolic = 95. These kinds of semantics may also specify constraints on the specification of some data such as maximum values, number of digits, occurrences, etc.
- The second type is **workflow semantics**, i.e. the semantics that allow specifying the order and status of stages in a specific process. For example, which stage occurred before, what was the initial stage or entry point, what is the termination stage, which activities terminated successfully, which stages did not occur or terminated partially etc.
- The third type is **contextual semantics** that allow specifying the provenance of a particular event. These semantics specify, for example, the parties involved, the institution, the department, the devices used for a particular procedure, the date where it occurred etc. An example is the place of measurement for the blood pressure, the device used, the identifier of the nurse performing the measurement, etc.

The reader should note that these semantics are often not clearly separated and they are often interlinked at different levels in health information systems [34].

In order to enable developing a LHS, Process Mining will require the clear definition of all three types of semantics for enabling cross-institutional interoperability. The last decade has seen many initiatives for enabling interoperability in healthcare. Examples are the well-known Meaningful Use initiative in the US that promoted the adoption of EHRs [9], and the epSOS project in Europe communicating continuity of care data from different countries [42]. However, these initiatives have been mostly limited to data and contextual semantics interoperability. Data and contextual semantics interoperability is necessary, but not sufficient for enabling cross-institutional Process Mining. Process interoperability builds on data and contextual semantics for further specifying the intra-organizational processes, but it also requires workflow semantics in order to make sense of EHR data at a process level.

Clinical information standards have extensively worked on the definition of data and contextual semantics leading to the definition of various data interoperability standards (e.g. openEHR, HL7 CDA, FHIR, CDISC, to name a few). These standards also provide the connection with biomedical terminologies for the precise specification of clinical information. Process interoperability standards have also been proposed by CCDS researchers for CIG implementations as explained before. Among these standards, openEHR was created for defining the full structure of the EHR allowing for version control and dynamic management of the application domain model [16]. This is done by relying on a two-level information architecture. The first level acts as a reference meta-model that specifies the EHR structures that do not vary over time originally defined in the GeEHR Australia and GEHR EU projects [17, 27, 30]. The second model allows for the definition of more complex constraints for developing health information schemas known as archetypes defined by Beale [6]. Archetypes are combined to form complex information schemas to represent full EHR data-sets known as templates. OpenEHR repositories allow the import of templates in a dynamic way without the need for performing changes at software level [6]. This boosts the scalability of openEHR systems since health is a complex domain in continuous evolution that often requires the redefinition of models for accommodating new evidence and supporting new procedures. OpenEHR has traditionally focused on the representation of data and contextual semantics. However, in the last few years, the openEHR community has developed the openEHR Task Planning Specification that allows for the specification of workflow semantics [3, 5].

With the addition of the Task Planning Model, the openEHR specifications cover most of the semantics needed to build on process mining methods for specifying rich process definitions after using Process Mining discovery algorithms.

In the following, we specify the model governance of archetypes and establish the link between clinical processes and the openEHR task model. There are other standards available for describing clinical information models (data and contextual semantics) in combination with terminologies. However, in this chapter we will present openEHR because it allows us to represent the full EHR structure, not only extracts, which is needed for providing the most complete information to PM algorithms. In addition, a workflow model built on openEHR archetypes will be precisely defined and seamlessly executed over various EHRs if they use the same set of archetypes for defining their model.

6.3   Data and Contextual Semantics with openEHR

As mentioned before, data and contextual semantics are specified in openEHR by means of Archetypes. Archetypes are commonly agreed models that represent (aspirational) maximum data sets of a specific reusable section of the electronic health record. For example, the Norwegian CKM develops archetypes as a nationally coordinated effort. These archetypes are reviewed by means of a Web application among clinicians from all over the country and, when consensus is reached, they are published openly so vendors can base their developments on these models [26]. Sharing a common library for clinical information models allows Norwegian vendors to rely on robust validated information models to build their applications. Since these models are common to all the vendors that implement openEHR, interoperability is granted as long as they rely on the same set of archetypes.

Archetypes are defined by means of the Archetype Definition Language (ADL). ADL can be visualized as a highly expressive language that was conceived for the specification of reusable information schemas known as Archetypes. Archetypes are defined in ADL instead of other well-known languages for expressivity reasons, since, for example, it provides properties such a rich set of leaf types (particularly intervals, date/times, coded terms, slots, and external references), and it provides a regular structuring (like JSON) for human readability. ADL models can be exported losslesly to other machine-readable formats such as XML, JSON, YAML etc.

Current openEHR-based systems allow for dynamic storage of data models. This means that their persistence model is not directly based on a proprietary database (e.g. relational or documental), but rather on the openEHR reference model and the templates (defined by combining archetypes). Therefore, when support for new functionality needs to be provided, they can obtain the archetypes published by their national CKM, localize them as openEHR templates, and use these templates as persistence schemas. This allows for directly storing and retrieving data in an openEHR compliant manner. This facilitates scalability and reduces the burden on the development of new functionality because the evolution of the models does not require modifying the software for enabling their persistence and management. Furthermore, this allows building open platforms in the sense that the transition from one vendor to another requires little effort since the information schema is shared across all of them.

6.3.1   Governance of Clinical Models

In order to develop a common interoperable model, governance of the archetypes that build these models is needed. As stated before, clinical information models specified as archetypes are (aspirational) maximal data sets formally specified in the ADL language. The process for publishing archetypes varies from country to country, but in general terms it is made by sharing the archetypes in a common national or regional repository where revisions with both clinical and technical experts are performed [10, 23]. This is an iterative process. The first step of the process is to create a draft archetype that covers a minimum set of requirements. The second step is to produce iterative reviews with clinicians that are users of the model (e.g. cardiologists for echocardiography report). Reviewers participate by commenting on the different elements that constitute the archetype and iteratively evolve it into a stable model that contains the requirements that satisfy the reviewers. The result is a clinical information model (CIM) that has been carefully validated by domain experts. Thus, it is a valuable information schema to drive the development of health information systems that defines an implicit ontology of the concepts that are required to represent a section of the EHR [24].

6.3.2   The Connection of Process Mining with OpenEHR

Figure 6.3 depicts the archetype for body temperature. One may attempt to redefine the archetype in a compliant manner with the XES model but this would end up in a replication of the work performed for developing the archetype which is, in fact, very costly due to the amount of time that clinicians have invested for implementing it. It makes more sense to keep the archetype model, which is actually a rich model since it is intended for storing all the attributes in the EHR, and reuse it for process mining performing queries to filter data. If these queries are defined using the Archetype Query Language, they will be interoperable

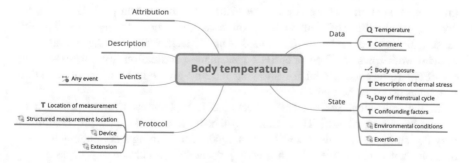

Fig. 6.3 Mindmap of the archetype body temperature

across openEHR EHRs, thus opening the door to apply the same process mining discovery strategy over different EHRs with the same openEHR model and therefore comparing and unveiling differences in the processes across hospitals. In addition, processes need to understand complex patterns such as events, intervals etc. that are actually modeled in openEHR taking care of covering the majority of clinical use cases. Besides, most clinical semantics cannot be represented only with semantic expressions since biomedical ontologies do not possess context rich semantics and the connection among them is still immature [37, 38]. The XES specification allows for performing extensions, some of them called semantic extensions that allow for referencing an external ontology. However, these extensions and how to deal with the specification of complex concepts that require the use of several ontological entities and relationships among them is not defined. The semantic link of XES allows for using a URI to refer to an ontology concept to specify its semantics. However, the way of expressing the semantics of complex entities that encompass a specific context, performer etc. is not elucidated. This is not a flaw in XES, since it was not designed for that purpose, but as a pragmatic format for sharing logs and events specifications. However, in the clinical domain the precise specification of both data and context semantics related to a process is needed if one wants to obtain valid inferences from the analysis of EHR information. Otherwise, confusing or erroneous conclusions may be derived from the analysis of clinical process data [34, 51].

6.4   Workflow Semantics with openEHR

Modern EHRs, and particularly Computerized-Provider Order Entry (CPOE), often define groups of activities or tasks that should be executed following a clear time pattern in a particular context [1, 43, 55]. Examples are chemotherapy regimes or preoperative tests.

From a temporal perspective, several types of plans appear in healthcare such as scheduled tasks, long running tasks, and coordinated activities [5]. OpenEHR uses two main classes to define what are commonly known as order sets in health information systems. These classes are Instruction and Action [15]. However, the precise specification of clinical logic often requires more expressivity. For this reason, Beale et al. recently developed a new specification for the definition of clinical workflows [5]. The openEHR task plan specification aims to extend the openEHR Reference Model for allowing the fine-grained definition of workflow semantics using archetypes.

In the following, we present an example from Process Mining provided by Ibanez-Sánchez et al. [25]. This example will be used to explain how process mining may be combined with the openEHR task model for defining a continuous learning loop. In their study, Ibanez-Sánchez et al. present the application of process mining to emergency units showing the flow of stroke patients in the emergency unit and detecting possible improvements such as the need for more triage units. In the

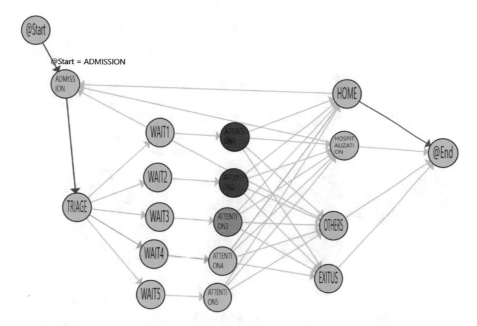

Fig. 6.4 Graph diagram inferred by Process Mining algorithms

emergency service presented, triage is performed using the Manchester Scale [33]. The Manchester scale is a triage method that classifies patients with a color and assigns a maximum waiting time depending on their priority. The code of colors is: red for cases requiring immediate attention, amber for very urgent cases, yellow for urgent cases, green for standard cases, and blue for non-urgent cases. The under-triage rate of the Manchester scale has been reported to be around 20% [56]. The study shows how Process Mining can help to understand a complex workflow and contribute to its improvement [25]. From left to right, Fig. 6.4 shows the path of patients across the emergency service generated by the process mining visualization tool PM App. The path starts in the hospital admission stage (on the left side of the figure), after it, patients go over triage and wait for medical attention. During medical attention, medical personnel examine them and they may undergo some tests while staying at the emergency department. Once they have gone through the medical attention stage, three scenarios may occur: (a) patients can be diverted to the stroke treatment unit, if stroke is suspected; (b) they may be admitted to other areas of the hospital; or, (c) they may be discharged home if their health problem does not require hospitalization.

A compelling finding by the Process Mining method used in the study presented is that young adults (20–40 years old) and adults (40–65 years old) classified in the same priority group had waiting times (after triage and before receiving medical attention) that did not significantly differ from older adults (65+) [25]. However, older adults (+65) showed differences of up to two hours during the

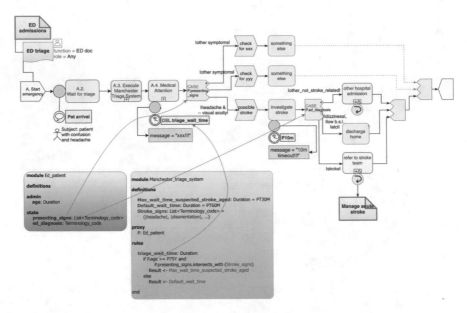

Fig. 6.5 Openehr Task Plan example for emergency service

medical attention stage with respect to young adults. This indicates that older adults required more time and resources in the medical attention stage, but their waiting time was the same as younger adults. In the case of stroke, the fast detection and treatment of stroke is needed in order to maximize survival and avoid cognitive damage. Waiting times among these patients represent an important issue since patients under-diagnosed with stroke (that are more prevalent in older adults) may suffer cognitive decay during that time.

In Fig. 6.5, we show an openEHR Work Plan defined from the process-mining chart generated with PM App. The emergency activities are grouped as a task group represented by the activities between the symbols named "Start Emergency" and "CASE" figure in green that diverts the patient to the adequate procedure after he has received emergency attention. The task plan defines the entrance of patients into the emergency service, where the patient waits for triage. When triage starts, a logic module triggered from the task workflow is activated to execute the Manchester Scale classification which assigns the patient a priority. The work plan also enhances the triage by activating a reminder in 10 min when the patient is an older adult. The new workflow aims to tailor the triage by helping the staff performing triage to be alert of possible stroke in those patients that are >65 years old and that often require more time during medical attention. In this way, the task plan acts as an alert system for triage services which are under high pressure by reminding them of possible stroke cases and monitoring the waiting time when patients are >65 years old. In the latter case, they alert attention personnel about them in the waiting lists. This improves the triage taking care of those patients that need more urgent care despite being classified in a group that does not precisely indicate their urgency. Thus, it uses knowledge from Process Mining output for providing a specific level of local adaption for this emergency service that can be combined with more standard protocols and scales such as the Manchester Scale. Once the emergency task group finishes an XOR logic is followed for determining which other tasks plans may be executed. In this case, three alternatives are available. If stroke is suspected, the stroke task plan starts its execution for the patient; if other hospitalization is needed, other task plans represented as other-hospital-admission can be triggered; if the patient is discharged because the health problem does not require hospitalization, the activity discharge-home is executed.

The reader should be aware that the example task plan is presented with illustration purposes only. It does not intend to represent a deployable task plan in an emergency department. In addition, the example shows the specific case for early detection reducing waiting times in patients with risk of stroke, but this should be leveraged with many other diseases and evaluated in a real environment determining the effect of the workflow.

Noteworthy, the main potential of the openEHR Task Model in combination with Process Mining Techniques lies in cases where one specific clinical guideline cannot be directly applied. Often, these cases are much more complex than the example presented and require the involvement of many more actors and departments of the hospital. An example of cases that can benefit from using process mining in combination with the openEHR task model are multimorbid patients where patterns and new cohorts need to be discovered in order to optimize their treatment [8]. OpenEHR allows for combining Process Mining with more patient specific information based on its descriptive and highly structured format. Also, it allows for cross-institutional process mining if the same set of archetypes are used.

So far, these techniques are in a very early stage of application, but they can make a significant contribution to the LHS paradigm if they are correctly leveraged. Figure 6.6 depicts an abstraction of an LHS cycle performing continuous improvement in the example previously presented. The figure is based on the concepts of Friedman and Macy [21, 22]. In the figure, the initial iteration starts by the motivation of understanding and improving the emergency service (1). In a second stage (2) resources are allocated and a multidisciplinary task force is assembled. Clinical experts should lead the task force working closely with process mining engineers. The task force studies process logs, meets all participant stakeholders and prepares data for the next stage. In stage (3), process-mining algorithms (e.g. PALIA) [14] are run on the data gathered. The task force analyzes the outcomes on stage (4) interpreting the outcomes and designing filters for better observing specific process flows. Stages (3) and (4) are iterative; the gray arrows between them in the picture represent the iterative behavior. Once the process is understood, all relevant ramifications observed and the areas that could be improved have been identified, the task force designs a task plan that aims to deliver advise and monitor the process making a specific intervention in the areas where improvement was considered necessary. Again, this is an iterative process that occurs between stage (5) and stage (6) where the advice from the task plan is delivered to the clinical

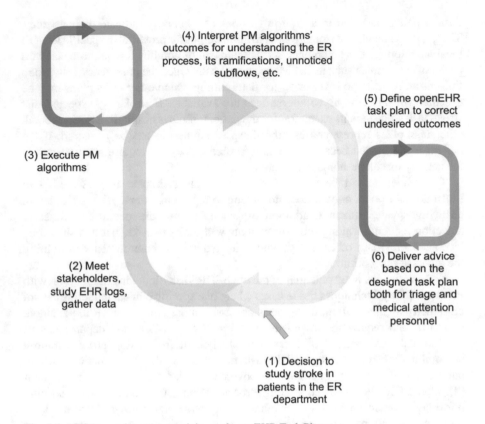

Fig. 6.6 LHS loop using process mining and openEHR Task Plans

personnel working in the emergency department and some adaptions requested by the clinical staff may be required. The cycle finishes with stage (6). However, since clinical staff uses the work plan in their daily activities, they generate new events stored in the EHR as openEHR compliant data. These new data can be used to measure if the intervention performed has improved the process and identify new areas that may be improved starting a new learning cycle and effectively implementing continuous improvement.

6.5 Privacy and Legal Framework

Since Process Mining in healthcare is based on clinical data reuse, special attention must be paid to compliance with privacy, legal, and ethical regulations. Interactive Process Mining, as well as other process mining techniques, uses real data as input in order to generate a workflow that describes reality, e.g. how a treatment has been applied to a large proportion of a population. The workflow model generated by means of Process Mining algorithms (such as the one depicted in Fig. 6.4) includes personal data from every subject. Since unveiling hidden subprocesses is one of the Process Mining objectives, it is important for the model not to exclude rare cases, because those often are the ones with co-morbidities and other complications. In Fig. 6.6, the LHS loop for the integration of Process Mining and openEHR was presented. This loop includes some stages that lead the user to access personal data: In stage (2), personal data is gathered, in stage (3) the Process Mining algorithms are executed, and in stage (4) the outcomes of the algorithms are interpreted.

This general data access vision from Process Mining contrasts with the EHR profile-based access. When accessing the EHR, most of the actors in a medical institution cannot see the whole EHR from any person, e.g. a traumatologist is not allowed to see the psychiatric record from the patients (this is known as data minimisation). However, for process discovery more complete data access may be required to unveil hidden workflow paths. Therefore the use of Process Mining imposes extra care over the data: Who will be able to act in each stage, what information will be available for each user and how it will be treated, should be defined.

In the European Union, through the General Data Protection Regulation (GDPR) [13], a new fundamental right has been created, the protection of personal data (Article 1, n.2). Clinical data, specifically, belongs to the special category -a type of data that is defined as the most sensitive data and thus extremely protected, as defined in Article 9 of the GDPR. The Regulation does not focus on research, but rather on protecting people from unethical use of personal data, mainly by companies. The importance of protecting personal data from EU citizens appears mainly related to the economy, with little information about the implementation of data protection practices in research ("Because the GDPR was intended as a law of general applicability that would offer protection to personal data when processed in all sectors of the EU economy, the unique challenges it has created for the research enterprise were likely unanticipated and unintended") [40]. In this line, some authors claim that there are too many uncertainties in the regulation around research and that research-friendly regulation should be created [49]. Since the research that is conducted in the stages (2) to (4) in the LHS is oriented to enhance the medical system already in place, the data processing could be deemed as compliant with the GDPR, as Article 9 in n. 2(h) and n. 3 state.

When Process Mining is to be conducted, the normal restrictions that apply to data in the medical field would still be valid: Data minimisation, accuracy, and so on. One important factor is data anonymization. In the context of the Regulation, there is the process of pseudonymization. In fact, the word anonymization does not appear in the whole GDPR document. Pseudonymization consists on removing personal information so the data cannot be traced back to the original person. A pseudonym is generated instead, so the person could be identified if necessary, but with some safeguards. If data was completely anonymized (i.e. it was not possible to trace the original user by any means) then it would not be personal data anymore, so the GDPR would not apply. However, if data from a subject such as post code and age were stored, it could be traced back to the person in some cases: e.g. if there were few people in the area within that age range, or in case another subject or company could make him/her stand out by crossing information with other sources [12]. Thus, complete anonymization as such is nearly impossible, and pseudonymization (rendering data with maximized anonymity) will be performed on data, reducing the risk of identification.

In order to conduct the research that will lead to a better medical system, the submission to an Ethical Review Board is needed. The same principles as in any other research apply here, but one: when "processing is necessary for the purposes of preventive or occupational medicine, for the assessment of the working capacity of the employee, medical diagnosis, the provision of health or social care or treatment or the management of health or social care systems and services on the basis of Union or Member State law or pursuant to contract with a health professional and subject to the conditions and safeguards referred to in paragraph 3" (Article 9, n.2). In this case, processing could be considered as necessary, since it allows preventive medicine and especially it is a means of management of the health systems.

Process Mining initiatives must therefore be careful to follow these regulations and be performed as a joint effort for healthcare improvement with organizational, ethical, and legal stakeholders backup. In particular, when involving data from various institutions.

References

1. Aarts J, Ash J, Berg M. Extending the understanding of computerized physician order entry: implications for professional collaboration, workflow and quality of care. Int J Med Inform. 2007;76:S4–13.
2. Bates DW, Kuperman GJ, Wang S, Gandhi T, Kittler A, Volk L, Spurr C, Khorasani R, Tanasijevic M, Middleton B. Ten commandments for effective clinical decision support: making the practice of evidence-based medicine a reality. J Am Med Inform Assoc. 2003;10(6):523–30.
3. Beale T. Decision support language (DSL) and Model, Feb 2020.
4. Beale T, Kejžar M, Polajnar M, Naess B, Santos D, Fabjan B. Task planning specification, May 2020.
5. Beale T. Task Planning Specification. https://specifications.openehr.org/releases/PROC/latest/task_planning.html#_task_planning_specification.
6. Beale T. Archetypes: constraint-based domain models for future-proof information systems. In: OOPSLA 2002 workshop on behavioural semantics, vol. 105, Citeseer, 2002, p. 1–69.
7. Beale T. FHIR vs the EHR, May 2019.
8. Berntsen GKR, Dalbakk M, Hurley JS, Bergmo T, Solbakken B, Spansvoll L, Bellika JG, Skrøvseth SO, Brattland T, Rumpsfeld M. Person-centred, integrated and pro-active care for multi-morbid elderly with advanced care needs: a propensity score-matched controlled trial. BMC Health Serv Res. 2019;19(1):682.
9. Blumenthal D, Tavenner M. The "meaningful use" regulation for electronic health records, Aug 2010.
10. Bosca D, Marco L, Moner D, Maldonado JA, Insa L, Robles M. Detailed clinical models governance system in a regional ehr project. In: XIII mediterranean conference on medical and biological engineering and computing 2013. Springer; 2014. p. 1266–9.
11. Boscá D, Marco L, Burriel V, Jaijo T, Millán JM, Levin AM, Pastor O, Robles M, Maldonado JA. Genetic testing information standardization in hl7 cda and iso13606. In: MedInfo, 2013. p. 338–42.

12. de Montjoye Y-A, Radaelli L, Singh VK, Pentland AS. Unique in the shopping mall: on the reidentifiability of credit card metadata. Science. 2015;347(6221):536–9.
13. European Commission. Regulation 2016/679 of the european parliament and of the council of 27 april 2016 on the protection of natural persons with regard to the processing of personal data and on the free move- ment of such data, and repealing directive 95/46/ec. general data protection regulation. http://data.europa.eu/eli/reg/2016/679/2016-05-04.
14. Fernandez-Llatas C, Valdivieso B, Traver V, Benedi JM. Using process mining for automatic support of clinical pathways design. In: Data mining in clinical medicine. Springer; 2015. p. 79–88.
15. Open EHR Foundation. Common Information Model. https://specifications.openehr.org/releases/RM/latest/common.html#_common_information.
16. Open EHR Foundation. openEHR – Working Baseline. https://specifications.openehr.org/.
17. Open EHR Foundation. OpenEHR Related Projects, May 2020.
18. Fox J. Cognitive systems at the point of care: the credo program. J Biomed Inform. 2017;68:83–95.
19. Fox J, Alabassi A, Patkar V, Rose T, Black E. An ontological approach to modelling tasks and goals. Comput Biol Med. 2006;36(7–8):837–56.
20. Friedman C, Rigby M. Conceptualising and creating a global learning health system. Int J Med Inform. 2013;82(4):e63–71.
21. Friedman CP, Flynn AJ. Computable knowledge: an imperative for learning health systems. Learn Health Syst. 2019;3(4):e10203. LRH2-2019-08-0027.
22. Friedman CP, Macy Jr J. Toward complete & sustainable learning systems. University of Michigan, 2014.
23. Garde S, Chen R, Leslie H, Beale T, McNICOLL I, Heard S. Archetype-based knowledge management for semantic interoperability of electronic health records. In: MIE, Citeseer, 2009. p. 1007–11.
24. Goossen W, Goossen-Baremans A, van der Zel M. Detailed clinical models: a review. Healthcare Inf Res. 2010;16(4):201–14.
25. Ibanez-Sanchez G, Fernandez-Llatas C, Celda A, Mandingorra J, Aparici-Tortajada L, Martinez-Millana A, Munoz-Gama J, Sepúlveda M, Rojas E, Gálvez V, Capurro D, Traver V. Toward value-based healthcare through interactive process mining in emergency rooms: the stroke case. Int J Environ Res Public Health. 2019;16(10):1783.
26. Oceans Informatics. Clinical Knowledge Manager. https://arketyper.no/ckm/.
27. Ingram D. The good european health record. In: Laires MF, Ladeira MF, Christensen JP, editors. Health in the new communication age. IOS, 1995. p. 66–74.
28. Guidelines Institute of Medicine Committee to Advise the Public Health Service on Clinical Practice. Institute of Medicine Committee to Advise the Public Health Service on Clinical Practice, Guidelines. The National Academies Press, 1990.
29. HL7 International. Profiling – FHIR v4.0.1. https://www.hl7.org/fhir/profiling.html.
30. Kalra D. Medicine in Europe: electronic health records: the European scene. BMJ. 1994;309(6965):1358–61.
31. Kawamoto K, Hongsermeier T, Wright A, Lewis J, Bell DS, Middleton B. Key principles for a national clinical decision support knowledge sharing framework: synthesis of insights from leading subject matter experts. J Am Med Inform Assoc. 2013;20(1):199–207.
32. Kinsman L, Rotter T, James E, Snow P, Willis J. What is a clinical pathway? Development of a definition to inform the debate. BMC Med. 2010;8(1):31.
33. Mackway-Jones K, Marsden J, Windle J, Harris N. Manchester triage group. and England Advanced Life Support Group Manchester. Wiley: Emergency triage; 2014.
34. Marco-Ruiz L, Malm-Nicolaisen K, Pedersen R, Makhlysheva A, Bakkevoll PA. Ontology-based terminologies for healthcare, 2017.
35. Marco-Ruiz L, Budrionis A, Yigzaw KY, Bellika JG. Interoperability mechanisms of clinical decision support systems: a systematic review. In: Proceedings from the 14th scandinavian conference on health informatics 2016, Gothenburg, 6–7 Apr 2016. Linköping University Electronic Press; 2016. p. 13–21.

36. Marco-Ruiz L, Malm-Nicolaisen K, Makhlysheva A, Pedersen R. Towards a national clinical decision support framework for Norway: expert assessment and proposed architecture. In: eTELEMED 2020: the twelfth international conference on ehealth, telemedicine, and social medicine, 03 2020.
37. Marco-Ruiz L, Pedersen R. Challenges in archetypes terminology binding using SNOMED-CT compositional grammar: the Norwegian patient summary case. In: Proceedings of the 16th world congress on medical and health informatics (MedInfo2017), volume in press, page in press, Hangzhou, Aug 2017. IOS Press.
38. Marco-Ruiz L, Pedersen R. The patient summary case: challenges in archetypes terminology binding using SNOMED-CT compositional grammar. In: eTELEMED 2019: the eleventh international conference on ehealth, telemedicine, and social medicine, Athens, 2019. p. 49–55.
39. Marco-Ruiz L, Pedrinaci C, Maldonado JA, Panziera L, Chen R, Gustav Bellika J. Publication, discovery and interoperability of clinical decision support systems: a linked data approach. J Biomed Inform. 2016;62:243–64.
40. McCall B. What does the GDPR mean for the medical community? Mar 2018.
41. Middleton B, Sittig DF, Wright A. Clinical decision support: a 25 year retrospective and a 25 year vision. Yearb Med Inform. 2016;25(S 01):S103–16.
42. Nalin M, Baroni I, Faiella G, Romano M, Matrisciano F, Gelenbe E, Martinez DM, Dumortier J, Natsiavas P, Votis K, Koutkias V, Tzovaras D, Clemente F. The European cross-border health data exchange roadmap: case study in the Italian setting. J Biomed Inform. 2019;94:103183.
43. Novak LL. Making sense of clinical practice: order set design strategies in cpoe. In: AMIA annual symposium proceedings, vol. 2007. American Medical Informatics Association, 2007. p. 568.
44. Olsen L, Aisner D, McGinnis JM. Institute of medicine (US). Roundtable on evidence-based medicine. The learning healthcare system: workshop summary, 2007.
45. Patel VL, Arocha JF, Kaufman DR. A primer on aspects of cognition for medical informatics. J Am Med Inform Assoc. 2001;8(4):324–43.
46. Pedrinaci C, Domingue J, Sheth AP. Semantic web services. Handbook of semantic web technologies. Berlin/Heidelberg: Springer; 2011.
47. Peleg M. Computer-interpretable clinical guidelines: a methodological review, Aug 2013.
48. Peleg M, Tu S, Bury J, Ciccarese P, Fox J, Greenes RA, Hall R, Johnson PD, Jones N, Kumar A, Miksch S, Quaglini S, Seyfang A, Shortliffe EH, Stefanelli M. Comparing computer-interpretable guideline models: a case-study approach. J Am Med Inform Assoc. 2003;10(1):52–68.
49. Peloquin D, DiMaio M, Bierer B, Barnes M. Disruptive and avoidable: GDPR challenges to secondary research uses of data, Mar 2020.
50. Rector A, Sottara D. Chapter 20 – formal representations and semantic web technologies. In: Greenes RA, editor. Clinical decision support. 2nd ed. Oxford:Academic; 2014. p. 551–98.
51. Rector AL, Johnson PD, Tu S, Wroe C, Rogers J. Interface of inference models with concept and medical record models. In: Proceedings of artificial intelligence in medicine Europe (AIME-2001), Jan 2001. p. 314–23.
52. Rocha RA, Maviglia SM, Sordo M, Rocha BH. A clinical knowledge management program. In: Clinical decision support: the road to broad adoption. 2nd ed. Elsevier Inc., 2014. p. 773–817.
53. Sheth A. Internet of things to smart IoT through semantic, cognitive, and perceptual computing. IEEE Intell Syst. 2016;31(2):108–12.
54. Sheth A, Anantharam P, Henson C. Semantic, cognitive, and perceptual computing: paradigms that shape human experience. Computer. 2016;49(3):64–72.
55. Sordo M, Boxwala AA. Chapter 18 – grouped knowledge elements A2- Greenes, Robert A. In: Clinical decision support. 2nd ed. Oxford: Academic; 2014. p. 499–514.
56. Storm-Versloot M, Ubbink D, Kappelhof J, Luitse J. Comparison of an informally structured triage system, the emergency severity index, and the manchester triage system to distinguish patient priority in the emergency department. Acad Emerg Med. 2011;18(8):822–29.

57. Valero-Ramon Z, Ibanez-Sanchez G, Traver V, Marco-Ruiz L, Fernandez-Llatas C. Towards perceptual spaces for empowering ergonomy in workplaces by using interactive process mining. Trans Ergon Personal Health Intell Workplaces. 2019;25:85.
58. Van der Aalst W. Process mining: data science in action. Berlin/Heidelberg: Springer; 2016.
59. XES Working Group and others. IEEE Standard for eXtensible Event Stream (XES) for Achieving Interoperability in Event Logs and Event Streams. IEEE Std 1849-2016, 2016. p. 1–50.

Part II
Interactive Process Mining in Health

Chapter 7
Applying Interactive Process Mining Paradigm in Healthcare Domain

Carlos Fernandez-Llatas

7.1 Dealing with Digital Transformation Paradigm in Healthcare

Healthcare is one of the most challenging problems that our society is currently facing. The life expectancy is increasing thanks to the new advances and the better quality of health solutions. According to demographic studies, the population over 60 was around 11% of the global population, and it is expected that in 2050 it will reach 22% [21]. It is a fact that people are reaching older ages, that implies more chronic illnesses, with more co-morbidities. This supposes a great increase in the complexity of the illnesses. Also, thanks to the new age of the internet, patients are more aware of their illnesses having larger expectations of the health systems, causing a great impact in the healthcare sustainability, which should cover this scenario with the same budget. This critical juncture is demanding the necessity of a new paradigm that will be able to deal with the drift of the health domain in the next years, to avoid the collapse of the system.

In this line, currently, the Digital Transformation paradigm is changing how health is distributed in society [17]. This profound revolution is stressing the system pushing health stakeholders to adapt not only their computer systems but also their culture and the way of working. According to Kawamoto et al. [23], to achieve successful clinical decision support systems, their application should be integrated into the clinical workflow, involving the physician and providing actionable actions.

C. Fernandez-Llatas (✉)
Process Mining 4 Health Lab – SABIEN – ITACA Institute, Universitat Politècnica de València, Valencia, Spain

CLINTEC – Karolinska Institutet, Sweden
e-mail: cfllatas@itaca.upv.es

© Springer Nature Switzerland AG 2021
C. Fernandez-Llatas (ed.), *Interactive Process Mining in Healthcare*, Health Informatics, https://doi.org/10.1007/978-3-030-53993-1_7

However, the use of Information Technologies (IT) for supporting the processes management in the healthcare domain is not a crucial task [24].

In healthcare, there are huge efforts to try to adopt business and industrial methodologies that have been successfully applied in other fields, like Lean Six Sigma or Change Management [6, 38]. However, these techniques have not achieved successful results in healthcare domains [7]. The engagement of healthcare professional stakeholders that should understand the current process and the effects expected by the processes optimization is the key factor that supposes the success or not in the application of these technologies [7].

To create scenarios where the processes may be optimized, it is critical to have methods for measuring and analyzing the processes. The definition of Evidence-Based Health Informatics (EBHI) [28], in close relationship with the definition of Evidence-Based Medicine (EBM) [29], shows the importance of Information and Communication Technologies (ICT) and Big Data in the health field. Information systems in hospitals should provide enough data for measuring the processes and to analyze their efficiency and efficacy. Traditionally, the lack of data was one of the classically defined barriers for creating evidence that would allow the improvement of care processes to patients. With the arrival of new mobile personal technologies and wearable sensors, the amount of data available to monitor the people's behaviour is dramatically growing [3]. The rapid digitization of society leads to the exponential growth of data from Internet of Things (IoT) devices [2]. According to statistical forecasts of the Institute for Humane Studies (IHS), the number of connected devices on the Internet will rise to 75.4 billion by 2025 [4]. All this information, added to the information already stored in Electronic Health Records (EHR), social media or/and patient portals, among others, suppose a great opportunity to extract valuable knowledge that will help improve the quality of life of citizens [25].

7.2   Data Science for Medicine: Filling the Gap Between Data and Decision

On the one hand, there exist methodologies for improving processes and on the other hand, there are data available for measuring and analyzing processes. So, the next step is to find the appropriate methods and technologies to support health professionals in understanding, measuring, and optimizing their processes. In this line, Artificial Intelligence and Machine Learning are called to be the paradigms in charge of providing the next generation of smart tools, methodologies and solutions in the world of medicine [34].

As already shown in previous chapters, the design of medical processes rules is not trivial due to difficulties in the formalized consensus among the medical doctors. In Fig. 7.1 we can see in a very abstract way how Machine Learning techniques work. While traditional medicine uses both the patient's signs and

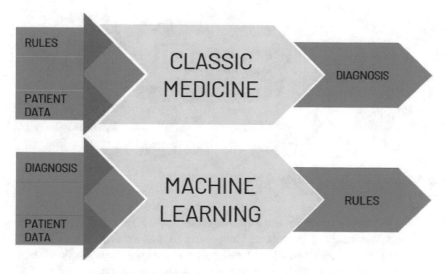

Fig. 7.1 Abstract view of Machine Learning diagnosis analysis compared with traditional medicine

symptoms and the medical knowledge rules for providing adequate diagnosis for specific patients, Machine Learning uses the signs and symptoms, with the set of diagnoses previously made by traditional medicine, to discover, by using advanced mathematical methods, the intrinsic rules behind the diagnosis model.

There is a wide quantity of Machine Learning systems that are applied to clinical Medicine [10, 33, 34]. There are real-time decision support systems that help physicians in a wide variety of medical fields [22], there is a continuous appearance in literature of Risk models covering all clinical disciplines [18, 19, 36], intelligent systems for supporting Epidemiological surveillance [20], technologies that are looking for providing individualized through personalized medicine [30] among others.

Machine Learning techniques can support Medical Doctors in the formalization of medical protocols by inferring these rules from the data available from cases. Thanks to that, Machine Learning techniques can reduce the time and workload in the definition of clinical protocols, increasing the quality of care, reducing the variability and, then, promoting prevention medicine by creating best practices that can be universally published [25].

7.2.1   Will the Doctors Be Replaced by Computers?

The impact of Artificial Intelligence and Machine Learning techniques is getting so big that some researchers are starting to argue that probably one solution would be to replace the doctors in some specific medical fields [13]. These researchers

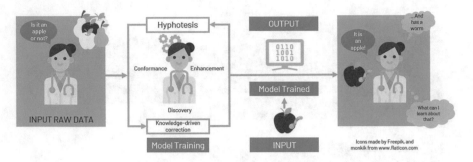

Fig. 7.2 Machine Learning techniques flow

defend that Artificial Intelligence systems make fewer errors than human doctors. The futuristic concept of Perceptual Computing [31] as an evolution of Cognitive computing [26] bets for an Artificial Intelligence where computers mimic the human brain and are able to act as humans being aware of their environment, understanding the human problems and acting accordingly. However, these paradigms require that actual models have, at least, the same computational power than the human brain. Otherwise, Artificial Intelligence and Machine Learning systems will never be able to mimic human decisions. There is not a mathematical model able to describe the capabilities of the human brain, but we have bounded the capacities of actual computational systems thanks to the work of Alan Turing [5]. So, in theory, it seems that intelligent computers are far from replacing humans with the current computation framework.

As long as this new revolutionary intelligent framework finally comes, we should use the techniques that we have at hand. Currently, Machine Learning techniques are not acquiring the expected presence in actual medical field [8]. Figure 7.2 shows the flow followed by a typical Machine Learning research. First, the question to be answered should be translated to a machine language, normalizing and pre-processing data to obtain the best accuracy in the results. As an example, a set of fruits with different sizes and colours is presented and it is required to create a system able to classify the fruits and determine which are apples and which are not. After that, a set of mathematical tools is applied to train a model only understandable by computers that is able to perform this classification. This model, given a set of data from the fruits measures (colour, size,..), processed in the same way than trained one, can automatically classify new elements eliminating the noise (variability) in them. In the example, the model can differentiate apples from other fruits, and removing the noise, worms, that makes it different from the prototypical apple.

Currently, the application of innovative algorithms and apps to patient diagnosis and treatments should prove that they work in the specific real conditions in which they should be applied using clinical cases. That means that it is mandatory to obtain enough evidence of the validity of the methods used prior to be deployed in a real scenario. Due to the appearance of Precision Medicine paradigm, each time the assessment of medical applications is harder. Health applications are each time more accurate and focused in a more reduced group of patients, even, one patient in case of Personal Medicine. This makes more complex to find a sufficient cohort of patients that produce enough statistical significance to make health professionals confident of the results of the case. Due to that, the accuracy of clinical automated systems decreases their utility in real scenarios.

Besides, Machine Learning techniques can infer complex models, but with some limitations. While Machine Learning algorithms are deterministic, human behaviour is not. Protocols that humans follow are affected by the variability of the human being. They are affected by beliefs, attitudes, and other external factors that usually can't be taken into account by mathematical algorithms. That means that while Machine Learning assumes that the same inputs provide the same outputs, in medicine it is possible that two patients with the same illness and the same treatment have different results due to differences in variability and external factors. These models can't be perfectly inferred by Machine Learning techniques and can only be an approximation.

But, probably the most limiting problem is that no Machine Learning system is error-free. Even in those applications where the full automation paradigm might make sense, Machine Learning developments often require an additional step of post-edition where a human expert corrects errors produced by the system. However, full automation often proves elusive or unnatural in many applications where technology is expected to assist rather than replace the human agents. In the case of Machine Learning applied to medicine, models are becoming *black boxes* for practitioners. The full automation will provide only the final decision, and health professionals should trust the result achieved by the intelligent system, even though all of those systems are not error-free and the error in the health domain might suppose dangerous situations for the patient. This provokes some suspicions in health professionals that, usually, suppose unsurmountable barriers for applying technology in daily practice. Because of this, the figure of a human expert who supervises the outcome of the process is unavoidable.

On the other hand, human error is an important problem to take into account in clinical medicine. Any mistake made by a physician could potentially suppose a life. Clinical errors might be due to different situations. Machine Learning techniques are supposed to support better decisions avoiding human errors. However, there are situations where the use of Machine Learning can increase clinicians' errors [32]. Medical errors happen every day in the health domain due to the influence of statistics misunderstandings in medical evidence [15]. *Zebra Retreat* errors are referred to rare diseases that have low evidence. These techniques tend to select the most common situations over the less probable. That means that these technologies are much less accurate in rare cases than in standard cases. However, physicians usually do not need help in the standard case, because in these cases the standard treatment works. But, in rare cases, Machine Learning systems can point to erroneous diagnosis or treatments that can, even, increase the human error. Other related examples are *Diagnosis Momentum*, this error is related to the correct or incorrect diagnostics that have been diagnosed in the past and perpetuated over time producing an error in the current treatment. This *Diagnosis Momentum* is produced by the assumption of the doctor that the clinical history is correct. This is the same feeling, or even worse, that a physician can face when he or she is working with a *black box* Machine Learning system. In a real situation with a high load of patients,the physician might have an overconfident position with the system and accept Machine Learning results as the reality.

Furthermore, these models also are *black boxes* for the Data Scientist who is selecting the Machine Learning techniques for the data. Algorithms selected by Data scientist are usually based on decisions that are not medical. Sometimes, models selection depends on its popularity amongst the data science community; its accuracy; its speed to return results; its ease of use compared to other options. This adds more limitations for the selection of the best tools for each problem.

7.2.2 Towards an Interactive Pattern Recognition Approach

There is not new knowledge without medical understanding. That means that, in current medicine, doctors should understand the illness processes to add evidence to medical knowledge. Machine Learning systems based in cognitive computing theory are not human-understandable, and for that, they can't offer knowledge to medical doctors. In this way, instead of use paradigms that mimic the human brain, why not create models that cooperate with humans taking advantage of the processing capabilities of human brains? This paradigm aims the promotion of interaction between human and intelligent systems. The idea is creating Machine Learning algorithms that produce human-understandable models allowing the extraction of evidence from the intelligent models.

In past works, we presented the Interactive Pattern Recognition (IPR) [12] as an alternative to the *black box* Pattern Recognition approach in health environments. Interactive Pattern Recognition is an iterative probabilistic approach that incorporates the expert in the middle of the inference process. IPR algorithms assume the priority of the human understandability over the accuracy of the findings achieved on the inference. This allows the expert, on the one hand, to correct the model in each learning iteration, avoiding undesirable errors, and on the other hand, converge to a solution iteratively, allowing the closely adaption to the real problem.

IPR has been applied to some classical PR problems such as interactive transcription of handwritten and spoken documents, computer-assisted translation, interactive text generation and parsing, among others [35]. In this new IPR framework, the most important factor to be minimized is the human effort that has to be applied to transform the system's potentially incorrect output into validated and error-free output. Given that the user effort is usually inversely proportional to the quality of the system output, most research related to this IPR framework ends up minimizing the system error rate as well. In this IPR framework, four main advantages have also been found:

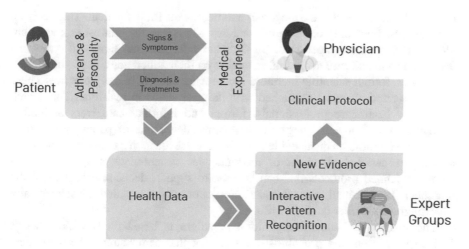

Icons made by Freepik, Vectors Market and Icon Pond from www.flaticon.com

Fig. 7.3 Interactive pattern recognition

- **Feedback**: Take direct advantage of the feedback information provided by the expert user in each interaction step to improve raw performance,
- **Multimodality**: The expert user can correct the system output in the most comfortable and closest modality. This characteristic arises as a natural property of an interaction. By properly acknowledging this fact, improved overall system performance and usability can be achieved.
- **Adaption**: Use feedback-derived data to adaptively (re-)train the system and tune it to the expert user behaviour and the specific task considered.
- **Comprehension**: Since the expert user is actively involved in developing the system output, this increases his/her understanding of the process and allows to export this development to other potentially less experienced users.

Figure 7.3 shows a graphical description of the Interactive Pattern Recognition Approach. The patients or citizens produce *health data* not only from the signs and symptoms of their illnesses but also from their treatments followed and their lifestyle data. This data represents the user status in a moment or a period. Using this data, Interactive Pattern Recognition algorithms can present findings over the data in an understandable view to experts' groups. These represent formal views of the user behaviour that can be used by those experts to provide formally described scientific literature. The findings achieved by IPR algorithms can be corrected by experts and are stored in databases representing the new medical evidence, updating the current clinical protocols in iterative iterations. This formal scientific literature is different from the traditional one because it is described in a human and machine-understandable way. This allows expert humans not only to correct by hand all the inaccuracies but also, to apply all the advantages and available frameworks for formal methods, like analysis of completeness, incoherence or ambiguity, among others. Physicians decide the diagnosis and treatments for the patient. This decision is taken based not only on the signs and symptoms and the clinical protocols but also on their medical experience. On the other side, patients' signs and symptoms are based on the disease evolution, as well as on their adherence and personality.

Besides, formal scientific literature can be used directly in daily practice. These formal descriptions can be matched with the user status in real-time. This match will allow healthcare professionals, formal and informal caregivers and other stakeholders to know the negative or positive deviations of patient status over the most common medical evidence. Using these data, it is possible to create a computer-assisted treatment or recommender systems, which allow creating formally defined protocols that can be used to support decision processes of the healthcare professional, any other stakeholder or even the patient in his/her daily life, improving his/her quality of life.

The Interactive Pattern Recognition paradigm is based on Bayesian theory. In [12] we presented a probabilistic framework that demonstrates the theoretical convergence of the model. In other words, if the problem follows the iterative paradigm, the system will find, in the limit, the most adequate lifestyle and care protocol for users and patients.

It is also important to highlight the importance of experts in the process. In the Interactive paradigm, the experts can correct the findings inferred by the algorithms, this allows the elimination of critical errors in the protocols applied to users. Also, these expert' corrections are very useful to accelerate the convergence of the pattern recognition paradigm [35]. In that way, the methodology not only uses the theoretical power of pattern recognition paradigms, but it is also used in combination with the knowledge of human experts as well as their common sense, allowing the creation of more robust and effective interventions.

7.2.3   Through Explainable Models

The main problem in the use of Interactive Paradigm is that it require the use of human-understandable models. Classical Machine Learning tools like Neural Networks, Support Vector Machines, or Hidden Markov Models, are aimed at learning the best accurate models, but the internal rules that are behind the models are not able for being human-understandable by. Thus way, in order to be interactive, it is needed to select new tools and algorithms that aim at the best accuracy but taking into account human readability.

This need for a new way to support experts in the understanding of Machine Learning decisions, is providing new research frameworks seeking to translate Machine Learning models to human language. As a result of this, the *Explainable Artificial Intelligence* appear in literature [9]. These techniques are trying to make human-understandable the results obtained by Machine Learning algorithms [1].

Explainable Models change the way of Machine Learning traditional flow, by creating a translation action after the Training phase that support human experts in the understanding of the models inferred by the system. This translation is made by a computerized system that is composed by an Explanation Interface that can show the results in a human-understandable fashion by using advanced process analytic tools, creating conversational recommender systems explaining that justify the decision taken by the system. This idea enables the expert to understand the reason of these decisions. In general, Explainable Models can communicate with experts in four ways [16]:

- **Explainable Statements**: The system provides natural language statements that explain to the expert the reasons for the selections made by the system.
- **Process Analytic View**: If the model was trained to allow a partial human understanding, the system can highlight some parts of the general model to strengthen the hypothesis by providing clues about the decisions taken in the raw model.
- **Similar cases**: The system provides similar cases that reinforce the decision.
- **Dissimilar cases**: The system provides cases that are not suitable in that case for reinforcing the decision taken.

In this line, some tools try to translate the models produced by Machine Learning Techniques. One of the most known is Local Interpretable Model-agnostic Explanations (LIME). LIME [27] is a model explainer that tries to explain the prediction of classifiers independently of the method used in a human-understandable way.

Using explainers, it is possible to bring the Machine Learning tools closer to Interactive methodologies. However, explainable models need to have a translator in order to provide knowledge. This allows a unidirectional interaction, with the system. The user can understand why the decisions are taken, but it is difficult to discover other alternatives to the decision taken. Besides, if the expert modifies the model to optimize it, the model should be retrained and the structures created can be different and incomparable. So the expert can understand the decisions, but the expert can´t easily correct the actions taken by the next decisions.

7.3 Interactive Process Mining

The Interactive Pattern Recognition approach has clear advantages over other methodologies due to its integration with experts. As said, the main disadvantage of this paradigm is that the Pattern Recognition framework requires to have a human-understandable focus. This allows professionals to analyze and correct the evidence inferred by algorithms. However, most Pattern Recognition algorithms are machine-oriented and are not human-understandable. In this way, it is necessary to find an adequate Pattern Recognition framework that allows the application of Interactive Pattern Recognition thesis. In this chapter, we propose the use of Process Mining Technologies as an adequate framework for the application of the Interactive Pattern Recognition Paradigm.

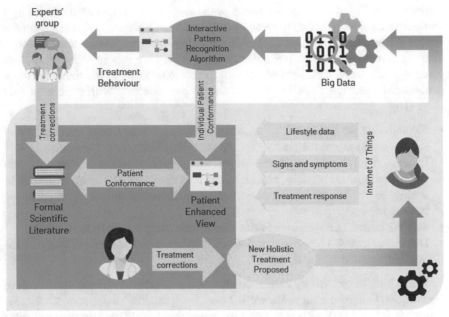

Icons made by Freepik, Vectors Market, Pixel perfect and Icon Pond from www.flaticon.com

Fig. 7.4 Interactive process mining

Process Mining [37] solutions can offer a clear care process understanding in a better way compared to other data mining techniques that are seen as *black box* systems. Process Mining can build human-understandable models without the need for an intermediate translation language. This allows, on the one hand, the direct understanding of the medical processes, and on the other hand, the direct modification of processes and permits the objective measurement of the effects of the changes. This enables the medical expert in the understanding of the models that explain the behaviour of their patients. Besides, it allows to modify the models according to their experience and measure their effects in an iterative way of optimizing the clinical protocols, empowering them in the use of fully bidirectional interactive systems.

Applying process mining through the Interactive Pattern Recognition approach allows an iterative way to control the process of care holistically. Figure 7.4 shows the authors' proposal for the application of Process Mining techniques over the Interactive Pattern Recognition paradigm. Process Mining algorithms can take advantage of available Big Data to infer the lifestyle and care processes followed by patients and citizens. This information is adequately presented as formal workflows. Based on this, experts can filter and analyze data looking for evidence using discovery and enhancement algorithms. By correcting possible errors and applying their professional knowledge, expert groups can create formal libraries of evidence and publish lifestyle and care protocols. These protocols support general practitioners in their daily practice as well as formal and informal caregivers or the patient him/herself. These stakeholders can have an enhanced view of the patient, highlighting the most interesting issues in their flow. To do this, they can apply conformance algorithms with formal scientific evidence, showing deviations of the process followed by the user with the ideal protocol. Furthermore, it is possible to analyze the patient's individualized behaviour change by comparing the current status with past inferred workflows. Using this information, it is possible to measure, for example, changes in treatment adherence by using individualized process mining conformance algorithms or even detect behaviour changes due to psychological illness [11]. Moreover, comparing patient's individual behaviour and response with other patients' flow, lets us find *similar patients* or patients who have a similar response to a specific treatment. Analysis of the effectiveness of treatments and recommendations on *similar patient*, can be valuable information to decide the best treatments to future patients.

With this information, as well as the knowledge about it, the health care stakeholders can modify the protocol or care processes to follow. As the protocols are formally described, it is possible to automate the cares using computerized systems as workflow engines [14]. Furthermore, since the execution of lifestyle and care protocols can be computerized, the digital data collection is easier, improving the formal evidence iteratively and progressively. This methodology allows professionals to infer initial formal processes from the available data. This facilitates the configuration of the system from scratch, allowing to discover and formalize the real processes that occur in reality, to optimize and correct them in an iterative way, without the necessity to manually create formal care protocols. Besides, this methodology is self-adapted to the population in which it is applied. Thanks to the acquired evidence and the current knowledge of the experts, in each iteration, the system improves the care protocols and, finally, the quality of life of the patients. By avoiding the *black box* concept in the pattern recognition paradigm, physicians can correct the protocols in each iteration, preventing critical errors due to automatic learning errors and extracting evidence from the results presented by intelligent algorithms.

7.4   Discussion and Conclusions

The presented methodology proposes a model for the continuous integration of human knowledge and the common sense of experts with the learning power of Pattern Recognition frameworks. This represents a new alternative to support the application of Evidence-Based Medicine in real combination with daily practice of physicians, formal and informal caregivers as well as the proper patient, providing a holistic system of care to improve their quality of life. In addition, thanks to the use of Process Mining technologies to provide formal evidence protocols as workflows, direct deployment of care and continuously learned recommendations is possible.

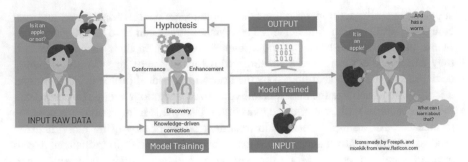

Fig. 7.5 Interactive process mining flow

These protocols can be automated over the emerging cloud of personal devices, anytime and everywhere thanks to computerized systems.

To meet this challenge, it is crucial to engage clinical experts, who demand solutions to real problems in daily practice. For that, to build real solutions, it is necessary to advance in new methodologies that involve the medical expert and can be incorporated in the workflow of medical professionals.

Applying Interactive Process Mining Solutions has some advantages over Classical Machine Learning. Figure 7.5 shows how Interactive Process Mining paradigm can be applied analogously to Fig. 7.2. The human person can provide a question to the system that is evaluated with the human in the loop, taking advantage of the human-understandable Process Mining techniques. While this model training is performed, the human being has access to the information provided by the system and this can inspire him/her to have new ideas or questions that may indicate new lines of research. This supposes that Interactive Process Mining not only provides answers to questions but can also empower medical doctors in a deeper understanding of medical processes leading to new questions that provide new knowledge. After training the model, the resultant one is human-understandable and provides a view of the clinical process that allows conclusions to be drawn. And when a new element enters with some noise, like an apple with a worm, the expert can not only detect the apple but also see and quantify the noise (the worm).

Table 7.1 summarizes the advantages of the application of Interactive Process Mining in several health fields. Interactive Process Mining brings the expert into the middle of the learning process making it more effective. This allows experts to become involved in the findings achieved by the global system, minimizing the rejection of findings due to the *black box* effect. In addition to that, since all the processes are continuously moderated by a human expert, and the learned and automated protocols can be corrected by them at any time, the system is potentially free from learning errors. This provides continuous monitoring and traceability of the process for healthcare professionals and caregivers, increasing confidence in the improved protocols.

Table 7.1 Advantages of interactive process mining

Field	Advantages of the use of interactive process mining
Value based healthcare	Support the measurement of the chain of value in clinical protocols
Evidence-based medicine	Incorporates the expert in the middle of the process of generating knowledge
	Support the definition of formal evidence for easier use in daily practice
	Incorporates the running knowledge of health experts
	Break the *Black Box* concept in statistical-based evidence
Precision medicine	Allows individualized inference of the behaviour of the patient
	Patient can be compared in different timelines to measure his/her behavioural changes
	Patients with a similar behaviour can be found to support the treatment decisions (Patient Twins)
Integrated care	It allows a direct matching of formal evidence with daily cares
	The use of Formal Evidence (Workflows) makes the automation and deployment of care protocols easier
	The patient is holistically tracked and the physician has a complete view of the status of the patient in each moment
Preventive medicine	Learn formal best practices to be applied to population
	Automated protocols can be widely deployed over healthy population
	Use all the information available for creating individualized protocols and measure behavioural changes

In this way, this methodology can be used to apply Precision Medicine in a more individualized and precise way, supporting the experts in the evolution of care protocols in parallel to the continuous evolution of patient behaviour. Process Mining technologies can build individualized behaviour models [11]. Thanks to Process Mining conformance algorithms, these models can be compared to the current status, detecting and highlighting differences in the patient behaviour at any time. Experts can use these differences to detect psychological changes in the early stages and deploy prevention protocols to avoid potential complications. This human understanding of individualized protocols allows us to provide insight that is difficult to obtain with databases queries or other different techniques.

Interactive Process Mining is an emerging paradigm that offers a broad range of capabilities in the healthcare field. This framework promotes a data-driven approach, like machine learning techniques, but offering a human-understandable vision such as knowledge-driven techniques, combining the best parts of both worlds. The next step is to provide appropriate tools and methodologies to help professionals put this paradigm into practice.

References

1. Adadi A, Berrada M. Peeking inside the black-box: a survey on explainable artificial intelligence (xai). IEEE Access. 2018;6:52138–60.
2. Atzori L, Iera A, Morabito G. The internet of things: a survey. Comput Netw. 2010;54(15):2787–805.
3. Chen M, Mao S, Liu Y. Big data: a survey. Mobile Netw Appl. 2014;19(2):171–209.
4. Columbus L. Roundup of internet of things forecasts and market estimates. https://www.forbes.com/sites/louiscolumbus/2016/11/27/roundup-of-internet-of-things-forecasts-and-market-estimates-2016/. 2016.
5. Cooper SB. Incomputability after alan turing. Not AMS. 2012;59(6):776–84.
6. Bonome Message Costa L, Godinho Filho M. Lean healthcare: review, classification and analysis of literature. Prod Plan Control. 2016;27(10):823–36.
7. Brandão de Souza L, Pidd M. Exploring the barriers to lean health care implementation. Public Money Manage. 2011;31(1):59–66.
8. Deo RC. Machine learning in medicine. Circulation. 2015;132(20):1920–30.
9. Došilović FK, Brčić M, Hlupić N. Explainable artificial intelligence: a survey. In: 2018 41st International convention on information and communication technology, electronics and microelectronics (MIPRO). IEEE, 2018. p. 0210–15.
10. Fernandez-Llatas C, Garcia-Gomez J-M. Data mining in clinical medicine, volume methods in molecular biology, vol. 1246. Humana Press, Springer; 2015.
11. Fernández-Llatas C, Benedi J-M, García-Gómez JM, Traver V. Process mining for individualized behavior modeling using wireless tracking in nursing homes. Sensors. 2013;13(11):15434–51.
12. Fernández-Llatas C, Meneu T, Traver V, Benedi J-M. Applying evidence-based medicine in telehealth: an interactive pattern recognition approximation. Int J Environ Res Public Health. 2013;10(11):5671–82.
13. Goldhahn J, Rampton V, Spinas GA. Could artificial intelligence make doctors obsolete? BMJ. 2018;363:k4563.
14. Gooch P, Roudsari A. Computerization of workflows, guidelines, and care pathways: a review of implementation challenges for process-oriented health information systems. J Am Med Inform Assoc. 2011;18(6):738–48.
15. Groopman JE, Prichard M. How doctors think, vol. 82. Springer; 2007.
16. Gunning D, Aha DW. Darpa's explainable artificial intelligence program. AI Mag. 2019;40(2):44–58.
17. Haggerty E. Healthcare and digital transformation. Netw Secur. 2017;2017(8):7–11.
18. Hou X-H, Feng L, Zhang C, Cao X-P, Tan L, Yu J-T. Models for predicting risk of dementia: a systematic review. J Neurol Neurosurg Psychiatry. 2019;90(4):373–9.
19. Ibrahim MS, Pang D, Randhawa G, Pappas Y. Risk models and scores for metabolic syndrome: systematic review protocol. BMJ open. 2019;9(9):e027326.
20. Jiomekong A, Camara G. Model-driven architecture based software development for epidemiological surveillance systems. Stud Health Technol Inform. 2019;264:531–5.
21. Kanasi E, Ayilavarapu S, Jones J. The aging population: demographics and the biology of aging. Periodontology 2000. 2016;72(1):13–8.
22. Kaplan B. Evaluating informatics applications—clinical decision support systems literature review. Int J Med Inform. 2001;64(1):15–37.
23. Kawamoto K, Houlihan CA, Balas EA, Lobach DF. Improving clinical practice using clinical decision support systems: a systematic review of trials to identify features critical to success. BMJ. 2005;330(7494):765.
24. Lenz R, Reichert M. It support for healthcare processes–premises, challenges, perspectives. Data Knowl Eng. 2007;61(1):39–58.
25. Mamlin BW, Tierney WM. The promise of information and communication technology in healthcare: extracting value from the chaos. Am J Med Sci. 2016;351(1):59–68.

26. Modha DS, Ananthanarayanan R, Esser SK, Ndirango A, Sherbondy AJ, Singh R. Cognitive computing. Commun ACM. 2011;54(8):62–71.
27. Ribeiro MT, Singh S, Guestrin C. "Why should i trust you?" explaining the predictions of any classifier. In: Proceedings of the 22nd ACM SIGKDD international conference on knowledge discovery and data mining, 2016. p. 1135–44.
28. Rigby M, Ammenwerth E, Beuscart-Zephir M-C, Brender J, Hyppönen H, Melia S, Nykänen P, Talmon J, de Keizer N. Evidence based health informatics: 10 years of efforts to promote the principle. Joint Contribution of IMIA WG EVAL and EFMI WG EVAL. Yearb Med Inform. 2013;8:34–46.
29. Sackett DL, Rosenberg WMC, Gray MJA, Haynes BR, Richardson SW. Evidence based medicine: what it is and what it isn't. BMJ. 1996;312(7023):71–2.
30. Schleidgen S, Klingler C, Bertram T, Rogowski WH, Marckmann G. What is personalized medicine: sharpening a vague term based on a systematic literature review. BMC Med Ethics. 2013;14(1):55.
31. Sheth A, Anantharam P, Henson C. Semantic, cognitive, and perceptual computing: paradigms that shape human experience. Computer. 2016;49(3):64–72.
32. Stone EG. Unintended adverse consequences of a clinical decision support system: two cases. J Am Med Inform Assoc. 2017;25:564–7.
33. Szolovits P. Artificial intelligence in medicine. Routledge; 2019.
34. Topol E. Deep medicine: how artificial intelligence can make healthcare human again. Hachette Book Group; 2019.
35. Toselli AH, Vidal E, Casacuberta F. Multimodal interactive pattern recognition and applications. Springer Science & Business Media; 2011.
36. Usher-Smith JA, Walter FM, Emery JD, Win AK, Griffin SJ. Risk prediction models for colorectal cancer: a systematic review. Cancer Prev Res. 2016;9(1):13–26.
37. van der Aalst WMP. Process mining: data science in action. Springer; 2016.
38. Van Rossum L, Aij KH, Simons FE, van der Eng N, ten Have WD. Lean healthcare from a change management perspective. J Health Organ Manag. 2016;475–93.

Chapter 8
Bringing Interactive Process Mining to Health Professionals: Interactive Data Rodeos

Carlos Fernandez-Llatas

8.1 Introduction

As we have argued in previous chapters, the application of new emerging computer technologies is causing a major earthquake in the healthcare field, promising a new era of digital health [31]. In past years, in the middle of a new fever of Artificial Intelligence and Machine Learning, there is a growing interest in the application of Process Mining techniques in the health domain [15, 34, 39]. However, this domain has some barriers that must be overcome to provide usable tools and methodologies [18].

In the world of digital health, there is a continuous change in methodologies, treatments and protocols. The high variability of medical treatments, local ethics and data protection laws, the suspicions of medical staff about the use of new emerging technologies, among a large set of other variables, significantly affect the success of the application of Information and Communication Technologies. This is because, in health, the success of a technology application is due, not only to the quality and new advances it provides, but also to the trust, use and acceptance that health professionals profess for it [25].

The creation of an appropriate Process Mining methodology is crucial to achieve good results. Some inspiring methodologies have appeared in the literature [44, 48] providing a new framework for the application of Process Mining techniques in a wide way in a large number of scenarios. In the case of health, due to the characteristics of the field, the penetration of these techniques has more difficulties than

C. Fernandez-Llatas (✉)
Process Mining 4 Health Lab – SABIEN – ITACA Institute, Universitat Politècnica de València, Valencia, Spain

CLINTEC – Karolinska Institutet, Sweden
e-mail: cfllatas@itaca.upv.es

© Springer Nature Switzerland AG 2021
C. Fernandez-Llatas (ed.), *Interactive Process Mining in Healthcare*, Health Informatics, https://doi.org/10.1007/978-3-030-53993-1_8

in other fields. Because of this, new methodologies specifically designed for their application in health are appearing in the literature. Most of these methodologies, based on questions [40] or goals [14], are trying to involve the professional in the learning process, in an interactive way [19], looking for a better understanding, trust and user experience, which are crucial for the success of the application of a new way of providing health.

Health is a very complex domain where the expert is the only recognized voice to decide whether the results provided are adequate or not. Therefore, to create a full interactive methodology it is essential to have a high commitment from professionals. This commitment depends on the personal interest of health staff, the added value that they expect to achieve with new technologies and the burden that these methodologies cause in their daily practice. The main priority of health professionals is to take care of their patients. In this line, physicians, who generally have little time, are not interested in techniques that do not provide added value to their main objective. Even in cases where Data Science can provide a clear improvement over the current state of the art, if this value is not properly presented to the expert, in an adequate time, or if the expert does not trust it, the probability of rejection is very high. This is because, in the case of health, the most precious resource that must be rationalized is the time dedicated by the health professional. Process Mining practitioners must provide the quality of results in the same way that the expert is expending time.

For that, in each iteration of the data analysis, especially in the firsts ones, each contact with the health professional must be productive. These iterations must follow a perfectly programmed strategy that requires special skills for the Data Scientist who is in charge of extracting the knowledge from professionals and providing the results that they are looking for. For example, in [40], Data Scientists use questions to interact, while in [14], the strategy is based on the definition of goals. However, in these methodologies, there is no analysis of what are the best tools to solve specific situations in the case of health.

In this chapter, we analyze some available frameworks, techniques, and algorithms in the process mining literature, to provide guidelines based on the multidisciplinary interaction of health professionals, with the intention being prepared to offer the best process indicators in the most optimal way.

8.2 Interactive Process Mining Data Rodeos

The main objective of a Process Mining methodology is to provide solutions for experts that help them understand how their processes behave. Thus, Process Mining should provide tools and algorithms to empower experts with understandable Process Indicators. An Indicator is an *information that helps to understand or measure the characteristics or intensity of one fact, or even to evaluate its evolution*. A Process Indicator is a *Process representation that can be used as an indicator to understand or measure the behaviour of a process*. To create Process Indicators that support health professionals in their daily practice, it is necessary to have data analysis interactions that transform raw data into understandable information. We named each of these interactions *Interactive Process Mining Data Rodeo* (or Data Rodeo, for simplicity). A Data Rodeo is a *highly coupled multidisciplinary interactive data analysis aimed at building process indicators that allow understanding, quantifying and qualifying processes and their changes in an objective, comprehensive and exploratory way.* Data Rodeos can range from a session of a couple of hours to complete researches that can take up to one month. Analogously to the concept of *Sprint* in the SCRUM development methodology [42], a Data Rodeo must provide results in short periods that need to be validated iteratively, by healthcare professionals.

8.2.1 Data Rodeo Sessions

The objective of a Data Rodeo session is to create Process Indicators that are useful for experts to understand, evaluate and optimize their processes. For each Data Rodeo session,the contribution of all stakeholders involved in the process is required. In the medical domain, there are, mainly, three kinds of professionals who have a role in the adequate implantation of digital health processes; Managers, Clinicians, and Information Technology (IT) professionals.

- Contrary to what may be thought, most of the time, managers are one of the main recipients of Process Mining systems applied in healthcare domains. Not only because managers are usually the ones who make the decisions about the possible deployment, or not, of new technologies, but also because they are the ones who have a wider view of the general processes in a health centre. Managers want tools that allow them to understand and control hospital processes. Managers can use Process Mining tools to analyze the general administrative behaviour of the hospital to gain insight into cross services, such as pharmacology or logistics, or to analyze specific areas, and to optimize their Quality of Service [26].
- Clinicians are the main holders of medical information. They can also be subdivided into two main groups, which are medical doctors by one side, and nursing and auxiliary staff by another. On the one hand, medical doctors are the ones who have the medical knowledge and evidence and have a broad vision of how treatments should be deployed. Besides, medical doctors decide on changing treatments. On the other hand, nursing and auxiliary staff are the professionals in charge of the daily operational actions. From a process perspective, constructing medical dashboards that do not reflect the knowledge, requirements, and concerns of doctors, could result in panels that do not provide useful medical information for professionals, and, consequently, reject their use. Furthermore, creating medical indicators that do not take into account the knowledge of nurses runs the risk of not reflecting the real operative that occurs

in a hospital and, as a result, the information that reaches managers and clinicians may be erroneous.

- IT professionals are the ones who control access to data. Most of the times, managers and clinicians have a partial idea of how the data is stored in the Hospital Information Systems (HIS), and its availability. For that, the involvement of IT Professionals is crucial for real support in data extraction and having a realistic scenario of how a process mining system can be integrated into the health centre.

In summary, to prepare an effective data analysis interaction in the healthcare domain it is necessary to have the agreement and interaction of all the stakeholders in the process. It is necessary that in the Data Rodeo session there be, at least one representative from each group. Otherwise, the results of the Data Rodeo session could fall on deaf ears.

As already stated, the objective of a Data Rodeo Session is to find process indicators that support health professionals in the real understanding, measurement, and assessment of the health processes that occur in clinical centres. By interactively involving professionals in the creation loop these process indicators, the risk of rejection and/or misuse of the provided tools can be significantly decreased. For the method to be interactive, it is crucial to use models that medical doctors understand [18, 36]. Otherwise, the feedback from health professionals will be erroneous, reducing the usability of the systems, and increasing the risk of rejection by the user.

These process indicators should be created to provide operational information that can be checked against the HIS, thereby increasing professionals' confidence in the indicators provided. These indicators should allow the health professional to have a real interaction with the system. They could navigate through the data having a real understanding of the behaviour of their processes and patients. This should cover from the general process to the individual patient analysis, detecting patients who do not conform to the standard case and discovering where in the process there are differences.

To achieve these process indicators, it is needed to provide the appropriate measurement tools that can quantify in an objective, comprehensive and exploratory way the health process as well as their changes.

8.2.2 Data Rodeos in an Interactive Process Methodology

Taking into account the life cycle of the implantation of new medical infrastructure, and the necessity of making that interactive,it is possible to divide this deployment into three main phases:

- **Shakedown**: This phase is the first contact of professionals with the methodology. In this phase, the main objective is to show to health professionals the potential of using Process Mining in their area. In this phase, professionals may have some suspicions and prejudices from previous experiences. Therefore, this phase is critical to building trust between health practitioners and data scientists. This phase is usually very short and generally provides throw-away process indicators that are used as the basis for the indicators that are generated in subsequent iterative phases.

The most effective way to implement Data Rodeos in this phase is to create short face-to-face Data Rodeo sessions with managers, clinicians, IT professionals, and the Process Mining Data Scientist (Interactive Process Miners). To avoid Data Privacy issues, meetings can take place in the data environment, with anonymous data being deleted from the system after each session. This session should be performed by an experienced Health Interactive Process Miner who could apply different Process Mining solutions to create specific indicators.

Each session must be especially time effective. Each meeting must finish with a view of the data to demonstrate what process mining technologies can offer them. In this phase the importance is not the accuracy of the content, so it is possible to use tools that can reduce noise, working with ideal data. This is because the focus is not to find medical evidence. The aim is to make health professionals aware of the possibilities in the use of Process Mining techniques. If this phase is successfully accomplished, the professionals' expectations soar and the next phase can be tackled.

- **Research**: After the shakedown phase a research project begins with the aim of developing a Process Mining dashboard that supports health professionals. In this phase, the main aim is to use all the process mining tools available to create accurate Process Indicators that provide adequate ways to measure and understand the processes and their changes. Assuming professionals are highly interested, we can schedule offline multi-session Data Rodeos to apply a more standard Process Mining methodology [44] that includes: understanding the real process, analyzing what data is available to show in the process and its quality (applying corrections if necessary); preparing the logs; and applying process Mining discovery, conformance and enhancement techniques to achieve the best process indicators for the problem at hand.

  At this stage, we should request the approvals of the Ethical Committees in accordance with the current laws depending on the country in which the system is implemented. Then, depending on the possibilities of accessing to the data, Interactive Process Miners can perform the Research actions using different models:

  - **Secure Environments**: In this model, Interactive Process Miners can access the data environment. This access can be full or partial, depending on the rights provided by the ethical committees. Interactive Process Miners can access the data physically entering the health centre or accessing the system through a Virtual Private Network (VPN) if this is possible according to the IT system of the health centre. This model is usually in close collaboration with units where a framework agreement is signed between the parts.
  - **Anonymous Data**: In the case that the access to secure environments is not available, it is possible to create Process Mining indicators by using

Anonymous data. This model requires a pre-process that makes the data free of personally identifiable information. The main disadvantage of this model is that professionals cannot navigate to the individual level to better understand the process of single patients.

- **Simulations**: Sometimes, when anonymizing the data is not possible, or even while the ethical committees are in the evaluation process, it is possible to start the research phase with simulated data. In this scenario, the data used is fake, so there are no privacy laws to comply with. This model is useful to test Process Mining methods before installing the tools in the hospital. However, this data is not enough to extract any kind of conclusions. Even if this data has been simulated based on statistical information of real data, the relationship among the different measures, dates, doctors, etc. are lost. Moreover, the models to simulate are always abstractions of reality, and for that, the results can be significantly different from real data analysis.

The importance of this phase is not the efficiency of the techniques to be used. The aim is to select the best algorithms to show the data in the best possible way. For that, complex research algorithms that require high computation capabilities are acceptable in this phase.

- **Production**: Once the research phase has finished, the next step is to put in production the identified Process Indicators in production. In this phase, a Process Mining dashboard should be deployed in the hospital that allows health experts to analyze the indicators. The efficiency of algorithms is of critical importance at this stage. The system response must be adequate to deliver the results to experts on time.

  The integration of the systems should now be complete. It can be direct, connecting the system to the HIS or through an Integration Engine. It can also be indirect, creating a specific Process Mining Data Warehouse that has the logs specified appropriately. The direct way allows just-in-time mining to permit a real-time vision of the process, on the contrary, the indirect version should periodically update the middleware database used for Process Mining. This version could be more efficient because a specific Process Mining Log-based Data Warehouse can be composed in advance to improve access to the data in terms of events.

Inspired in the well-known Hype Cycle Gartner Curve [29] the behavioural process of implantation of a new Interactive Process Mining system in a health centre can be represented. Figure 8.1 shows the curve of expectations depending on the phases. The *Shakedown* phase is the first contact with the methodology that increases the expectations of the expert in an exponential way. After the first moment, the expert can enter a psychological stage of disappointment due to the lack of quality data, the difficulties in accessing it, as well as the difference between the perceived and the actual process. Before reaching user rejection, a new *Research* Data rodeo can suppose a new impulse to the expectations of health professionals. Repeating this process in several iterations allow us to achieve an adequate set of process indicators in the *Production* phase that can perfectly cover

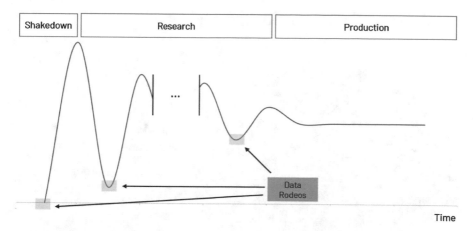

Fig. 8.1 Phases in the application of a Interactive Process Mining Methodology

the expectations of the experts and provide the correct view to analyze, measure and optimize their processes.

8.3 Interactive Data Tools for Data Rodeos

To perform adequate Data Rodeos, it is necessary to have adequate process mining tools depending on the phase. Figure 8.2 shows the characteristics of the tools that can be used in each of the phases.

Mature general Process Mining algorithms that are widely used in different areas and fields, and can be used in all the phases of the stages. Examples of those tools are General Process Discovery algorithms, like Inductive Miner [28], Heuristic Miner [50], or PALIA [21], as well as filters, conformance and enhancement tools, that are widely tested in different scenarios [15, 39, 44].

Quick research tools are those that are not mature enough to ensure their accuracy, but can show views that can provide interesting clues about the processes behaviour. Examples of those are techniques to make quick over-abstractions that can easily show easily models with low noise, that might have accuracy problems in some cases [45]. These tools can be used on Shakedown and in research phases.

General automated Views are complete views that have a demonstrated utility in other scenarios and can be applied directly in some similar cases. For example, Indicators that have been used to analyze emergency processes can be used in sub-processes like Stroke in emergencies [26]. These views can be used in the Research and Production Phases. Their use is not recommended in shakedown phases because this automation usually requires a complete data cleaning that is not desirable in quick Data Rodeos.

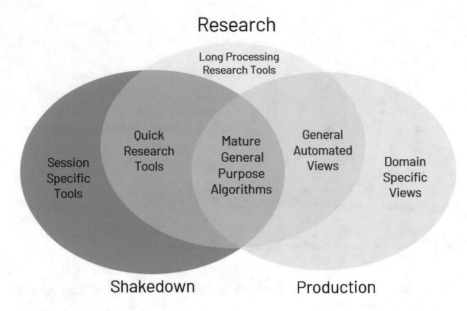

Fig. 8.2 Tools used in Phases of a Process Mining system deployment

In Quick Data Rodeos in the Shakedown phase, *Session Specific tools* can usually be created to quickly correct data, eliminate data quality issues that produce an excess of *spaghetti* in the models, or remove outliers, among a vast amount of different situations. These tools are usually created using quick scripts to prepare the logs prior to the discovery. These algorithms can be discarded in the next stages and changed for more detailed, mature and accurate data correction techniques.

Long Processing Research Tools that require a long processing time are not usually suitable for daily practice due to their low usability. However, these techniques can be used in research phases, e.g. to train classification systems, to stratify some models, or even create trace clusters that show different behaviours in a huge quantity of patients [11].

Finally, *Domain Specific Views* can be created for a better understanding of processes in the production phase, for example specific colour maps can be created to highlight precise situations that are only valid for a specific domain.

The selection of the tools to be used depends on the decisions of Interactive Process Miners who manage Data Rodeos, according to the problems to solve at each moment. Interactive Process Miners must build their own Data Rodeo Toolkit depending on their experience and programming skills. There is a big set of tools available on the literature, for Python Programmers [1], R [22], as well as complete

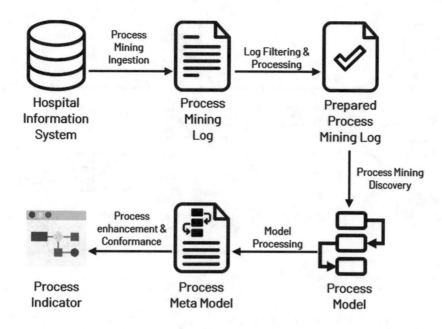

Icons made by Freepik, Good Ware, and Pixel perfect from www.flaticon.com

Fig. 8.3 General Purpose Data Rodeo flow

suites to perform Data Rodeos, some are open-source, like ProM [47] or Apromore [27] while there are other commercial ones such as Celonis[1] and DISCO.[2]

Figure 8.3 shows the flow of a general-purpose Data Rodeo. The first stage is the *Process Mining Ingestion*. At this stage, the data is extracted from the HIS and a Process Mining log is created by collecting the available events. In the second stage, called *Log Filtering & Processing*, the log is processed with the objective of filtering, correcting, or grouping activities among others. This will produced a refined Process Mining log that shows more adequately the process, according to what the professional wants. Once the log is prepared, the process model is inferred using *Process Mining Discovery* algorithms. In the third stage, after the discovery, in the *Model Processing* stage the model can be enriched with more data to construct a meta-model that contains not only nodes and edges but also the statistical information about timings, frequency and the events referred to each of the structures in the visual model. Finally, *Process Enhancement & Conformance* stage, produces the final Process Indicators that highlight the specificities that health experts needs to understand, measure and compare their clinical processes.

In the next subsections, each one of the stages is detailed.

---

[1] https://www.celonis.com/
[2] https://fluxicon.com/disco/

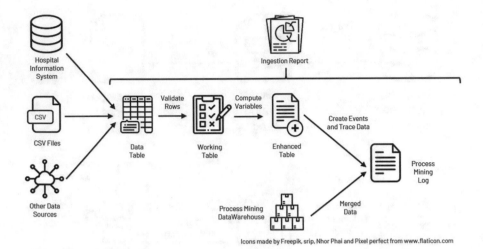

Fig. 8.4 Process Mining ingestion flow

8.3.1 Process Mining Ingestion

The ingestion process is in charge of providing the Datalog to start the Process Mining flow. In the Process Mining flow, several stages can be identified that are shown in Fig. 8.4. In a health IT system, the data is usually stored in a Hospital Information System. In case that access to the raw databases is possible, and to build Query languages to access the available data. In the case of informal data rodeos, usually in the Shakedown phase, the experts generally provide the data in Comma-Separated Values (CSV) files. In both cases, the data can be represented in a set of rows and columns that represent the available data. Most Data Science tools use this way of representing data, but in case of data sources available in other formats, it is recommended to transform these data to facilitate its processing. Therefore, in an Interactive Process Miner toolkit, it is highly recommended to have tools to manage CSV Files or SQL Connections to facilitate data access.

Once raw data tables have been collected, it is time to start selecting the relevant data for creating process indicators. The first action is the validation of the rows. With the help of clinicians and IT professionals, the Interactive Process Miner can select the adequate rows that will be processed in the next stages. In an example, suppose that we are accessing a database with all the laboratory data (which can be a large amount of data) that in each row has a different kind of value. To create a process indicator for diabetes and be only interested in glycosylated values, we can skip the rest of the data by ignoring all the rows that are not interesting. This can be implemented through IF-THEN tools that allow Interactive Process Miners to greatly reduce considerably the amount of data to process in the following stages. In case of query sentences to access databases we can usually tune the queries to avoid this data previously, but this option is not always possible (e.g. in CSV files), and this selection of data is easy to understand by physicians that can follow the process of ingestion process more easily.

After reducing the data table to process, we need to convert the data to compute the variables that are used to create the events and trace data that will be used on the Process Mining log. The idea of this stage is to create new values, which are not available on the working data but provide a semantic vision that facilitates the understanding of the clinical process semantically. For example, Temporal Abstractions [20, 41] can provide a temporal semantic interpretation that can be inferred from the data to provide a high-level view of the medical process that will facilitate it understandability. Besides, the creation of discrete values from numerical data [43] using the adequate medical standards that can provide a semantically health professional understandable view. Also at this stage, format corrections (e.g. dates), variable aggregations, variable renaming,... etc. are performed. The resulting table is called *Enhanced* table.

Once the data is processed and the variables updated, the next stage is the creation of events and trace data. The event data is made up of the timestamp information, the node name, the identification of the trace, and some metadata associated with the event. On the other hand, the trace data are a set of metadata associated with the same case. Depending on the nature of the data, and the expectations of health professionals three kinds of events can be created, *Named* events, whose name is defined by the clinician according to the mapping of the process, *Variable* events, whose name depends on the value of a computed (or not) value of one of the variables existing in the Enhanced table, or *Mixed* events, which have a named part and a variable part that is linked in the event name. For example, in case of Emergency Rooms [26] the *Admission* event is named by the expert and represents the moment when the patient entered in the system; in the case of the discharge it is interesting to split it in different nodes depending on the destination (*Home, Exitus, Transfer...*); and in the case of Attention, health professionals prefer to have separated nodes depending on the level of triage (*Attention1, Attention2...*). Figure 8.5 shows a process model with the three types of events in the example.

Depending on where the data needed to create the events is, the actions to be performed can be divided into two groups:

- One Row – One or multiple Events: All the information to create one or more events is located in each one of the rows. This schema allows efficient creation of the events. Processing of all the table is not required to create the events and each row and event can be deleted from memory after being processed.
- Multiple Rows – One or multiple Events: The information to create events is not in one row and it's needed to process several rows to create each event. For example, the name and the start date are in different rows. This schema requires full processing of the rows, before creating each event. This supposes to keep in memory rows and events to create the log. This can be a problem when working with a big quantity of data. It is possible to save memory by creating mechanisms to update the events in the log with each row, but that usually affects directly to the computation time.

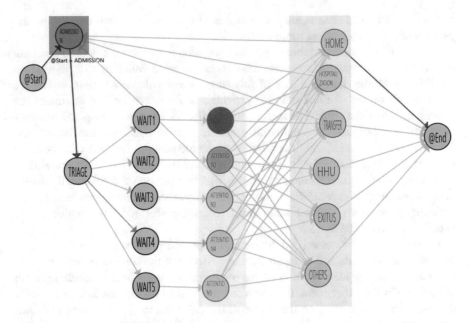

Fig. 8.5 Process indicator for emergency rooms

Also at this stage, data quality is evaluated and the interactive data cleaning process is performed [35]. By analyzing the obtained results, Interactive Process Miner can detect, in combination with the IT professionals and clinicians, what the data problems are and what the possible solutions are. All the quality issues should be reflected in the Ingestion Report (errors in dates, incomplete logs,...). This is a document that shows all the corrections performed over the rows to construct the final log, ingestion stats and relevant information. This document is crucial to show the health and IT experts the possible limitations of the Process Indicators that can be constructed with this log. Not only the base quality of the data can be shown but also the report can be used as the starting document to detect problems in the IT system of the hospital that can be corrected interactively. For Interactive Process Miners, it will be recommendable that this report is automatically or semi-automatically created by their toolkit after the application of each one of the correction algorithms.

In a Shakedown phase it is suitable to use rude data denoising tools to limit spaghetti effect [18]. For example, removing all the infrequent data [7] or all the traces that do not conform to a given model [4]. In Research and Production phases, there is time to analyze the data quality and perform the adequate corrections to create a clean log, using the knowledge given by health and IT professionals iteratively and interactively. In that way, it is recommended to create specific filters for production or to even correct the data in the HIS source logs if possible.

Once a clean log has been created, it can be merged with already existing Process Mining logs to create a Process Mining Data Warehouse to create a more efficient way of applying Process Mining techniques to create Process Indicators for the production phase. This process can be automated using Extract, Transform and Load (ETL) systems that can incrementally create these Data Warehouses.

8.3.2 Log Filtering and Processing

After creating the log, the next stage filters and processes the data to select the adequate log to construct the process indicators.

One of the most common tools that can be used in this phase is stratification filters, which are tools that extract sub-logs from the main log, representing a sub-population depending on a specific characteristic. For example, filters to select patients based on their age, gender, or specific illnesses. These filters can be developed using algorithms that process the log and select only the patients (traces) that have the specified characteristics. The trace variable could be discrete, where only a set of possibilities is valid. For example, gender can be male or female; or numeric, for example, age. In this case, in the filter, the maximum and minimum value should be specified. Furthermore, using the adequate discretizers in the ingestion phase, numerical values can be converted into semantically understandable terms based on medical algorithms existing in the literature [43]. The use of these medical terms facilitates the understanding of the medical experts, making the interaction with them easier.

Doctors might explore new ideas to stratify patients. Sometimes, looking to facilitate the understanding of the process due to excess of Spaghetti Effect [18], or trying to discover a new stratification based on different behaviours of patients [6]. Clustering techniques [12] are classic pattern recognition techniques that allow creating partitions of the log based on the similarity of its elements. One of the main disadvantages that clustering techniques have in the field of pattern recognition is the selection of the best distance and configuration to ensure the validity of the partitions [24]. However, interactive methodologies have the advantage of integrating an expert in the loop. Using the adequate distances, the expert can interpret the partitions giving them a semantic sense that provides a very interesting view to health professionals [19]. This technique, known as Trace clustering, has been used several times in literature; to analyze the behaviour of cardiovascular patients depending on its risk model [38], or analyzing the obesity dynamics to create new risk models that can increase the medical knowledge [43], or analyzing behaviours of different hospital circuits [33]. The selection of the adequate distance is crucial to provide proper groups, there are classic distances available for general sequential analysis [2], distances that take into account the topological similarity between the models [6, 16] or distances that take not only into account the topology, but also the metadata available (length of stay, frequency,..) to compute the distance [11].

Besides, filters that split the log by dates, or daily times can be very useful to detect the behaviour of the process over time.

Moreover, not only filters can be applied in this phase, but also, processing algorithms that can correct or simplify the log according to the information that the expert is giving us. For example, algorithms that fuse sequential events that are equivalent, that group or rename specific events, that assume that the completion of one activity is the start of the next one, or other specific algorithms that are semantically described by the expert, and provided support in the better definition of the Process Mining log, thanks to interactive methodology.

8.3.3 Process Mining Discovery

Process Mining Discovery algorithms are the ones that, given a log, provide a model that represents them. Discovery algorithms are the most common, representative and differentiating technique of Process Mining paradigm.

There are several Discovery algorithms available in literature [15, 39, 44]. Also, there are some works in literature dealing with Interactive Process Discovery techniques. These techniques are thought to use experts' feedback to increase the effectiveness of Process Discovery algorithms [10]. While automatic Process Discovery algorithms provide models using different statistical strategies, Interactive Process Discovery algorithms take advantage of the know-how and common sense of human experts for a better and quicker convergence [19]. Interactive Process Discovery not only provides solutions to support humans in models corrections but also provide conformance checking algorithms for the measurement of the accuracy of the human modifications suggestions [9] and Model Repair solutions that support the experts by suggesting modifications in the models to achieve more accurate ones. [5, 8]. Also, there are discovery algorithms specifically designed to try to cover special features of medical models, where the results of the activities can be a reason for the selection of the next event. For example, after a diagnosis test activity, depending on the result of the test, there is a selection of the adequate treatment. Activity-Based Process discovery algorithms, like PALIA [21], enrich the logs with the results of the activities to tag the edges with the reason for the transitions.

In the interactive methodology, the selection of one adequate model is crucial to collect human expert feedback. In case of health, physicians have difficulties to understand complex models [36]. The use of these models, not only have important limitations in the use of process indicators but also, by using interactive process discovery techniques, it is necessary a translation from the model to the expert language that should be performed by the Interactive Process Miner. In this translation, some important information can be lost and the feedback could be erroneous. In that way, it is recommended to use field understandable models, assuming some loss of expressivity, instead of complex models that can cause erroneous feedback and rejection from the user.

8.3.4   Model Processing

After the discovery process, the models that represent the logs can be processed to compute the metadata associated with the model. To create useful solutions, models should be beyond topological processes where only nodes and edges are being taken into account. Two processes can have the same events, but their timing and frequency can be different. The analysis of those differences, can support medical doctors in the understanding of the dynamical characteristics of the process and, then, allowing them to optimize the processes. In this line, metadata associated with the process is key to assess experts in the dissimilitudes among processes. In an Interactive Process Miner toolkit, algorithms should be available to process models to compute common and specific metadata and associate it to models.

Three kinds of metadata associated with models can be defined.

- **Computing Nodes and Edges Metadata**: Statistical information associated with model structures is crucial to understand how the executions of models have been performed. Statistics like frequency, average or median duration, unique number of patients, . . . provide vital information to understand the behaviour of the process. Also, it is possible to compute specific statistics depending on the problem. For example, in [26] a new variable is computed measuring the adequacy of the waiting states in emergency rooms according to the Manchester gold standard.

  Besides, it is possible to add semantic information associated with model structures to increase the interactivity of the models. For example, identifying semantic task structures [23], or Workflow Patterns [46] can facilitate the understanding of the models not only for their syntactical behaviour but also, for the semantics associated with nodes.

- **Computing Model Abstractions** Sometimes, the simplification of the models can be a good option to provide quick views. Usually, Process Mining applications offer simplifications of models via removing infrequent behaviour. Although this can be an adequate solution in some cases, these techniques should be managed with care and guarantee the correctness of the information presented, because otherwise it could create some confusion in the expert [45]. In the case of clinical data, infrequent behaviours sometimes are more interesting than standard cases. While standard cases are covered by standard treatments, infrequent cases are the ones that doctors consider of interest. Adverse effects are one of the most interesting cases in several clinical domains [30]. For that, before applying these abstraction techniques, an Interactive Process Miner should ensure that confusion is not created in the health professionals. Another option to simplify models is, instead of removing infrequent behaviour, to group nodes hierarchically to present the model with the required granularity in each case. Guided by the expert, the whole process can be divided into sub-processes, making the model more readable.

- **Event References**: Nodes and edges represent actions and transitions that have been produced. Storing the relationship between topological structures of the model with the log events allows the complete navigation from the process to the individual. This enables medical doctors to analyze all the events associated to a specific structure. That, for example, permits the evaluation of the specific patients that follow a specific path, or allows the computing of specific statistics such as statistical significance when comparing two models [26]. Supporting the navigation from the model to the individual, has a positive effect on the understandability of the model and the trust of the professional in the tool. Sometimes, medical doctors have problems to understand some transitions to actions that might have no sense in the model, due to process inefficiencies or data quality issues. In these cases, analyzing the events associated with strange edges allows the understanding of the unexpected behaviour. However, keeping the event references associated with the model can suppose a high computing and memory cost that, is some cases, cannot be viable.

8.3.5 Model Enhancement

Once the model has been discovered, and their metadata computed, it is the moment to present the result to experts. In the Interactive Paradigm, having the expert in the loop requires a complete communication between the expert and the data science algorithms [19]. So far we have analyzed tools to access, collect and process the data. However, the success of an interactive system lies not only in its capability to extract information but also in the way it is presented to the human expert. In that way, although very relevant information is extracted, if the Interactive Process Miner fails in the selection of visual tools for the adequate presentation of data, the experts will probably not understand the final result and, as a consequence, the complete model will be useless.

The Model Enhancement phase is the last one and its result is the Process Indicator that will be presented to the user. The tools used by Interactive Process Miners should provide very expressive and flexible solutions to show enhanced models in different ways. In the Process Mining literature, there are a huge quantity of works that create useful process indicators by using enhancement models. These provide an augmented model view where the model is presented highlighted with the available metadata information. The selection of highlighting tools depends on the characteristics of the process to be presented.

One of the most used techniques in the literature to show statistical data in the model is the creation of maps that reflect some characteristics in the model like the colour [17, 26, 32], size [37], tags or transparency of nodes and edges. Figure 8.6 shows an example where the nodes have been coloured with a gradient that represents the median length of stay, and gradient for arcs represents the number of patients that, proportionally, follow this transition. In this example, the redder the colour, the greater the proportion. Also, tooltips can be used to show the whole stats offering detailed information to the user, that can easily detect the most common paths and in what activities the patient stay more time than in others. Other solutions

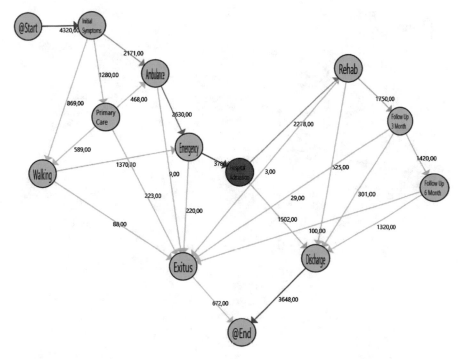

Fig. 8.6 Process Inferred using a Process Mining Discovery algorithm and Enhanced with gradient colors representing stats

can tag the transitions with the number of patients or the average time of the transition [45].

Furthermore, it is interesting to combine process information with business intelligence statistics that can be obtained from the cohort of patients selected to infer the Process Indicator. Creating Dashboards combining both informations can provide a richer view for the health professional. There are a huge quantity of process analytic views that can show medical processes [13, 33] and business intelligence systems applied to healthcare [3, 49]. Besides, it numerical information can be used in Process analytic tools to create abstractions that can show models as single points in a graph that can be presented as a point in a two-dimension graph [33], as a curve representing the change in time [16] or as an enhanced calendar to show different kinds of behaviours depending on the period in the year [11].

The comparison of groups can help health professionals to discover their differences and this can allow them to understand groups characteristics. In medicine, a classic trust measure to discover differences between two cohorts of patients is Statistical Significance. This technique can be used to highlight the differences between the two models referring to two cohorts. This approach can not only discover when a process is different but also in which parts of the models the differences lie [26]. Also, we can simply subtract the values showing

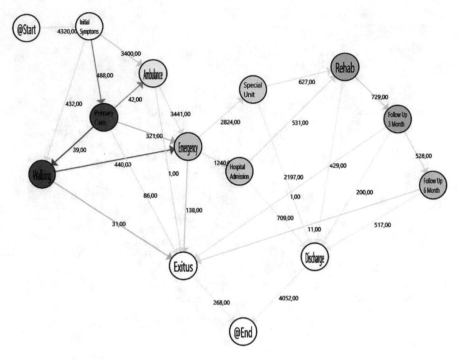

Fig. 8.7 Difference enhancement model

maps that highlight the differences between the process nodes and edges and their degree. Figure 8.7 shows a Process Indicator with enhancement showing negative differences in red colour and the positive ones in green colour. The saturation of the colour reflects the degree of difference in negative or positive respectively.

Moreover, the model can be enriched with figures that ease the understanding of the map. Figure 8.8 shows an example of a Real-Time Location System Process Indicator that uses a map of the building for a better understanding of movement behaviour of a patient at home.

There are more options in the literature to enrich the models, like showing the cases associated with nodes and edges [26], or displaying the traces as relational Social networks [33].

8.4   Conclusions

Process Mining has a high quantity of algorithms and tools that can be used to provide Process Indicators that can support Health professionals in understanding clinical processes. Interactive Process Miners should analyze the process and select the best algorithms in each phase to provide the best Process Indicators that maximize the Medical Professionals' understanding of the process.

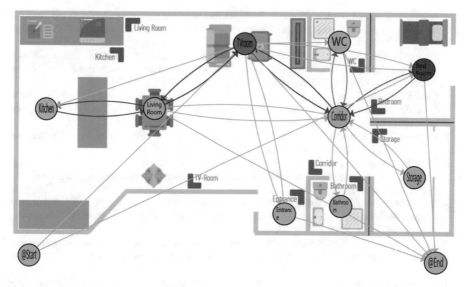

Fig. 8.8 Process with maps methaphors

This formalization of processes allows the creation of tools for Data Rodeos that facilitates the process of learning interactively. The selection of enhancement models is as important as the algorithms used to extract the information. In this case, it is very important not only to select the best algorithms and enhancement tools but also to select the best possible models, with the adequate meta-model information, and choose the adequate cohort after ingestion that deals with the data quality in the best possible way.

The final result are Process Indicators that can show the actual behaviour of the process. However, the creation of Process indicators should take into account the previous experts' knowledge about the medical process, comparing it with existing medical evidence, algorithms and gold standards. This allows comparing the behaviour of the actual process with the ideal one.

References

1. Berti A, van Zelst SJ, van der Aalst W. Pm4py web services: easy development, integration and deployment of process mining features in any application stack. BPM Demo Track, 2019.
2. Bose RPJC, Van der Aalst WMP. Context aware trace clustering: towards improving process mining results. In: Proceedings of the 2009 SIAM international conference on data mining. SIAM; 2009; p. 401–12.
3. Brandão A, Pereira E, Esteves M, Portela F, Santos MF, Abelha A, Machado J. A benchmarking analysis of open-source business intelligence tools in healthcare environments. Information. 2016;7(4):57.

4. Carmona J, van Dongen B, Solti A, Weidlich M. Aligning event data and process models. In: Conformance checking: relating processes and models. Springer International Publishing, 2018. p. 125–58.
5. Cervantes AA, van Beest NRTP, La Rosa M, Dumas M, García-Bañuelos L. Interactive and incremental business process model repair. In: OTM confederated international conferences "on the move to meaningful internet systems". Springer; 2017. p. 53–74.
6. Conca T, Saint-Pierre C, Herskovic V, Sepúlveda M, Capurro D, Prieto F, Fernandez-Llatas C. Multidisciplinary collaboration in the treatment of patients with type 2 diabetes in primary care: analysis using process mining. J Med Internet Res. 2018;20(4):e127.
7. Conforti R, La Rosa M, ter Hofstede AHM. Filtering out infrequent behavior from business process event logs. IEEE Trans Knowl Data Eng. 2016;29(2):300–14.
8. Dixit PM, Buijs JCAM, van der Aalst WMP. Prodigy: human-in-the-loop process discovery. In: 2018 12th international conference on research challenges in information science (RCIS). IEEE; 2018. p. 1–12.
9. Dixit PM, Buijs JCAM, Verbeek HMW, van der Aalst WMP. Fast incremental conformance analysis for interactive process discovery. In: International conference on business information systems. Springer; 2018. p. 163–75.
10. Dixit PM, Verbeek HMW, Buijs JCAM, van der Aalst WMP. Interactive data-driven process model construction. In: International conference on conceptual modeling. Springer; 2018. p. 251–65.
11. Dogan O, Martinez-Millana A, Rojas E, Sepulveda M, Munoz-Gama J, Traver V, Fernandez-Llatas C. Individual behavior modeling with sensors using process mining. Electronics. 2019;8(7):766.
12. Duda RO, Hart PE, Stork DG. Pattern classification. Wiley; 2012. Google-Books-ID: Br33IRC3PkQC.
13. Erdoğan T, Tarhan A. Process mining for healthcare process analytics. In: 2016 joint conference of the international workshop on software measurement and the international conference on software process and product measurement (IWSM-MENSURA). IEEE; 2016. p. 125–30.
14. Erdogan TG, Tarhan A. A goal-driven evaluation method based on process mining for healthcare processes. Appl Sci. 2018;8(6):894.
15. Erdogan TG, Tarhan A. Systematic mapping of process mining studies in healthcare. IEEE Access. 2018;6:24543–67.
16. Fernández-Llatas C, Benedi J-M, García-Gómez JM, Traver V. Process mining for individualized behavior modeling using wireless tracking in nursing homes. Sensors. 2013;13(11):15434–51.
17. Fernandez-Llatas C, Lizondo A, Monton E, Benedi J-M, Traver V. Process mining methodology for health process tracking using real-time indoor location systems. Sensors. 2015;15(12):29821–40.
18. Fernandez-Llatas C, Martinez-Millana A, Martinez-Romero A, Benedi JM, Traver V. Diabetes care related process modelling using Process Miningtechniques. Lessons learned in the application of InteractivePattern Recognition: coping with the Spaghetti Effect. In: 2015 37th annual international conference of the IEEE engineering in medicine and biology society (EMBC), 2015. p. 2127–30.
19. Fernandez-Llatas C, Meneu T, Traver V, Benedi J-M. Applying evidence-based medicine in telehealth: an interactive pattern recognition approximation. Int J Environ Res Public Health. 2013;10(11):5671–82.
20. Fernandez-Llatas C, Sacchi L, Benedí JM, Dagliati A, Traver V, Bellazzi R. Temporal abstractions to enrich activity-based process mining corpuswith clinical time series. In: Proceedings of the international conference on biomedical and healthinformatics (BHI2014), 2014.
21. Fernandez-Llatas C, Valdivieso B, Traver V, Benedi JM. Using process mining for automatic support of clinical pathways design. In: Fernández-Llatas C, García-Gómez JM, editors. Data mining in clinical medicine, number 1246 in methods in molecular biology. New York: Springer; 2015. p. 79–88.

22. Gatta R, Lenkowicz J, Vallati M, Rojas E, Damiani A, Sacchi L, Berardino De Bari, Dagliati A, Fernandez-Llatas C, Montesi M, et al. pminer: an innovative r library for performing process mining in medicine. In: Proceedings of the conference on artificial intelligence in medicine (AIME 2017). Springer; 2017.
23. Gatta R, Vallati M, Fernandez-Llatas C, Martinez-Millana A, Orini S, Sacchi L, Lenkowicz J, Marcos M, Munoz-Gama J, Cuendet M, de Bari B, Marco-Ruiz L, Stefanini A, Castellano M. Clinical guidelines: a crossroad of many research areas. challenges and opportunities in process mining for healthcare. In: Di Francescomarino C, Dijkman R, Zdun U, editors. Business process management workshops. Cham: Springer International Publishing. 2019. p. 545–56.
24. Halkidi M, Vazirgiannis M. Clustering validity assessment: finding the optimal partitioning of a data set. In: Proceedings 2001 IEEE international conference on data mining. IEEE; 2001. p. 187–94.
25. Holden RJ, Karsh B-T. The technology acceptance model: its past and its future in health care. J Biomed Inform. 2010;43(1):159–72.
26. Ibanez-Sanchez G, Fernandez-Llatas C, Celda A, Mandingorra J, Aparici-Tortajada L, Martinez-Millana A, Munoz-Gama J, Sepúlveda M, Rojas E, Gálvez V, Capurro D, Traver V. Toward value-based healthcare through interactive process mining in emergency rooms: the stroke case. Int J Environ Res Public Health. 2019;16(10):1783.
27. La Rosa M, Reijers HA, Van Der Aalst WMP, Dijkman RM, Mendling J, Dumas M, García-Bañuelos L. Apromore: an advanced process model repository. Expert Syst Appl. 2011;38(6):7029–40.
28. Leemans SJJ, Fahland D, van der Aalst WMP. Discovering block-structured process models from event logs containing infrequent behaviour. In: Lohmann N, Song M, Wohed P, editors. Business process management workshops. Springer International Publishing; 2014. p. 66–78.
29. Linden A, Fenn J. Understanding gartner's hype cycles. Strategic Analysis Report N° R-20-1971. Gartner, Inc, 2003. p. 88.
30. Loke YK, Price D, Herxheimer A. Adverse effects. Cochrane handbook for systematic reviews of interventions version, 5(0), 2008.
31. Mamlin BW, Tierney WM. The promise of information and communication technology in healthcare: extracting value from the chaos. Am J Med Sci. 2016;351(1):59–68.
32. Mannhardt F, Blinde D. Analyzing the trajectories of patients with sepsis using process mining. In: RADAR+ EMISA@ CAiSE, 2017. p. 72–80.
33. Mans RS, Schonenberg MH, Song M, van der Aalst WMP, Bakker PJM. Application of process mining in healthcare–a case study in a dutch hospital. In: International joint conference on biomedical engineering systems and technologies. Springer; 2008. p. 425–38.
34. Mans RS, van der Aalst WMP, Vanwersch RJB. Process mining in healthcare. SpringerBriefs in business process management. Springer International Publishing; 2015.
35. Martin N, Martinez-Millana A, Valdivieso B, Fernández-Llatas C. Interactive data cleaning for process mining: a case study of an outpatient clinic's appointment system. In: Di Francesco-marino C, Dijkman R, Zdun U, editors. Business process management workshops. Cham: Springer International Publishing; 2019. p. 532–44.
36. Martinez-Millana A, Lizondo A, Gatta R, Vera S, Salcedo VT, Fernandez-Llatas C. Process mining dashboard in operating rooms: analysis of staff expectations with analytic hierarchy process. Int J Environ Res Public Health. 2019;16(2):199.
37. Partington A, Wynn M, Suriadi S, Ouyang C, Karnon J. Process mining for clinical processes: a comparative analysis of four Australian hospitals. ACM Trans Manag Inf Syst. 2015;5(4):1–18.
38. Pebesma J, Martinez-Millana A, Sacchi L, Fernandez-Llatas C, De Cata P, Chiovato L, Bellazzi R, Traver V. Clustering cardiovascular risk trajectories of patients with type 2 diabetes using process mining. In: 2019 41st annual international conference of the IEEE engineering in medicine and biology society (EMBC). IEEE; 2019. p. 341–4.
39. Rojas E, Munoz-Gama J, Sepulveda M, Capurro D. Process mining in healthcare: a literature review. J Biomed Inform. 2016;61:224–36.

40. Rojas E, Sepúlveda M, Munoz-Gama J, Capurro D, Traver V, Fernandez-Llatas C. Question-driven methodology for analyzing emergency room processes using process mining. Appl Sci. 2017;7(3):302.
41. Sacchi L, Larizza C, Combi C, Bellazzi R. Data mining with temporal abstractions: learning rules from time series. Data Min Knowl Disc. 2007;15(2):217–47.
42. Schwaber K, Beedle M. Agile software development with Scrum, vol. 1. Prentice Hall Upper Saddle River; 2002.
43. Valero-Ramon Z, Fernandez-Llatas C, Martinez-Millana A, Traver V. A dynamic behavioral approach to nutritional assessment using process mining. In: 2019 IEEE 32nd international symposium on computer-based medical systems (CBMS). IEEE; 2019. p. 398–404.
44. van der Aalst W. Data science in action. In: Process mining: data science in action. Berlin/Heidelberg: Springer; 2016.
45. van der Aalst WMP. A practitioner's guide to process mining: limitations of the directly-follows graph. Proc Comput Sci. 2019;164:321–28.
46. van Der Aalst WMP, Ter Hofstede AHM, Kiepuszewski B, Barros AP. Workflow patterns. Distributed Parallel Databases. 2003;14(1):5–51.
47. Van Dongen BF, de Medeiros AKA, Verbeek HMW, Weijters AJMM, van Der Aalst WMP. The prom framework: a new era in process mining tool support. In: International conference on application and theory of petri nets. Springer; 2005. p. 444–54.
48. van Eck ML, Lu X, Leemans SJJ, van der Aalst WMP. PM^{2}: a process mining project methodology. In: Zdravkovic J, Kirikova M, Johannesson P, editors. Advanced information systems engineering. Springer International Publishing; 2015. p. 297–313.
49. Watson HJ, Jackson M. Piedmont healthcare: using dashboards to deliver information. Bus Intell J. 2016;21(3):5–9.
50. Weijters AJMM, van Der Aalst WMP, De Medeiros AKA. Process mining with the heuristics miner-algorithm. Technische Universiteit Eindhoven, Tech. Rep. WP, 2006;166:1–34.

Chapter 9
Interactive Process Mining in Practice: Interactive Process Indicators

Carlos Fernandez-Llatas

9.1 Approaching the Process Assessment to Health Professionals

In the previous chapter, we analyzed algorithms and tools that can be used in Data Rodeos for constructing Process Indicators. With the objective of supporting Medical professionals, we should also provide dashboards that present the best indicators to understand, measure and optimize the processes.

In current systems, the analysis and evaluation of processes are usually addressed using numerical indicators that represent the status of the process in a moment in time. These are known as Key Performance Indicators (KPI) [16] and are compared with previously defined values that represent the expected value in the execution of the processes. These KPIs should be defined before the start of the processes and are directly related to specific goals required to measure the success of a specific process. This success indicator can be related to different concepts to be evaluated such as finance, quality of service (QoS), efficiency, efficacy, adherence...among others. Adequate KPIs should be Specific, Measurable, Achievable, Relevant and Timely (SMART).

Thinking about Perceptual Computing, the application of KPIs is not always easy. The lack of contextual information, the difference between the perceived and the real processes, the indeterminacy of human behaviour make the use of KPIs insufficient to provide an adequate vision to experts. They are still more inadequate in processes such as ergonomics, which involve human beliefs, mood

C. Fernandez-Llatas (✉)
Process Mining 4 Health Lab – SABIEN – ITACA Institute, Universitat Politècnica de València, Valencia, Spain

CLINTEC – Karolinska Institutet, Sweden
e-mail: cfllatas@itaca.upv.es

© Springer Nature Switzerland AG 2021
C. Fernandez-Llatas (ed.), *Interactive Process Mining in Healthcare*, Health Informatics, https://doi.org/10.1007/978-3-030-53993-1_9

and attitudes. Sometimes, KPIs are approached by using subjective questionnaires due to the difficulty of having objective measures that represent the correct execution of interventions of ergonomists. Also, the reasoning behind KPIs is not always easily interpretable by humans.

To implement KPIs that can provide a contextual and personalized view, to support the evaluation of perceptual questions and supporting ergonomist in the real understanding of the process, it is necessary to bring a new KPIs framework that, on the one hand, provides more rich and human-understandable indicators and, on the other hand, can be automatically formalized and learned. In this chapter, we propose Interactive Process Indicators (IPIs) as the way to overcome the limitations of KPIs.

9.2 Interactive Process Indicators (IPIs)

Interactive Process Indicators (IPIs) are Process Indicators produced as a result of the application of the interactive paradigm with professionals. IPIs not only provide a way to understand, measure, and optimize the process but also allow the expert to navigate behind the model discovering the features and specificities of the process.

This means IPIs use the benefits of the Interactive framework to create process-based indicators that provide human-readable and contextualized KPIs. IPIs can be created using Process Mining technologies via Interactive Data Rodeos. The capabilities of Interactive Process Mining technologies can support not only the characterization of general process-based KPIs, which show how the process is executed in an organization, but also the analysis of individual and personalized aspects of the processes going to the general to the individual. IPIs are not numbers but advanced views in the form of enhanced processes that provide a human-understandable view that supports the expert in the better perception of the processes for an advanced assessment.

To support the evaluation of processes in a predictive, contextual and person-alized way, IPIs take time into account. For example, using IPIs to compare the evolution of the processes, it is possible to evaluate the degree of completion of the objectives. Furthermore, this evolution should be processed to convert the acquired data into formal knowledge. In this way we propose the following hierarchy of IPIs:

- **IPIs** take the raw information acquired as log events (e. g. from the Internet of Things systems) and provide an enhanced Process view that supports a better understanding of the current status of the worker. For example, by applying Process Mining Technologies a view of the flow of a surgery area can be provided [6], or to discover the usual behaviour of a human [10].
- **IPIs Evolution**. These are IPIs that make a timely or stratification comparison between two IPIs to support experts in the understanding of the produced changes. In that case, flows can be produced that highlight the changes by

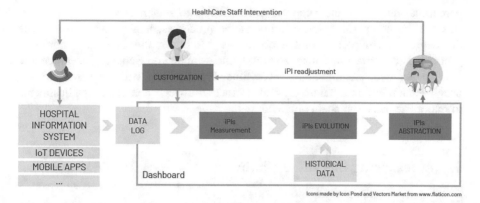

Fig. 9.1 IPIs hierarchy

comparing different stratification of patients or measuring the changes produced on the process after an organizational change [12].

- **IPI Abstractions**. These are IPIs aimed to provide a high semantic view of the findings to support experts in the easy analysis of the general findings. They can be numbers describing an objective measure acquired from the flows that can be represented by graphics [5], or even semantic sentences like *The user is adherent to the treatment*. The IPI Abstractions are computations performed over other IPIs that summarize the achieved findings. In that way, it is always possible to access the origin of the results in a human-understandable way. So, if an expert has doubts about an IPIs Abstraction he/she can access the IPIs that have been used for this reasoning and discover the reality behind these results.

Figure 9.1 shows how experts can use IPIs to apply interactive methodology [8] in their daily practice. The expert can create IPIs in iterative Data Rodeos creating IPI definitions that can be computed with the data available in the system. IPIs offer a view of the status of the current processes.

When the expert wants to make a change in the process in order to improve it, the effects of these changes affect the data collected and, after computing the IPI, they can show the effects of this change in the process. Furthermore, the evolution of the process can be compared, highlighting the differences between the processes in time, to measure the value chain of the performed actuation. Having this evolution in time, models can compute abstraction and be shown as process analytics views (for example, histograms or curves) that can display the evolution in time of the process. The expert should be able to interact with these Process Analytic views to access the processes that are behind these abstractions and from the processes, the expert should be able to access to individuals. This interaction capability from general to individual is called *Full Crawling*. Full Crawling allows experts to navigate models, allowing them to discover the reasons for the differences among processes.

The Data Rodeos performed in different iterations will produce rich IPIs that could provide a contextual and personalized view. This enables the evaluation of perceptual questions and supports professionals to understand the real process. Besides, by comparing the evolution of the processes, it is possible to evaluate the degree of completion of the objectives. Moreover, this evolution should be processed to convert the data acquired into formal knowledge. This procedure will be iterative and interactive over time. Professionals will keep the person's progression monitored iteratively and interact with the system making adjustments to maximize the value chain obtained by the patient.

9.3 Measuring the Value Chain

The Interactive Process Indicator is a view of the behaviour of the patients in the health system. To use this indicator in the Value-Based Healthcare paradigm [17], it should supply information about the different aspects that give benefits to the patient in the value chain. According to the Triple Aim paradigm, [2] three main aspects can be used to measure the value in a medical process:

- **Population Health:** Since ancient times, when the concept of medicine was born, the main interest of physicians was to keep the population healthy. According to the definition of the World Health Organization (WHO), *Health is a state of complete physical, mental and social well-being and not merely the absence of disease or infirmity* [14]. In this line, all the efforts in medicine would be intended to provide health to citizens, in all the aspects of their life. The objective measurement of healthy population has been one of the most challenging research activities of the medical community. The definition and computation of basic statistical medical variables, like prevalence and incidence, of the diseases, using bio-statistics [15], the development of the epidemiology research field [18], as well as the creation of risk models [3], are examples of attempts to model patients' health status.
- **Economical Cost:** Although the main interest in healthcare is to provide better health to patients, this is not always possible due to the lack of resources. The most classical way to measure the value in the medical process is to measure the economical costs of the process. The continuous population increase and the appearance of chronic illnesses associated with age, require the reduction of the general budget of the health service to make it sustainable. For that, it is crucial to optimize the health protocols, in order to provide the best results using as few resources as possible.
- **Patient Experience:** The traditional medical focus, intended to provide better health to patients, usually ignores the person behind the patient [11]. In this paradigm, the patient has no decisions about his/her health, in this approach the relationship between doctors and patients follows a paternalist model. In the last decades, a new vision of the patient as the main responsible of his/her disease has changed the concept of medicine to a patient-centred one [4]. The idea of patient-centred medicine takes into account the concerns, beliefs and attitudes

of the patient to select the best treatment. The personality of the patient has a big impact on patient health. An adequate adherence of the patient is crucial to improve the patient's health [13]. Besides, it promotes self-care as well as self-efficacy [1] to empower patients in the prevention and management of their illnesses. It not only supposes a more direct and better experience for the patient but also will imply an increase in the sustainability of health systems due to the better control of the patients [19].

9.4   Interactive Process Indicators by Example

In this chapter, we have designed an example with the objective of showing how to use IPIs in practice. As already stated in many occasions along the book, each medical problem requires specific solutions. However, going too deep into specific solutions can make it more difficult to understand the general purposes of IPIs. This example is based on simulations. In the third part of the book, we analyze specific cases and how Interactive Process Indicators work in real situations. However, in this chapter, we have designed a purely academic example whose objective is far from extracting medical conclusions.

For this example, we have designed a hypothetical disease where stabilization time is critical, not only for the survival of the patient but also for the posterior rehabilitation of the patient. In this case, the more time the patient is not stabilized, the more probabilities there are for the decease of the patient. In the same way, if the patient survives, the time to stabilization affects the time of rehabilitation and even death of the patient during the rehabilitation phase. If the patient survives for more than 9 months it is assumed that the patient is out of danger.

For the simulation, we have used an Ambient Assisted Living Simulation system [9] specifically designed to simulate complex situations to evaluate human behaviour. These simulations have been designed to illustrate how Process Mining technologies can show the value chain effects of the specific actions deployed by professionals.

The simulated disease has a different behaviour in different patients. The objective is to have a very complex illness with wide variability. Figure 9.2 shows a graphical representation of the problem. Using this distribution, we have simulated the behaviour of patients in the hospital. Patients should be stabilized in less than a predetermined time following a Gaussian distribution (Mean: 10 h, Standard Deviation: 5 h). If the patient is not stabilized during this time (*TimeToDeath*), the patient dies. No patient can die in less than 1 h, and if the patient has more than 24 h of *TimeToDeath* it's supposed that the patient is stabilized and always recovers, even if the stabilization occurred very late. The time of stabilization affects directly to the mortality of patients in the rehabilitation process. Patients with late stabilization have more probabilities of death on the rehabilitation stage. On the other hand, patients with quick stabilization have more probabilities to reach discharge without the need for a rehabilitation process (Fig. 9.3).

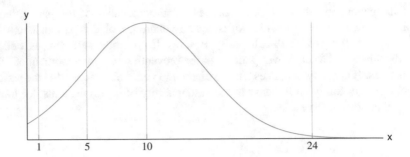

Fig. 9.2 Gaussian representing the behavior of the simulated illness

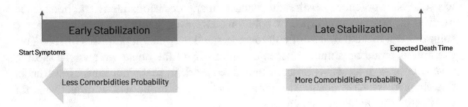

Fig. 9.3 Effects on stabilization of the disease

9.4.1 Analyzing the Hospital Process

In our example, this disease is treated in the health system as a common critical illness. This means that the patients follow the usual paths as general patients in a sanitary centre. Using the simulation system, we have reproduced how a usual health system covers this problem. In this line, we have assumed that the health system is digitized, and all the events can be recovered from the hospital Electronic Health Record (EHR). Besides, we have considered an ideal system, where the data quality errors are negligible.

Figure 9.4 shows the graphical representation of the process. After having the initial symptoms, the patient has three different possibilities to access the health system. He/she can call an ambulance to go to the hospital, can go to a primary care center or, can even decide to go to the hospital by his/her own (Walking). If the patient selects the Primary Care way, Primary practitioners detect the anomalies in the patient status and can recommend to the patient to go to the hospital. The variability of care or even the difference of experience of primary care doctors supposes that the recommendation of professionals might be the derivation to hospital emergencies, by his/her own means or, if the practitioner has suspicions, he/she can call an ambulance.

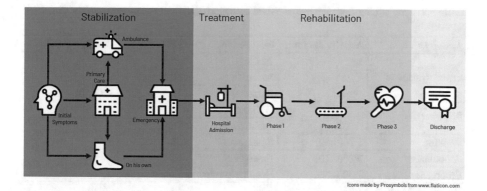

Icons made by Prosymbols from www.flaticon.com

Fig. 9.4 Hospital Protocol to cover the illness

Once the patient enters the emergency system, the professionals diagnose the illness and stabilize the patient. The patient can die (*Exitus*) at any moment in the process according to the model presented in Fig. 9.2. Once the patient has been stabilized, there is not an immediate risk of death for the patient. After being stabilized, the patient is moved to a bed in the hospital. When the patient is ready to leave the hospital the rehabilitation protocol begins. The rehabilitation lasts a maximum of nine months separated into three stages. At the end of each stage, the patient is evaluated and the rehabilitation doctor decides if the patient should continue the rehabilitation or not. Also, as a consequence of the co-morbidities acquired by the patient due to the effect of the disease, the patient might die during the rehabilitation stages. The co-morbidities of the patient are directly related to the stabilization time. The later the patient is stabilized, the higher the probability of his/her decease. On the other hand, the earlier he/she is stabilized, the less probable it is that the patient needs a new stage of rehabilitation.

Table 9.1 presents the base probabilities and timing (average and standard deviation) of the activities that we selected for the simulation. After the initial symptoms, *Walking* action has a probability of 0.3, *Ambulance* 0.5 and *PrimaryCare* 0.2. Besides, the selection of Primary Care requires some administrative actions (getting a pre-appointment) that suppose a delay of 1 Day (with 2 h 30 min of Standard Deviation) in the treatment. After *PrimaryCare* action, the patient is derived to the hospital *Emergency* by an *Ambulance* or by *Walking* with the same probability, depending on the criteria of the physician. After the patient has been stabilized in *Emergency*, he/she is admitted to the hospital. The *HospitalAdmission* action takes 8 days (1 day of standard deviation). When the patient exits the hospital, the appointment to the *Rehab* first visit takes 7 days (1 day of standard deviation). This starts the rehabilitation process that can have a maximum of three blocks of sessions of three months each.

These base probabilities are affected by the time of stabilization, i.e. the time between the initial symptoms and the admission in the hospital and the *timetodeath* computed for each patient. If the patient overcomes the *timetodeath* at any moment

Table 9.1 Base timing (average and standard deviation) and flow probabilities of the simulated experiment

Activity	Activity duration	Next action	Probability	Duration transition
Initial symptoms	–	Walking	0.3	–
		Ambulance	0.5	–
		PrimaryCare	0.2	1d(2:30)
PrimaryCare	0:30(0:10)	Walking	0.5	–
		Ambulance	0.5	–
Walking	1:30(0:30)	Emergency	1	–
Ambulance	0:20(0:10)	Emergency	1	–
Emergency	1:30(0:30)	HospitalAdmission	1	–
Hospital admission	8d(1d)	Rehab	1	7d(1d)
Rehab	2:30(1:30)	Rehab 3 months	1	90d(1d)
Rehab 3 months	1:30(0:30)	Rehab 6 months	1	90d(1d)
Rehab 6 months	1:30(0:30)	Discharge	1	90d(1d)
Discharge	–	–		

before the stabilization, the patient dies and passes to *Exitus* status. After the stabilization, if the patient is in the $latestabilization$ area, he/she can die in one of the three stabilization blocks depending on the difference between the $timeofstabilization$ and the $timeofdeath$. If this difference is bellowed the 5%, 10% 20%, or 30% the patient will die in the Hospital during the first, second or third Rehab phases, respectively. On the contrary, if the difference is in the early stabilization area and the difference is above 95%, 90% or 80% the patient will be discharged in advance from the hospital, without the need of rehabilitation, after the first or the second phase of rehabilitation, respectively. The third phase of rehabilitation is the last possible one and ends on Exitus or Discharge.

9.4.2 Base Process

Using this information, we have simulated a log with the events of the process. Figure 9.5 shows an Interactive Process Indicator that can represent the behaviour of the process in the hospital. Gradient colours show how the patient is treated in this health system. This IPI is the result of applying a Process Mining Discovery algorithm. For this example, we have used PMApp and the PALIA [12] algorithm to create the indicator. At first sight, the IPI on the Fig. 9.5 shows the current behaviour of patients at a glance. Most patients go to the emergency department of the hospital by ambulance (2171). About a third of the patients do not need rehabilitation(1502) and the majority of the patients that start Rehabilitation (2278) finish the three stages adequately (1320).

In our example, quantifying the health in case of a life-threatening illness, some measures like the number of exitus (Deaths), of reduction of co-morbidities

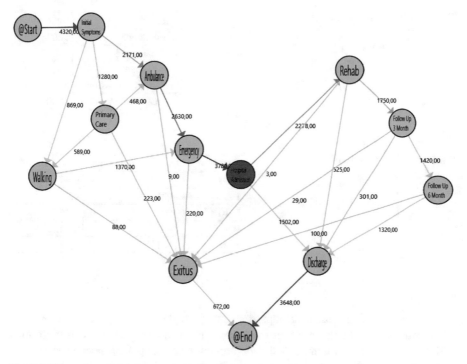

Fig. 9.5 Illness Interactive Process Indicator with Enhancement heat map

associated to the illness can be the main objective to cover to provide better health to population. By having an abstraction IPI of the Exitus ratio, we can get an idea of the mortality of the illness that is around 16% of the patients, that means that from 4320 patients, 3648 finish the treatment, while 672 die in the process. However, Fig. 9.5 provides a richer view of the process. In that enhanced model, we can easily see the status of the illness flow. Most of the patients follow the *Discharge* with the three phases of rehabilitation.

To measure the costs in Process Mining problems, it is only required to provide the cost associated with each one of the activities. This easily allows the computation of each trace cost. Table 9.2 shows the cost associated with the activities in our example. Some services have fixed costs like *Ambulance* or *PrimaryCare*, while others have a variable cost depending on the time spent in the activity, like *Emergency* and *HospitalAdmission*. This means that the start and the end events of the activity are needed for a precise cost measurement. XES [20] allows the incorporation of this information in the process of mining logs. Furthermore, Activity-Based Logs [7] store enough information to deal with this problem. PALIA is the discovery algorithm in this example. This has been selected because it is able to natively use Activity-Based Logs.

Having this table in mind, we can construct an abstraction IPI that shows the costs of the different patients according to the activities performed. In the example, the total cost of all the 4320 patients was around 51M €(51181590.6).

Table 9.2 Cost associated to
activities (in €)

Activity	Cost
Ambulance	500
Primary care	300
Emergency	300 X hour
Hospital admission	500 X day
Rehabilitation phase	6000

Table 9.3 Cost Groups of
illness (in €)

Cost group	Cost group number	Cost group %
>15 K	1749	0,40
1–5 K	921	0,21
5–10 K	690	0,16
10–15 k	499	0,12
<1 K	461	0,11

Moreover, we can make groups depending on the costs. Table 9.3 shows the
distributions of patients based on the costs. 40% of the patients expend more than
15K€ in treatments. Figure 9.6 shows the flow of patients that have an individual
cost above 15K€. As can be seen, the most critical cost path is the one that
represents the patients that require all the rehabilitation stages.

In our problem, patient experience is related to their expectatives and the contact
quality with the health system. In life-threatening diseases, patients want a diagnosis
as soon as possible, waiting as short as possible. Moreover, patients want to be
healthy as soon as possible with no secondary effects that affect their lifestyle,
having little rehabilitation time and with the fewer possible co-morbidities. Statistics
associated with IPI can show important information to evaluate the patient's
experience. Table 9.4 shows the percentage of patients (33%) that require the
maximum rehabilitation sessions (9 months) and Table 9.5 shows that most of the
patients (68%) are stabilized in less than 4 h.

9.4.3 Adding a Special Unit

After the first round of analysis, the managers intend to improve the flow of more
expensive patients to decrease their cost. To do that, by analyzing the literature, the
managers discover that improving the quality of care in the hospital, they can reduce
the mortality and, therefore, the co-morbidities of patients. Those co-morbidities
affect the number of needed rehabilitation phases, and consequently, make each
patient treatment more expensive. In our example case, we suppose that the medical
evidence demonstrates that the creation of a new Special Unit reduces the mortality

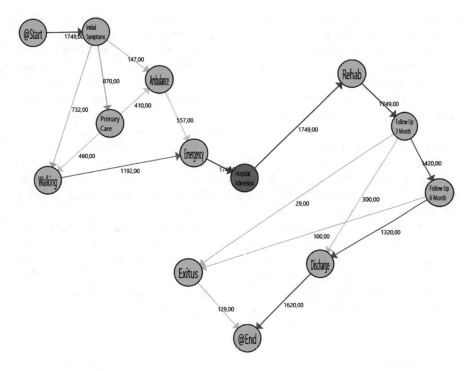

Fig. 9.6 Interactive Process Indicator of all the patients with a cost above 15K€

Table 9.4 Rehabilitation sessions need of patients

Rehab	Rehab number	Rehab %
No	2042	0,47
9 month	1420	0,33
3 month	528	0,12
6 month	330	0,08

Table 9.5 Stabilization time groups

Stabilization time	Stabilization time number	Stabilization time %
<4 h	2959	0,68
4–6 h	535	0,12
6–8 h	407	0,09
No stabilized	320	0,07
8–10 h	95	0,02
>10 h	4	0,00

of patients by a 3% in the hospital and a 5%, a 10% and a 15% in each rehabilitation phase. Also, these innovative treatments reduce the need of rehabilitation in a 5% in the hospital and a 10% in each one of the rehabilitation phases. The cost of this new unit is greater than a usual hospital admission (800€ per day) as well as the average length of stay in the unit (10 days with 2 days of standard deviation). Besides, the treatment proposed by this unit is only adequate for 70% of the patients. 30% of the patients, who have a specific type of this illness, should be treated as usual.

Having seen this, the hospital managers decide to deploy a new special unit to treat the disease in a more specific way. With the deployment of this new unit, the hospital expects to improve the population health by reducing the mortality; reducing the economical costs by decreasing the number of patients that require the maximum rehabilitation time; and increasing the patient satisfaction, by reducing the rehabilitation time.

Updating the simulator configuration with this information, we have simulated a new set of 4320 patients, the same number as in the first set. Figure 9.7 shows the new results. The most important change that can be seen is the appearance of a new node in the flow referring to the new *SpecialUnit*. As expected, the Special Unit patients have a greater Length of Stay (LoS) than usual patients, and the number of patients that are covered by this Unit is two thirds of the patients that are admitted

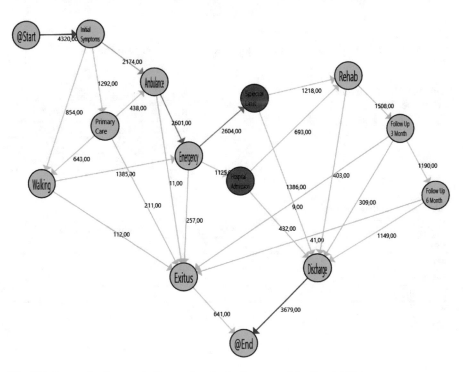

Fig. 9.7 Interactive Process Indicator after the deployment of the Special Unit

Table 9.6 Rehabilitation Phases patients after Special Unit Deployment

Rehab	Rehab number	Rehab %	Difference
No	2409	0,56	+367
9 month	1190	0,28	−230
3 month	403	0,09	+125
6 month	318	0,07	+12

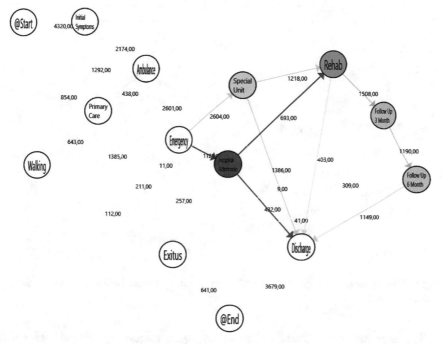

Fig. 9.8 Difference base Evolution Interactive Process Indicator between the Process with and without Special Unit

to the hospital. This can be seen by the colour gradient of the nodes and the colour gradient of edges, respectively.

Table 9.6 shows the rehabilitation groups. As expected, the number of patients that require the three phases of rehabilitation decreased (−5%), but the number of patients that requires none, one or two phases have increased. That means the change has adequately affected the rehabilitation needs.

Seeing this information as a process, Fig. 9.8 shows the number of patients difference between the base case and the Special Unit case. As can be seen (by the red colour gradient), all the rehab stages have decreased in the number of patients because in all stages there are more patients with fewer co-morbidities. In the same way, the normal hospital admission has dramatically reduced the number of patients since most of them were covered by the new unit. Special Unit colour remains grey because there is no previous information about this activity.

Table 9.7 Cost Groups after Special unit deployment

Cost group	Cost group number	Cost group %	Difference
>15 k	1611	0,37	−138
5–10 K	1226	0,28	+536
10–15 K	660	0,15	+161
<1 K	487	0,11	+26
1–5 K	336	0,08	−585

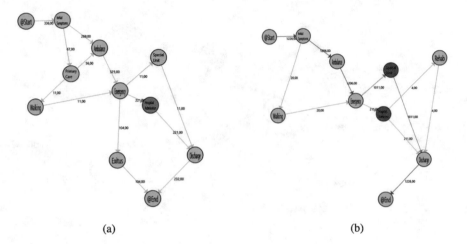

(a)   (b)

Fig. 9.9 Flows of cost groups. (**a**) Flow of patients with cost from 1–5K€ (**b**) Flow of patients with cost from 5–10K€

However, differently than the Hospital managers foresaw, the global economical costs were increased. The Economical-Cost in this second round was around 56M€ (56342436,35€) (an increased Cost in more than 5M€). Table 9.7 shows the cost changes depending on the groups. In the same line, although the number of patients that have a global cost greater than 15K€ has significantly decreased, the rest of the costs have increased, except the 1–5K€.

Analyzing the costs in detail, Fig. 9.9 shows the flow of patients with costs from 1–5K€ (Fig. 9.9a) and 5–10K€ (Fig. 9.9b). As can be seen, patients in the first group are the ones that stay less time in the hospital (that are the ones that decrease the number of patients), and patients in the second group are the ones that stay more time in the hospital (that are the ones that increase the number of patients). So, although the number of patients that make the three phases has decreased, it seems that the cost of maintenance of the special unit makes the total budget much more expensive than expected.

From the Patient Experience perspective, globally, the rehabilitation in the three phases has decreased a 5%. That supposes that patients have an increase in their quality of life after the acute event. On the other hand, Table 9.8 shows the differences in the Stabilization time with no significant changes.

Table 9.8 Stabilization Time after Special Unit Deployment

Stabilization time	Stabilization time number	Stabilization time %	Difference
<4 h	2921	0,68	+38
4–6 h	543	0,13	−8
6–8 h	415	0,10	−8
No stabilized	334	0,08	−14
8–10 h	104	0,02	−9
>10 h	3	0,00	1

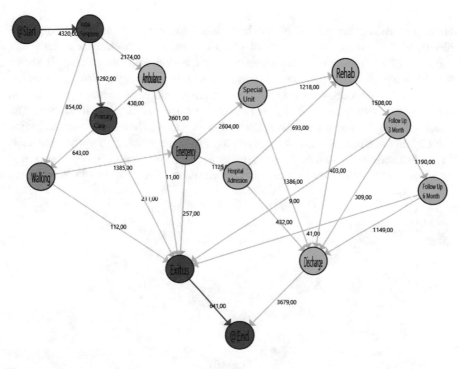

Fig. 9.10 Exitus Influence map after Special Unit deployment

Analyzing the population health improvement, the increase in costs has no significant changes on the patients' survival. In this case, 85% of the patients survived, which supposes a mere 1% increase in the survival rate.

At this moment, the hospital managers do not understand why the application of this new unit does not have effects in the survival rate of the patients. In order to get some clues, the Interactive Process Miners provide an Exitus influence map (Fig. 9.10). This Exitus Influence Map is a problem specific map, designed in a Data Rodeo, which shows the influence on the previous activities of deceased patients. In that way, the colours in the map are related to the percentual number of deceased patients that have visited the related activity. This Exitus Influence Map can be seen as a Bayesian Network. This map is very useful to detect the statistical causality based on a temporal relationship between the decease of the patient and the rest of the activities. This figure shows that most Exitus are related to the first activities after the emergency visit. After seeing this influence map, Hospital Managers realize that the key problem in the management of this disease is not at the hospitalization level. Most Exitus are dependent on the decisions taken at the first hours after the initial symptoms.

9.4.4 Creating an Information Campaign

Having analyzed the results of the last phase, the hospital managers prepare a new plan to improve the process of disease care. The IPIs obtained show that the mortality of patients is mostly related to the primary care process. It seems that Primary care protocols are not adequate to take care of this disease properly. Therefore, experts decide to start an information campaign to train patients and primary care professionals in the diagnosis and early stabilization of patients. The assumed cost of the Information Campaign is 1M€. Thanks to this campaign, the citizens are more aware of the symptoms and the number of ambulance calls increase from 50% to 80%. Also, Primary Care professionals are better prepared and have the instruments to make the stabilization of the patients in 80% of the

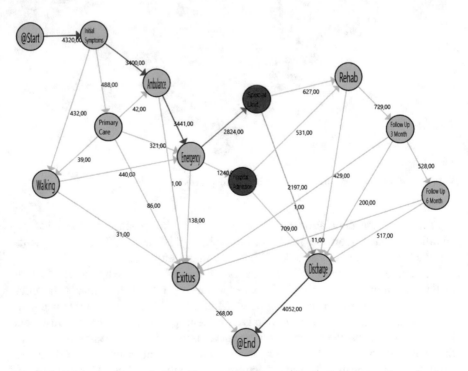

Fig. 9.11 Interactive Process Indicator between the Process after the Information Campaign

cases, allowing a quick derivation to emergencies. With these modifications in the probabilities, we simulated a new set of data.

Figure 9.11 shows the new discovered IPI. With the new configuration, the survival rate was increased until 94% (an increase of 9%). A quick visual comparison shows, as expected, that the flow of patients that call an ambulance has clearly increased and the patients that are discharged in the special unit without rehabilitation needs increase dramatically.

The global economic is now around 45M€ (45730803,74€) (Saving more than 10M€). Table 9.9 shows the new cost groups compared with the previous one. The number of High-Cost patients (>15K€) decrease dramatically (801 patients) and the medium-low cost patients (5–10 K) increased in the same way. It seems that the decrease in rehabilitation patients is positively affecting the economical cost.

Analyzing the stabilization time (Table 9.10), the patients that have been stabilized in less than 4 h have increased in a 21% (+876 patients), and the rest of groups have all decreased. This decrement seems to be related to the number of patients that comes in the ambulance and the improvement in primary care quick stabilization.

According to the rehabilitation needs (Table 9.11), the number of patients that needs some rehabilitation has decreased to 12% (−16%). The most important change is that people who do not need rehabilitation increase an 18% (+753

Table 9.9 Cost Groups after Information Campaign

Cost group	Cost group number	Cost group %	Difference
5–10 K	1976	0,46	+750
10–15 k	891	0,21	+231
>15 k	810	0,19	−801
1–5 K	437	0,10	+101
<1 K	206	0,05	−281

Table 9.10 Stabilization Time after Information Campaign

Stabilization time	Stabilization time number	Stabilization time %	Difference
<4 h	3797	0,88	+876
4–6 h	250	0,06	−293
6–8 h	135	0,03	−280
No stabilized	118	0,03	−216
8–10 h	19	0,00	−85
>10 h	1	0,00	−2

Table 9.11 Rehabilitation Phases Patients after Information Campaign

Rehab	Rehab number	Rehab	Difference
No	3162	0,73	+753
9 month	528	0,12	−662
3 month	429	0,10	+26
6 month	201	0,05	−117

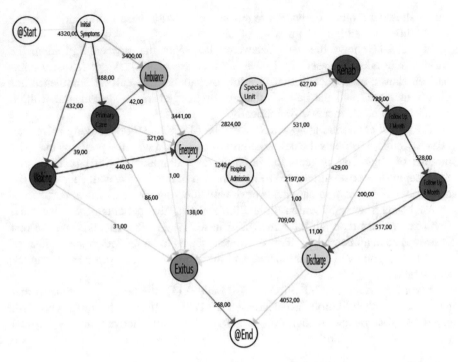

Fig. 9.12 Difference base Evolution Interactive Process Indicator after the Information Campaign

patients). This significant change seems to be due to the decrease of stabilization time that ease off the risk of co-morbidities, abating the needs of rehabilitation.

All this information can be easily shown using a Difference Map. Figure 9.12 shows the Difference map after the Information Campaign. This map clearly shows the differences in the evolution of the process after the improvement. There is a clear increase of patients coming to emergencies by ambulance that obviously suppose a decrease of patients going trough primary care by their own, showing the effects of the Information Campaign both qualitatively and quantitatively. This supposes an increment in the people that reach the Emergency Department that reach the Emergency Department without dying. Because of this, the number of patients that are treated in the hospital increase, but the patients that need rehabilitation significantly decrease, with a very highlighted red colour. Therefore, there is less mortality than in the previous stage.

Another interesting view can be the differences between the Exitus influence map. Figure 9.13 shows this Evolution IPI. As can be seen, the influence to mortality patient going to Primary care has decreased, as well as the presence in the hospital. This means that people that reach the admission in the hospital have less probability to die than in the previous scenario. However, it can be shown that people that come by ambulance have increased their probability of Exitus,

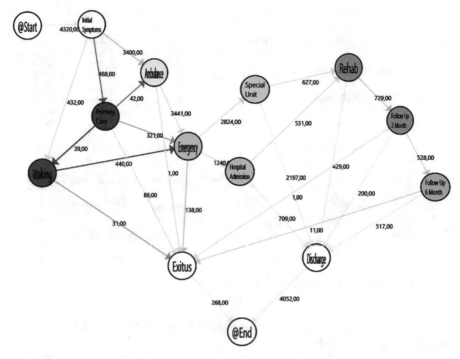

Fig. 9.13 Exitus Influence map Difference after Information Campaign

and more patients die in emergencies. If we see that as a complete process thanks
to IPIs, we can understand that the increase of effectiveness in the primary care
process has permitted that patients that have fewer probabilities to survive, that in
previous process configurations died on the way, can now reach the Emergency
Department, even in the case that stabilization was not possible. This is the cause of
the increase of mortality in the emergency. If we would have had these numbers as
individual KPIs we would have thought that there was a problem in the Emergency
Department, but IPIs can offer enriched and contextual information that can better
support the healthcare experts in their decisions, beyond simple numbers.

Each one of the IPIs can be abstracted to provide numbers that can provide a
high-level view of the main statistical results according to main goals. Figure 9.14
shows a possible basic dashboard with the most important values comparing the
three stages. According to the three main points in the Value Chain, we can infer
some general conclusions. The population health, related to mortality, has been
improved by increasing the survival rate in a 10%. The Economic Costs has been
decreased globally in 5M€. Regarding patient experience, the waiting time of

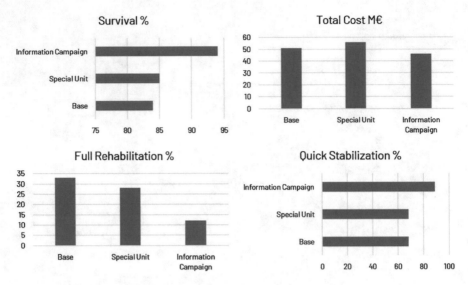

Fig. 9.14 IPI abstractions dashboard

patients, as well as the number of co-morbidities related to the rehabilitation needed, have been also decreased.

To enable a Full Crawling dashboard, the system should keep the relations between the abstractions and the associated processes to allow navigation from the Abstraction Dashboard to the IPIs and their evolution. This navigation is crucial to support health experts in understanding the reasons for the changes produced in the process over the different stages.

9.5   Conclusions

The use of IPIs to analyze the process in interactive iterations can offer a more enriched views, and more adequate to understand how the process is deployed in real scenarios. Experts can discover the processes based on the real one, and compare it with clinical pathways that are available in the literature. Also, process can be traced to provide performance indicators that can be used to measure the effects of the improvement actions over the patient value chain.

Figure 9.15 shows the flow of different kinds of IPIs. In each iteration Data from Hospital Information systems can be used to compute the base IPIs. Evolution IPIs can be used to measure qualitatively and quantitatively the impact of the process changes over time. It is also possible to provide high-level IPI abstractions that show a quick view of the process. These IPI abstractions can be used to create Process Analytic Dashboards, which can be combined with the other IPI views to offer a complete and navigable process view. These combined views are crucial to

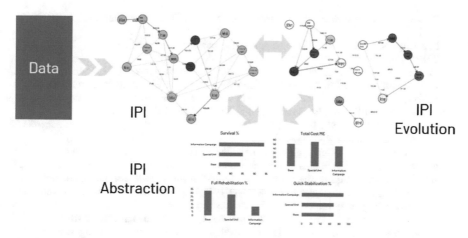

Fig. 9.15 IPI flow

show the process globally, supporting experts in taking better decisions than those based on numeric indicators.

References

1. Bandura A. Self-efficacy. The Corsini encyclopedia of psychology, 2010. p. 1–3.
2. Berwick DM, Nolan TW, Whittington J. The triple aim: care, health, and cost. Health Aff. 2008;27(3):759–69.
3. Covello VT, Merkhoher MW. Risk assessment methods: approaches for assessing health and environmental risks. Springer Science & Business Media; 2013.
4. Epstein RM, Street RL. The values and value of patient-centered care. Ann Fam Med. 2011;9(2):100–3.
5. Fernandez-Llatas C, Benedi J-M, Garcia-Gomez JM, Traver V. Process mining for individualized behavior modeling using wireless tracking in nursing homes. Sensors. 2013;13(11):15434–51.
6. Fernandez-Llatas C, Lizondo A, Monton E, Benedi J-M, Traver V. Process mining methodology for health process tracking using real-time indoor location systems. Sensors. 2015;15(12):29821–40.
7. Fernandez-Llatas C, Meneu T, Benedi JM, Traver V. Activity-based process mining for clinical pathways computer aided design. In: 32th annual international conference of the ieee engineering in medicine and biology society, vol. 2010, 2010. p. 6178–81. PMID: 21097153.
8. Fernandez-Llatas C, Meneu T, Traver V, Benedi J-M. Applying evidence-based medicine in telehealth: an interactive pattern recognition approximation. Int J Environ Res Public Health. 2013;10(11):5671–82.
9. Fernández-Llatas C, Mocholí JB, Sala P, Naranjo JC, Pileggi SF, Guillén S, Traver V. Ambient assisted living spaces validation by services and devices simulation. In: 33th annual international conference of the IEEE engineering in medicine and biology society. 2011;2011:1785–8. PMID: 22254674.
10. Fernandez-Llatas C, Rojas E, Benedí JM, Traver V. Making p-health feasible: automatic detection of personal behavioural changes through process mining analysis techniques. In:

Proceedings of the international conference on biomedical and healthInformatics (BHI2017), 2017.

11. Hamburg MA, Collins FS. The path to personalized medicine. N Engl J Med. 2010;363(4):301–4.

12. Ibanez-Sanchez G, Fernandez-Llatas C, Celda A, Mandingorra J, Aparici-Tortajada L, Martinez-Millana A, Munoz-Gama J, Sepúlveda M, Rojas E, Gálvez V, Capurro D, Traver V. Toward value-based healthcare through interactive process mining in emergency rooms: the stroke case. Int J Environ Res Public Health. 2019;16(10):1783.

13. Martin LR, Williams SL, Haskard KB, DiMatteo MR. The challenge of patient adherence. Ther Clin Risk Manag. 2005;1(3):189.

14. World Health Organization et al. Preamble to the constitution of the world health organization as adopted by the international health conference, New York, 19–22 June, 1946; signed on 22 July 1946 by the representatives of 61 states (official records of the world health organization, no. 2, p. 100) and entered into force on 7 Apr 1948. http://www.who.int/governance/eb/who_constitution_en.pdf. 1948.

15. Pagano M, Gauvreau K. Principles of biostatistics. Chapman and Hall/CRC; 2018.

16. Parmenter D. Key performance indicators: developing, implementing, and using winning KPIs. Wiley; 2015. Google-Books-ID: bKkxBwAAQBAJ.

17. Porter ME, Teisberg EO. Redefining health care: creating value-based competition on results. Harvard Business Press; 2006.

18. Rothman KJ, Greenland S, Lash TL. Modern epidemiology. Lippincott Williams & Wilkins; 2008.

19. Turner RM, Ma Q, Lorig K, Greenberg J, Andrea R. DeVries. Evaluation of a diabetes self-management program: Claims analysis on comorbid illnesses, health care utilization, and cost. J Med Internet Res. 2018;20(6):e207.

20. Verbeek HMW, Buijs JCAM, Van Dongen BF, Van Der Aalst WMP. Xes, xesame, and prom 6. In: International conference on advanced information systems engineering. Springer; 2010. p. 60–75.

Part III
Interactive Process Mining in Action

Chapter 10
Interactive Process Mining in Emergencies

Gema Ibanez-Sanchez, Maria Angeles Celda, Jesus Mandingorra, and Carlos Fernandez-Llatas

10.1 The Emergency Process

The Emergency Department(ED) is one of the most critical areas that exist in a hospital. ED is usually formed by a set of professionals that offers multidisciplinary assistance due to the high variability of patients that can be treated. This department is normally located in a specific area that follows a set of functional, structural and organizational requirements for guaranteeing the security, quality and efficiency of care to Emergency patients. The patients that are suitable to be treated by these units are those that have a sudden appearance of a health problem of diverse cause and variable severity that requires the imminent attention of a health professional.

According to the severity, we can separate the patients that are treated in emergency departments in three groups: Critical, Emergency, Urgent patients. Critical patients are those that require immediate reanimation measures and advanced life support, like, heart attack. Emergency patients are those that are in a life-threatening

G. Ibanez-Sanchez
Process Mining 4 Health Lab – SABIEN – ITACA Institute, Universitat Politècnica de València, Valencia, Spain
e-mail: geibsan@itaca.upv.es

M. A. Celda
Emergency Department at Hospital General de Valencia, Valencia, Spain

J. Mandingorra
IT Department at Hospital General de Valencia, Valencia, Spain

C. Fernandez-Llatas (✉)
Process Mining 4 Health Lab – SABIEN – ITACA Institute, Universitat Politècnica de València, Valencia, Spain

CLINTEC – Karolinska Institutet, Sweden
e-mail: cfllatas@itaca.upv.es

© Springer Nature Switzerland AG 2021
C. Fernandez-Llatas (ed.), *Interactive Process Mining in Healthcare*, Health Informatics, https://doi.org/10.1007/978-3-030-53993-1_10

situation, like upper gastrointestinal bleeding, and require a short time attendance for stabilizing the patient. Finally, urgent patients are those that are not in a life-threatening situation, but requires the correction of the situation as soon as possible, like for example acute pain patient.

Due to these differences in the process, the patient should follow a different circuit depending on the complexity of their illness. Then, one of the most critical processes occurring in the emergency process is triage. The triage is the first step in the emergency process, in which the patient severity is evaluated, classified and distributed to the most adequate circuit. There are some standards of triage [7] but, usually, the triage process has 5 levels depending on the attention priority:

- Level 1 (A.K.A. Red) that are the circuit reserved for critical patients. These patients usually skip the administrative phases of the process and receive the immediate attention of all the required ED staff, that can stop all their current activities to take care of the prioritized patient. Usually, these patients have reserved a specific care area, usually called Reanimation area or Box Zero, with the advanced equipment required for cardio-respiratory resuscitation and life support.
- Level 2 (A.K.A. Orange) Are the emergency patients. These should be treated in a short time, usually less than 10 min.
- Level 3 (A.K.A. Yellow) Are urgent patients. These should be treated in medium time, usually less than 30 min.
- Level 4 (A.K.A. Green) Are the minor urgent patients. These should be treated in a long time, usually less than 90 min.
- Level 5 (A.K.A. Blue) Are the non-urgent patients. According to some standards, these patients can wait until 120 min before being treated.

After the triage process, the patient stays in the waiting room until a physician takes care of their case. This instant is called *First Attention*. From this moment, the patient is considered officially attended by the doctor. The patient stays in the unit until the doctor considers that the problem of the patient is controlled and no more immediate actions are needed in a short time, or, due to the severity of the problem, the patient should be treated in a more specific unit. At this moment the doctors Signs a *Discharge* document, and the patient, officially, is considered out of the Emergency Department. The time elapsed from the entry of the patient in the ED and the Discharge is called Length of Stay (LoS). Depending on the situation the patient after the discharge, it can be admitted in the hospital for deeper care, sent to home, or derived to primary care or Home Hospitalization Units (HHU). If the severity of the patient is so high, producing the death of the patient, this fact is usually called *Exitus*.

Although after the Discharge the patient is considered free of urgent measures, it is possible that, in some hours, the patient can come back to the emergency department due to an increase in the complexity of their health problem. In the literature, usually, the return of patient in short-term is stated when is less than 72 h [17, 25], and in the long-term, in less than 30 days [27]. In these cases, the emergency visits are considered part of the same episode of the patient, even if the patient is admitted due to other different problem. These *Returns* are usually declared as adverse effects in the Emergency Department indicators. Also if, as a consequence of a Return, the patient is finally admitted in the hospital, this fact is called *Readmission*. The excessive Readmission rate of patients is considered an adverse effect in the emergency.

10.2   An Interactive Process Indicator for Emergency Departments

In emergencies, some Key Performance Indicators (KPI) have been used for evaluating the performance of Emergency Departments [24]. Measures like, Returns or Re-admissions in 72 h or 30 days, Length of Stay in the unit or Time of First Attention are usual indicators that are used in Emergency Departments. These numerical indicators can offer a way for measuring the process of key features objectively. However, these numeric indicators do not offer a complete view of the process of supporting experts in the evaluation of the value chain of the emergency process.

Using Process Mining technologies we can produce indicators, not only for providing a way for offering an evaluation of the Emergency Departments but also, for showing the behaviour of the process more completely and understandably, enabling doctors to better evaluate the differences among the processes.

In Fig. 10.1 we show a proposed Interactive Process Indicator (IPI) that uses the existing data in a real hospital that we have tested for a specific disease [13].

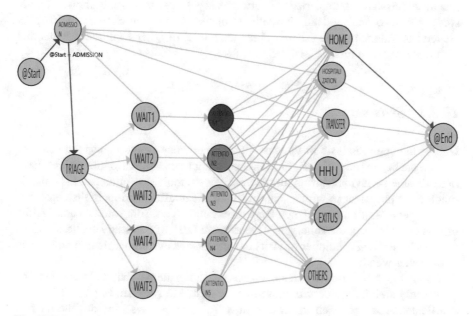

Fig. 10.1   Interactive Process Indicator in Emergencies

In this example, we have used a set of one year of data from the Emergency Department of the Hospital General in Valencia (Spain). We have identified five general stages in this IPI. *Admission* event, that is when the patient enters in the Emergency Department. This time is determined by the hour of the first registry of the episode of the patient in the Hospital Information System (HIS) at the hospital. The *Triage* corresponds to the event that occurs when the patient is classified and his/her seriousness is stated. The timing of this activity is determined for the start and the end of the triage in the computer application used by the nurse for this action. The *Wait* is the period since the triage of the patient until the first attention. This action is divided depending on the seriousness. When a doctor is free can call a patient in one of the priority queues, and the *Attention* activity starts. The action ends with the *Discharge* of the patient. In the IPI we have separated the discharge of the patient depending on the final destiny (Home, Hospitalization, Primary Care,...). If the patient returns in less time than the configured return limit (72 h or 30 days), the emergency flow is repeated. In other cases, the episode ends.

In Fig. 10.1 we have shown the nodes with a gradient of colour representing the medians of duration in each one of the stages, and the transitions with the number of patients. This set of colours represents the *footprint* of the behaviour of the Emergency Department of the hospital. This *footprint* is different depending on the behaviour of the hospital, the current status, the number and seriousness of the patients treated in the unit and all other the variables that affect the emergency process in a specific hospital.

This IPI can be compared with others to evaluate the effects of different features over the behaviour of the Emergency Department. In the next sections, some examples of how Interactive Process Mining technologies can be used for analyzing the most classical characteristics of Emergency Departments are shown. In our study, we have analyzed all the patients of the Emergency Service of Hospital General of Valencia during 2018. There are a total of 80,164 unique patients that visit emergencies a total of 218,965 times.

10.2.1 Seasons

One of the open analysis in the case of an Emergency Department is the case of the seasonality in the patients [19, 21]. According to this scenario, the patients have not the same behaviour during all the year. For example, the influenza [21], that is much more prevalent in winter than in summer, can affect seriously the capability of management of an Emergency Department unit. Also, some studies analyze the effects of weather in the Emergency Department [19]. In this study, the less serious patients have a larger number of visits to emergencies in summer than in winter due to the better weather.

Using the IPI base, we have compared the patients that have visited the Emergency area in winter with those that are treated in summer. Figure 10.2 shows a difference map between the two groups. This map shows in nodes the median

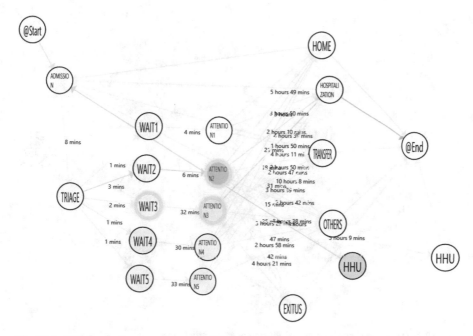

Fig. 10.2 Differences between Summer and Winter Flow

difference in the time of stay in each one of the areas. In the case of the edges, the difference represents the percentual difference in the number of patients. The redder the colour represents more ratio of patients in summer. The green colour represents winter. The nodes highlighted with a yellow ring are those that have significant differences (computing P-Value with a confidence of 95%) in the time spent in the stages. As can be seen, in general, the patients spend more time in the Emergency Department in winter. Especially, interesting is the node of attention of patients of level 2. However, in summer the number of hospitalizations increase.

10.2.2   Working Days and Weekends

The differences in the days are not only based on temperatures and environmental variables. In the literature, there are works that advice about the discrepancies in the Quality of Care in the Emergency Department in weekends [18]. Some of those works argue that the different experience of professionals that are active on weekends, or the decrease of them, or even the lack of activity of some services can delay or even change the usual care protocols that patients follow. Also, some works in the literature suggest that those differences can even increase the mortality in weekends [5, 22].

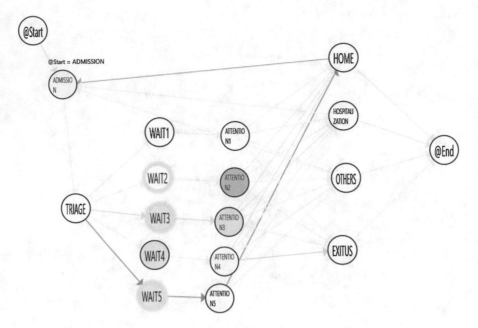

Fig. 10.3 Differences between weekends and working days

Figure 10.3 shows the differences between weekends and working days. Taking a look at the flow of patients, we realize that their normal path has changed. As it can be seen in the base IPI Fig. 10.1 the common patient is classified as Level 3, however, in weekends the percentage of level 3 patients decreases and the non-urgent patients increase. This might be because most primary care centres are closed on weekends. As has been mentioned, a measure of the quality of care is the number of returns to the hospital. As can be seen in the figure, there is an increase in the returns from home. As literature says, it seems that the Quality of Care has decreased on weekends, in this process. As it can be seen the time of waiting and attention decrease on weekends in comparison with working days. Especially interesting is the time of waiting for first attention that, in Waiting 2, 3 and 5 stages, has statistical significant differences. Also, it is important to notice that Level 1 patients, has not differences in their attention.

10.2.3 Age

One of the discriminators that traditionally have been used in the Emergency Departments is age. There are lots of studies that point out that older people have differences in the way to access the Emergency Department than young people [11, 20]. Some studies have discovered a difference in the priority achieved by

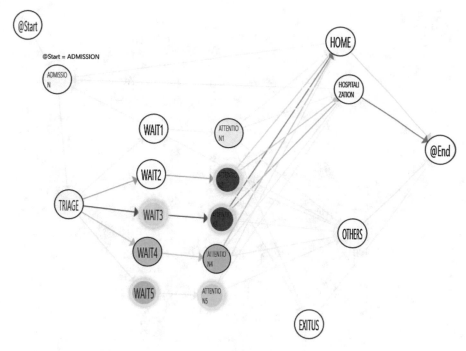

Fig. 10.4 Elderly patients(>65) compared with rest

elderly people in the emergency triage [26]. Other studies suggest that older people have a greater Length of Stay than young people, but shorter when they are admitted to the hospital [4, 16]. Also, we can found in the literature studies that indicate that elderly visit more the Emergency Department of the hospital than young people [16, 23]. However, other studies have not found any difference in age-related behaviors in Emergency Department [9]

Process Mining technologies can support us in the understanding of the behaviour of elderly people in each health department centre. Figure 10.4 shows the differences in the behaviours between the patients >65 and the rest of the patients. The red represents elderly people and green represent younger patients.

In our case, elderly patients have different geometry in the triage, but differently than other health centers [26]. In this hospital, elderly acquire a more priority in the triage phase. Also, this kind of patients, stay more time in attention than others and are more probability to be admitted in the hospital than younger people, as said in literature.

In case of the relation of age and the admission to the hospital, Fig. 10.5 shows a difference of the hospitalization influence map between elderly people and the rest. In this map, the gradients of colours at the arcs are computed using the ratio of patients that finally are hospitalized starting from this arc. As can be seen, elderly people with high priority have more probabilities to be admitted in the hospital. On the other hand, the patients with less priority (level 4) that are finally admitted in the

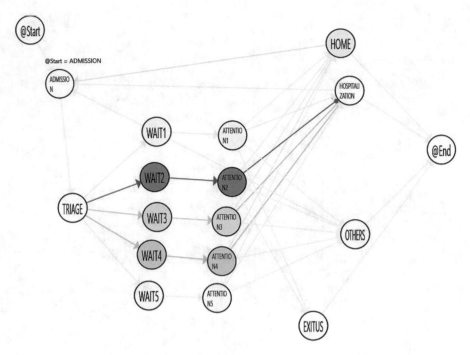

Fig. 10.5 Elderly patients(>65) Hospitalization Influence map difference with rest of patients

hospital, are more probable to be younger people. These views are more complex to acquire with other KPI that are not process-oriented.

10.2.4 Hyperfrequenters

Hyperfrequency is a well known common problem in Emergency Departments [2]. Hyperfrequenters are patients that visit the Emergency Department at a high rate. Usually, the rate that is used for considering a patient as hyperfrequenter is 10 visits per year. Usually, these patients are associated with psychological or chronic diseases, however, there is not a clear profile of these patients [2]. For that, there is a growing interest in the characterization of these patients and in the analysis of their impact over the health system [2, 3, 15].

Figure 10.6 shows the behaviour of hyperfrequenters. In our case, green colours refer to hyperfrequenters and red, for the rest. In nodes, it can be seen how the time of attention and the waiting time is fewer in hyperfrequenters than in the rest of cases. Also, in arcs, we can see that usually hyperfrequenters acquire a higher level of priority in the triage and have fewer probabilities to be hospitalized. As expected, these patients have more probability of return. Also, it's important to notice that if the patient is critical, there is no difference in the flow.

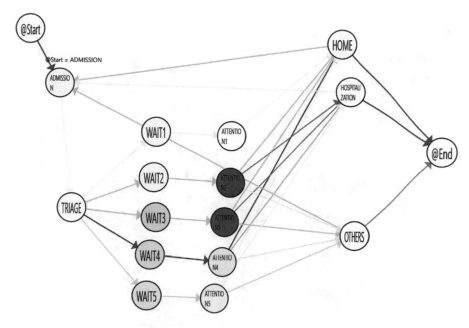

Fig. 10.6 Difference between not frequenters and hyperfrequenters

10.2.5 Returns and Readmissions

For analyzing the quality of care in an emergency we should the efficacy in the stabilization of the patient and the capability of suppression of the immediate necessity of care. One of the measures that are related to that point is the readmission. Readmissions are the patients that return to the emergency after discharge in less of a given time. Short term limits are around 72 h [17, 25] and are associated with a deficient resolution to the emergency. On the other hand, long term limits, around 30 days, are associated with the wrong management of chronic diseases like diabetes [27] or elderly people comorbidities [14].

In addition to the quality of care, those readmission visits, and even, only returns with no hospital admission, can affect the patient and health professional experience. This is because of the increase in the number of patients, imposing additional pressure in the unit that can produce delays in care.

Figure 10.7 shows the differences between the readmitted patients and those that not return in less than 72 h. As it can be seen the waiting time it's not affected by the return. The triage has a significant little increase of time (less than a minute) probably for the explanation of the previous history. However, the time of attention has big differences in non-critical episodes. Readmitted patients stay more time in attention than not returning patients.

Figure 10.8 shows the difference between *Returns* with no admission in the hospital and *Readmission*. The effect observed with no returns is even more marked.

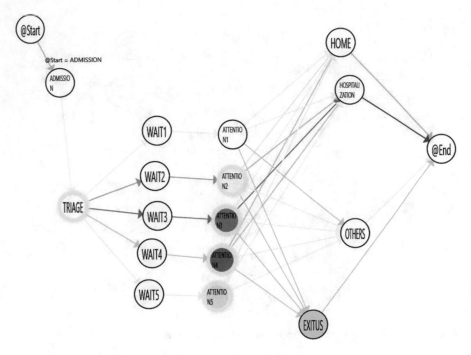

Fig. 10.7 Differences between Readmissions and No Return Flow

The returned patients wait for more time in the first attention than readmitted patients.

As patients that are finally admitted are supposed to have a greater seriousness than only returned, it seems that these patients are detected by health professionals and are quickly transferred to specific units for better care.

10.2.6 Length of Stay

The Emergency Department overcrowding is a problem that can produce critical situations in the hospital. One of the main effects that produce this circumstance is the increase in the length of stay of patients in the area. This is associated in the literature with patient experience [6] and with the care efficiency [28].

Some reasons make this time grows. The increasing of hospital occupancy can delay the admission of patients in the hospital. As a consequence of that, patients should stay in the Emergency area waiting for a bed, not only occupying space, but also consuming precious resources from emergencies like nurses, auxiliary personnel, or specific medical devices. This produces saturation in emergencies increasing the Length of Stay(LoS) [8].

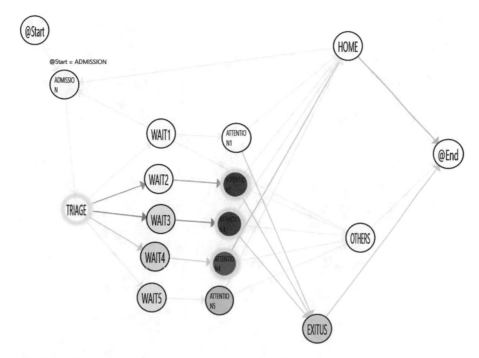

Fig. 10.8 Differences between Return and Readmission Flow

But the hospital occupancy is not the only variable that can affect the Length of Stay. The triage level, the test realized to the patients, and the efficiency in the care [28] or the delay in providing analgesic medication [12] are aspects that can affect to the Length of Stay.

Figure 10.9 shows the flow that indicates the differences between the patients that stay in the unit less than 4 h (green) compared with those that stay more than 4 h (red). As it is expected, the Length of Stay is directly related to the time of attention, that is the most durable activity in the unit. But also we can see that affects the time of waiting. It is important to notice that in critical and very urgent patients the time of waiting not to affect the patients. According to the arcs, as the literature says, there is a relationship and the triage with the LoS variable. There is a higher percentage of high LoS patients in higher priority triage levels, and, on the contrary, there is a higher percentage of low LoS patients in lower priority triage levels. Also, there is a higher relation on patients with lower LoS in returns and hospitalizations.

10.2.7   Exitus

One of the worst adverse effects that can occur in emergencies is mortality. In medical jargon, the death of a patient is usually named *Exitus*. The Exitus in

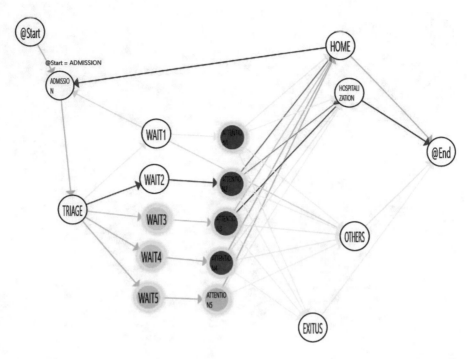

Fig. 10.9 Length of Stay (LoS) comparing >4h with <4h

an Emergency Department is infrequent [10]. This can be because highly critical patients are usually quickly derived to the Intensive Care Unit or Surgery areas. In Emergency Rooms, the Exitus is usually associated with the complexity of the disease of the patient at the admission to emergencies [1].

Figure 10.10 shows an influence map of the processes in the Exitus. The colour nodes in the influence map refer to the number of Exitus that have previously performed this stage. The higher number of patients has finally deceased after the activity, the redder is the colour in the node. As can be seen, the mortality is representative of critical and urgent people, as expected according to literature.

10.3   Discussion and Conclusion

The application of Interactive Process Mining methodologies and technologies can offer a new perspective for analyzing the aspects that should be taken into account to understand the behaviour of the processes in an Emergency Department.

In this study, we have analyzed different Key Performance Indicators that are being usually used in Emergency Department. From that starting, we have offered a new view, using Interactive Process Indicators, that not only offers the required

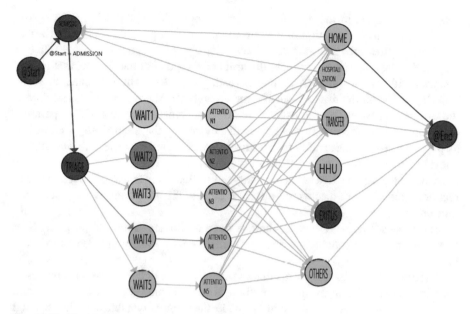

Fig. 10.10   Total Influence over Exitus

numerical view but also offers a process-oriented view that supposes a quick and understandable way for discovering the root causes behind of these indicators.

The Interactive Process Indicator has been created using minimum information that can be easily collected in a wide percentage from all digitally transformed Emergency Departments around the world. In our experience, it is possible that the quality of the data was not always optimum, but most of the times, the data that we have used in this study is usually available in most of Emergency Departments around the world. This supposes a better probability of acquiring quality data for the creation of these IPIs. Of course, complex situations like critical patients (Level 1) can have quality problems due to the fact that the priority is to take care of the patient above the administrative actions, and for example, the administrative admission of the patient can occur after the care. In any case, these cases are few and can be corrected assuming the adequate way of the emergency protocols. Also, some hospitals have not information to the time of triage, in these cases, the triage can be assumed as a fixed time. IPIs information also should be complemented with classical numerical stats, but, in this chapter, we are focused on the analysis of the information that Interactive Process Mining can provide to medical doctors. This statistical information is easy to achieve and is out of the scope of this work.

In our studies, we have verified that the number of patients and the time spent in each one of the stages depend directly not only in the capabilities of the hospital but also on the kind of the target population, demographics, weather.... This adds a high variability in the analysis of emergencies that difficult the comparison of the practices that are applied in each hospital. The application of a protocol can work properly in a specific moment for a specific population but fail in another case. In this way, in the application of new protocols and best practices, it is necessary to continuously measure their effects in their value chain focused on the patient. In that way, it is more effective to compare the unit before and after the change, that tries to compare different hospitals. Another interesting view is to split the behaviour of the unit depending on the disease-causing the emergency. There is a high variability of the different diseases that are usually treated in an emergency unit. This separation can increase the precision in the effects discovered by the methodology. However, as this information has usually difficulties to be recovered because is in free text or, has a low quality, we have left it out of the study.

Among the aspects that we have analyzed in this chapter using Process Mining technologies, we have discovered different facts in the behaviour of the emergency unit process.

In critical scenarios (Level 1), there is not a difference in the care of patients. It supposes that critic patients are always treated in high priority independently from environmental issues.

According to weather, it seems that in this case, although there are differences in the same way as seen in the literature, there is not too much gap between winter and summer. In Valencia, where the study is made, the weather is stable over the year and there are not the same high differences in temperature than other parts in the world. This is a possible cause of having not a big gap in seasons. This shows the variability in the evidence depending on the different hospitals. The age and other demographic variables have different effects in distinct hospitals. Hyperfrequenters are outlier patients and its behaviour is very interesting for medical staff. The reduction of noise has a direct impact on these patients. For that is very important to not denoise data log in order to keep the integrity of this information in the Emergency Department problems. We have also analyzed how influence maps can show the effects of the different circuits in the process.

These discoveries can suggest new questions to health professionals that should be validated with studies. The application of this methodology in an iterative way, allow the confirmation of the first of medical intuitions that allows a more efficient and effective way to improve the medical process.

References

1. Alimohammadi H, Bidarizerehpoosh F, Mirmohammadi F, Shahrami A, Heidari K, Sabzghabaie A, Keikha S. Cause of emergency department mortality; a case-control study. Emergency. 2014;2(1):30.
2. Alonso CF, Pareja RR, Mulet JMA, Martín-Sánchez FJ. Hyperfrequent users of Spanish hospital emergency departments. Eur J Emerg Med. 2016;23(3):236–7.
3. Alpern ER, Clark AE, Alessandrini EA, Gorelick MH, Kittick M, Stanley RM, Dean JM, Teach SJ, Chamberlain JM, Pediatric Emergency Care Applied Research Network (PECARN). Recurrent and high-frequency use of the emergency department by pediatric patients. Acad Emerg Med. 2014;21(4):365–73.

4. Baum SA, Rubenstein LZ. Old people in the emergency room: age-related differences in emergency department use and care. J Am Geriatr Soc. 1987;35(5):398–404.
5. Bhonagiri D, Pilcher DV, Bailey MJ. Increased mortality associated with after-hours and weekend admission to the intensive care unit: a retrospective analysis. Med J Aust. 2011;194(6):287–92.
6. Chang AM, Lin A, Fu R, McConnell KJ, Sun B. Associations of emergency department length of stay with publicly reported quality-of-care measures. Acad Emerg Med. 2017;24(2):246–50.
7. Farrohknia N, Castrén M, Ehrenberg A, Lind L, Oredsson S, Jonsson H, Asplund K, Göransson KE. Emergency department triage scales and their components: a systematic review of the scientific evidence. Scand J Trauma Resusc Emerg Med. 2011;19(1):42.
8. Forster AJ, Stiell I, Wells G, Lee AJ, Van Walraven C. The effect of hospital occupancy on emergency department length of stay and patient disposition. Acad Emerg Med. 2003;10(2):127–33.
9. Caro Fuchs, Bilge Celik, Steffie HA Brouns, Uzay Kaymak, and Harm R Haak. No age thresholds in the emergency department: a retrospective cohort study on age differences. PloS One 2019;14(1). https://www.ncbi.nlm.nih.gov/pmc/articles/PMC6353140/pdf/pone.0210743. pdf
10. Heymann EP, Wicky A, Carron P-N, Exadaktylos AK. Death in the emergency department: a retrospective analysis of mortality in a Swiss university hospital. Emer Med Int. 2019;2019. https://www.ncbi.nlm.nih.gov/pmc/articles/PMC6745091/pdf/EMI2019-5263521.pdf
11. Hughes JM, Freiermuth CE, Shepherd-Banigan M, Ragsdale L, Eucker SA, Goldstein K, Hastings SN, Rodriguez RL, Fulton J, Ramos K, et al. Emergency department interventions for older adults: a systematic review. J Am Geriatr Soc. 2019;67(7):1516–25.
12. Hughes JA, Brown NJ, Chiu J, Allwood B, Chu K. The relationship between time to analgesic administration and emergency department length of stay: a retrospective review. J Adv Nurs. 2020;76(1):183–90.
13. Ibanez-Sanchez G, Fernandez-Llatas C, Celda A, Mandingorra J, Aparici-Tortajada L, Martinez-Millana A, Munoz-Gama J, Sepúlveda M, Rojas E, Gálvez V, Capurro D, Traver V. Toward value-based healthcare through interactive process mining in emergency rooms: the stroke case. Int J Environ Res Public Health. 2019;16(10).
14. Koehler BE, Richter KM, Youngblood L, Cohen BA, Prengler ID, Cheng D, Masica AL. Reduction of 30-day postdischarge hospital readmission or emergency department (ed) visit rates in high-risk elderly medical patients through delivery of a targeted care bundle. J Hosp Med. 2009;4(4):211–18.
15. LaCalle EJ, Rabin EJ, Genes NG. High-frequency users of emergency department care. J Emerg Med. 2013;44(6):1167–73.
16. Latham LP, Ackroyd-Stolarz S. Emergency department utilization by older adults: a descriptive study. Can Geriatrics J. 2014;17(4):118.
17. Lee EK, Yuan F, Hirsh DA, Mallory MD, Simon HK. A clinical decision tool for predicting patient care characteristics: patients returning within 72 hours in the emergency department. In: AMIA Annual Symposium Proceedings, vol. 2012. American Medical Informatics Association; 2012. p. 495
18. Miró Ò, Sánchez M, Espinosa G, Millá J. Quality and effectiveness of an emergency department during weekends. Emer Med J. 2004;21(5):573–74.
19. Otsuki H, Murakami Y, Fujino K, Matsumura K, Eguchi Y. Analysis of seasonal differences in emergency department attendance in shiga prefecture, Japan between 2007 and 2010. Acute Med Surg. 2015;3(2):74–80.
20. Samaras N, Chevalley T, Samaras D, Gold G. Older patients in the emergency department: a review. Ann Emer Med. 2010;56(3):261–69.
21. Schull MJ, Mamdani MM, Fang J. Community influenza outbreaks and emergency department ambulance diversion. Ann Emer Med. 2004;44(1):61–7.
22. Sharp AL, Choi HJ, Hayward RA. Don't get sick on the weekend: an evaluation of the weekend effect on mortality for patients visiting US EDs. Am J Emer Med. 2013;31(5):835–7.

23. Strange GR, Chen EH, Sanders AB. Use of emergency departments by elderly patients: projections from a multicenter data base. Ann Emer Med. 1992;21(7):819–24.
24. Vanbrabant L, Braekers K, Ramaekers K, Van Nieuwenhuyse I. Simulation of emergency department operations: a comprehensive review of kpis and operational improvements. Comput Ind Eng. 2019;131:356–381.
25. Verelst S, Pierloot S, Desruelles D, Gillet J-B, Bergs J. Short-term unscheduled return visits of adult patients to the emergency department. J Emer Med. 2014;47(2):131–9.
26. Vilpert S, Monod S, Ruedin HJ, Maurer J, Trueb L, Yersin B, Büla C. Differences in triage category, priority level and hospitalization rate between young-old and old-old patients visiting the emergency department. BMC Health Serv Res. 2018;18(1):456.
27. Wei NJ, Wexler DJ, Nathan DM, Grant RW. Intensification of diabetes medication and risk for 30-day readmission. Diabet Med. 2013;30(2):e56–62.
28. Yoon P, Steiner I, Reinhardt G. Analysis of factors influencing length of stay in the emergency department. Can J Emer Med. 2003;5(3):155–61.

Chapter 11
Interactive Process Mining in Surgery with Real Time Location Systems: Interactive Trace Correction

Carlos Fernandez-Llatas, Jose Miguel Benedi, Jorge Munoz Gama, Marcos Sepulveda, Eric Rojas, Salvador Vera, and Vicente Traver

11.1 Introduction

The collection of adequate data is key not only for creating Interactive Process Indicators (IPIs) but also for analyzing and evaluating the evolution of the process for its posterior optimization. The quality of data gathered is crucial to have precise models. With the arrival of new mobile personal technologies, Internet of Things Paradigm and wearable sensors, the quantity of data available for monitoring the people's behaviour is dramatically growing [8]. Within this idea, a new generation of hospital room sensors, lab equipment, employee wearable and patient monitoring, among others, are generating Intelligent Environments spaces [30]. In these spaces,

C. Fernandez-Llatas (✉)
Process Mining 4 Health Lab – SABIEN – ITACA Institute, Universitat Politècnica de València, Valencia, Spain

CLINTEC – Karolinska Institutet, Sweden
e-mail: cfllatas@itaca.upv.es

J. M. Benedi
PRLHT, Universitat Politècnica de València, Valencia, Spain
e-mail: jbenedi@dsic.upv.es

J. Munoz-Gama · M. Sepulveda · E. Rojas
School of Engineering – Pontificia Universidad Católica de Chile, Santiago, Chile
e-mail: jmun@uc.cl; marcos@ing.puc.cl

S. Vera
MySphera, Valencia, Spain
e-mail: svera@mysphera.com

V. Traver
Process Mining 4 Health Lab – SABIEN – ITACA Institute, Universitat Politècnica de València, Valencia, Spain
e-mail: vtraver@itaca.upv.es

© Springer Nature Switzerland AG 2021
C. Fernandez-Llatas (ed.), *Interactive Process Mining in Healthcare*, Health Informatics, https://doi.org/10.1007/978-3-030-53993-1_11

the amount of data available for analysis, in terms of patient records, population health data and other databases, has massively increased, bringing a new complexity level. Moreover, it provides a new opportunity for creating new models to use more advanced analytic, visualizations and decision support tools, to improve accuracy in the diagnostics, allowing more effective and precise treatments [16]. Consequently, new algorithms and methods are appearing to analyze human vision [6], and human activity [4], among others. Below this umbrella, Real-Time Location Systems (RTLS) have been appeared to take advantage of tracking, navigation and positioning on indoor locations, to follow the behaviour of the business processes.

There are large quantity of RTLS solutions in the literature [9, 17, 18]. Some systems use the localization to support the activity recognition of human in smart homes [1]; systems that monitor the daily activity of elderly in Ambient Assisted Living (AAL) environments [27]; systems that create a movement behaviour model of users in smart places [13]; or systems that use location to support analysis and optimization of the organization processes, for example, for measuring unobtrusively the time of treatment on hospitals for better management and improvement of Quality of Service [3, 21, 25], or for tracking the surgery process inside a hospital [10].

In this context, Pattern Recognition and Machine Learning techniques can use this amount of data for automatically creating process models. Process Mining [29] is can discover models from RTLS logs that provide human-understandable models. Process Mining technologies [29] can support individual behaviour analysis not only for detecting behavioural changes, but also to offer a human-understandable view of the real changes of a user [13]. Maps of models extracted from RTLS can be used to build IPIs that shows the behaviour processes of patients in a precise way in an objective an unobtrusive way.

However, the deployment of RTLS is still under research [9, 17]. There are several problems to be addressed when an RTLS is deployed in a real scenario. Noisy environments and building structures can interfere with RTLS signals and can affect their accuracy. In this way, it is critical to perform a precise deployment of the RTLS to optimize the system and to avoid undesirable interference [18]. However, mobile elements of indoor spaces, like furniture and, even humans, as well as environmental factors, like humidity and temperature, can unpredictably affect the signal propagation due to reflection, refraction, diffraction and absorption [7]. This noise produces an undesirable effect on Process Mining algorithms called *Spaghetti Effect* [11]. This effect dramatically decreases the human understandability of Workflows produced by the Process Mining discovery algorithms.

This RTLS noise can be assessed by human experts that can correct the models obtained by the system, in an iterative and interactive way [12]. Error models can be built by professionals that can support automatic system in the better correction of results to provide clean systems that make fully understandable the models inferred. In this work, we present an Interactive Error-Correcting based method (EC) [2] using an Edit Distance framework, to correct the data and obtain an insight of the executed process. Error Correcting techniques have been successfully used to calculate distances between processes and RTLS traces [13], in previous studies involving process analysis. This method was tested in a hospital of Spain (who wants to remain anonymous) using the existing RTLS infrastructure deployed in that environment with 3915 patients collected between March 2012 and May 2013.

11.2 Background

In literature, there are several techniques thought to get the position of a mobile point in an area. Radio Frequency Identification (RFID) systems for Indoor Location are growing exponentially [7, 9, 15]. Due to the increase in the presence of WiFi networks in cities, WiFi triangulation [7] is a solution used for positioning. WiFi triangulation not only is used for indoor positioning problems, but most of the current mobile phones also use WiFi networks to enrich GPS signal to get more accuracy. However, one of the more important problems of WiFi-based systems that can suppose a barrier for its adequation to the problem is the batteries duration. WiFi signal requires a relatively high quantity of energy to perform communication among nodes. This made that objects to be located should recharge its batteries more regularly than other lower energy RFID protocols, and this is not desirable in some scenarios, where the recharge of batteries can affect the proper process itself. Other RFID protocols, like ZigBee or Bluetooth 4.0, can increase the time of life of the nodes without a battery recharge. In fact, with some configurations, these technologies can create nodes with an autonomy of years [13].

RTLS are valuable systems than can increase data gathered from hospitals, to automatically build models using Process Mining techniques [19]. Process Mining is a research field that focuses on extracting information from data generated and stored in the databases of the information systems; in this specific case, the Hospital Information Systems (HIS). These data are extracted to build events logs, to view all set of traces executed, each containing all the activities executed for a process instance [28, 29]. Events logs correspond to a series of traces of each executed case in the past for the studied process. The event log must contain the minimum required data (case id, timestamp and activity name [29]), to allow the application of the available methods, techniques and algorithms of Process Mining.

In the past, previous studies have used process mining in Healthcare with sensors and RTLS, obtaining significant insights about the executed processes [29]. Studies showed, through the use of Process Mining techniques, activities followed in a surgery process [10] and the personal process followed through the personalized healthcare sensor data [26]. Both studies demonstrate process mining ability to understand executed activities, but also that this directly depends on data quality, from the systems, in this case, sensors and RTLS.

However, the main problem of RTLS is the accuracy [9, 15]. The unpredictable reflections, refractions or absorptions of signals due to the heterogeneity of walls and furniture of rooms, environmental factors or, even, the position of human stakeholders, act as a signal attenuator that, depending on their position, can cause a large number of localization errors. This noise produced by RTLS produces an important spaghetti effect in the Discovery. This makes more difficult to understand the process and become complex even to visualize.

Those errors are very difficult to detect and evaluate. The most efficient way to deploy an RTLS is to integrate it into the infrastructure as an additional layer to the building construction. However, this is not always possible, and the beacons usually are not in the most efficient position to avoid signal problems. Also, the intended use of the room affects dynamically to the quality of the signals. There are not the same signal reflections when the room is void than when it is at full capacity. For that, it is necessary a continuous redesign of the RTLS network to ensure a correct accuracy [17]. One of the most common techniques performs this evaluation comparing the position of the object (got through the RTLS) with a manually collected log of the objects. However, the use of this invasive evaluation methodologies can affect the process that might produce unpredictable measurement errors, especially if the locating objects are humans that are affected by the presence of other humans that are auditing his movements [17]. For that, the use of non-invasive evaluation methods can suppose a great advantage to provide a more accurate log of the system.

In this chapter, we propose an unobtrusive correction of traces By using Error Correcting techniques Error Correcting (EC) [2] for reducing the Spaghetti effect in Process Mining. EC is based on the definition of edition primitives (Insertions, Deletions, etc.) for correcting syntactic patterns. EC algorithms are intended to discover the most probable sequence of edition primitives that should be applied to each trace to make it compatible with the ideal model. Using this method, the RTLS accuracy can be improved, resulting in better models to study and analyze through Process Mining techniques and tools. These clean models can be used as IPIs in the better understanding of medical processes.

11.3 Trace Correction

Formally, the aim of this paper is to provide an algorithm is to correct Traces $\mathcal{T}$ in the RTLS log according the model defined by the expert $\mathcal{M}$:

Definition 1 A Trace $\mathcal{T}$ is defined as a set of tuples $\mathcal{T} = (x_1, t_1) \ldots (x_n, t_n)$; Where x_i is the position and t_i the time spent

Definition 2 Given a Finite State Model $\mathcal{M}$ and Trace $\mathcal{T}$; a sequence $T_i, T_j \in \mathcal{T}$ is compatible ($\approx$) with a transition $(i \rightarrow j) \in \mathcal{M}$ if $\exists q_i \rightarrow q_j \wedge q_j = x_j$

In Pattern Recognition field, Error Correcting technique usually is based on the definition of an edit distance. Edit distance [14] defines a set of operations (Insertions, Deletions,...) that can be applied to a noisy input to correct it according to a goodness model. Formally:

Definition 3 Given a Finite State Model $\mathcal{M}$ and a Trace $\mathcal{T}$; an Edition Operation O is a function $O(i) = (i', c)$ Where $i \in \mathcal{T}$, i' is the corrected event and c is the cost associated to apply the function

Definition 4 O is the set of possible Edition Operations O

According to that, Edit Distance provides a dissimilarity measure between a given model M and an input trace T by calculating the set of operations ($\in O$) with the lower cost according to an error model. Formally:

Definition 5 The Edit Distance of the input trace T to a given model M, based on an operation set $f = \{o_1, .., o_n\} \in O \mid f(T) \approx M$ is:

$$ED_O(T, M) = ED_{\hat{f}}(T, M) = \min_{T \in O} ED(f, M)$$

$$\hat{f} = arg \min_{f \in O} ED_f(T, M)$$

where f is an error function for correcting the input T according the model M; and $\hat{f}$ is the optimal error function.

Error Correcting has been applied to several research fields; it have been used for manuscript text recognition [20]; Image and video Indexing [24] or DNA Analysis [5] among others.

For correcting an input Trace T using EC techniques it is needed a Model M that represent all the possible valid sequences. In our problem, RTLS provides the sequence of rooms in the user's trace (See Table 11.1). So, the most direct Model that can be used is the building's map. The building's map can be defined formally as a Finite State Automaton (FSA), where the nodes are the possible rooms that can be reached by the user, and the edges are the possible transitions among the different rooms. An example is shown in Fig. 11.1. In that case, only adjacent rooms have arcs between them. So according to that, a valid sequence of rooms is the one that is accepted by the automaton. For example, according to the figure, the sequence $Start \rightarrow Transfer \rightarrow OR1 \rightarrow Transfer \rightarrow End$ is accepted by the automaton, but the sequence $Start \rightarrow OR1 \rightarrow Transfer \rightarrow End$ is not valid, because $OR1$ node is not reachable from $Start$.

Also, a set of defined operations should be defined that could be used for correcting the sequence according to the automaton. According to the literature [14] we can select a minimum set of basic operations like Insertions, that suppose the addition of a Room in the sequence at a determined position; Deletions, that suppose the deletion of a Room in the trace; or Substitutions, that suppose the substitution of a Room to other in the sequence at a determined position, among others.

In the example, a possible valid correction sequence for $Start \rightarrow OR1 \rightarrow Transfer \rightarrow End$ is the addition of a $Transfer$ Node after $Start$. This solution is not unique, other solutions can be the deletion of $OR1$ Node or the addition of $WakeUp$ and $Transfer$ after $Start$.

According to that, an Error-Correcting algorithm for denoising of RTLS traces should find the optimal set of edition operations $\hat{f}$ that transforms the input trace T to one accepted by the language defined by the Model M. That means the calculation of the dissimilarity between the trace and the automaton. However, calculate the dissimilarity with an automaton is a complex problem [31]. As our problem can be shown as a simplification of Graph Edit Distance problem [14]. Due to the different set of valid sequences, that could be infinite, there is not possible to apply dynamic programming like in string comparisons [22]. In the literature, a similar problem has been approximated using A^* search algorithms [23] for calculating sub-optimal Edit Distance between two graphs. In our case, we propose a windowed correction between $-\mu_1$ to μ_2. When the trace fails, instead to perform a Breadth-first search, we limit the correction search to μ_1 positions before and μ_2 positions after. In that case, the expert will decide the quality of the correction. If the window is 0 the behaviour will be similar to a basic greedy algorithm and if the Window is $-\infty$ to ∞ the behaviour will be equivalent to a Full Breadth-first search. This is formally described in Algorithm 1.

Algorithm 1 Correct Trace Algorithm

1: **function** CORRECT TRACE($\mathcal{T}$, M, O Analysis Window (μ_1, μ_2))
2:     INITIALIZATION:
3:         $i = 0$; Last Event
4:         $j = 1$; Current Event
5:         S_0; Cost of Correcting Trace (Score)
6:         $\Delta = \emptyset$; Corrected Trace
7:     STEP1:
8:     **if then**$\exists (i \rightarrow j) \approx M$
9:         $S_j = S_i + C_0 + t_{i,j}$
10:        $\Delta = \Delta \vee \{(x_j, t_j, C_0)\}$
11:    **else**
12:        $O(i - \mu_1, i + \mu_1) = \forall O(l) \in O; l | [i - \mu_1, i + \mu_1]$
13:        $\beta = \{(x_l, t_l, c_l), \ldots, (x_m, t_m, c_m)\}$ where
14:            $arg\min_{f \in O(i-\mu_1, i+\mu_2)} \sum_{n=l}^{m} C(o_n) | \forall \beta \approx M$
15:        **if then**$\beta \leq i$
16:            $\Delta = \Delta - \{\beta, \ldots, i\}$
17:        **end if**
18:        $\Delta = \Delta + \beta$
19:        $S_j = S_i + C_\beta + t_\beta$
20:        goto STEP1
21:    **end if**
22: **end function**

Intuitively, for each event in the trace, the algorithm is evaluated. If $(i \rightarrow j)$ is according to the model, the event is not corrected and the Score is updated with the cost of no correction and a time adjustment cost. This time adjustment is dependent on the time spent in the activities. If $(i \rightarrow j)$ is not compatible the algorithm start a windowed search over all the possible correction operations between $i - \mu_1, i + \mu_2$ ($O(i - \mu_1, i + \mu_1)$) in order to find the minimum cost sequence that makes the transition compatible (β). After that, the resulting trace is corrected Δ and the Score is updated with the cost of the operation and the time adjustment. In our example, a short time position has not the same probability to be a reflection error than a long time position. For that, time adjustment should be different.

These traces are formatted as an ordered list of locations with their timestamp and duration, that are referred to the position of a user in a specific area at a determined moment. An example of raw observation stream is shown in Table 11.1.

Table 11.1 Sample of an RTLS log

Id	Start	End	Location
...			
57232	22/08/2013 9:37	22/08/2013 9:43	Transfer
57232	22/08/2013 9:43	22/08/2013 9:52	Operating Room 2
57232	22/08/2013 9:52	22/08/2013 10:47	Wake Up
56458	22/08/2013 9:57	22/08/2013 10:01	Transfer
56458	22/08/2013 10:01	22/08/2013 11:15	Operating Room 2
55859	22/08/2013 10:05	22/08/2013 10:06	Transfer
55859	22/08/2013 10:06	22/08/2013 11:02	Wake Up
57418	22/08/2013 10:48	22/08/2013 11:29	Wake Up
56164	22/08/2013 10:57	22/08/2013 11:00	Transfer
55859	22/08/2013 11:02	22/08/2013 11:04	Transfer
55859	22/08/2013 11:04	22/08/2013 13:02	Operating Room 5
56164	22/08/2013 11:13	22/08/2013 12:29	Operating Room 1
56458	22/08/2013 11:15	22/08/2013 11:15	Transfer
56458	22/08/2013 11:15	22/08/2013 11:53	Wake Up
...			

The result of the algorithm is the most probable ordered set of correctional operations that modify the input trace for producing the trace compatible with the structural model with the minimum total cost, that is the sum of all the correctional operations costs. The result might not be optimal if the window selected is not $(-\infty, +\infty)$.

11.4   Experiments

In this section, an evaluation of the method described in the previous section is presented. This evaluation was performed in a real scenario using prospective RTLS data of the Surgery Department of a Hospital in Spain. The corpus was collected real patients who have surgery programmed between mars of 2012 and may of 2013. All the patients wear a Zigbee bracelet that interconnects with a set of beacons that are installed in each one of the rooms of the Surgery area of the hospital. The RTLS collect all positions of patients during their intervention process in a corpus. In total, 3915 patients were studied for collecting the log that is formed by 22.315 location changes. For the experiments, we use PALIA Algorithm as Process Mining Discovery because it has a specific RTLS module [10].

In Table 11.1 a piece of the complete Log is presented. The corpus is stored in *csv* format and has five main fields that are used by the algorithm. *Id* represents the anonymized identification of the patient. *Start* is the moment when the patient enters in the specified area. *End* is the moment when the patient leaves the room.

Finally, *Location* represents the identification of the Surgery area where the patient is located at the specified period.

11.4.1   Interactive Pattern Recognition for Improving the Application of Error-Correcting Techniques to RTLS

The errors in the RTLS can suppose mistakes that add a layer of noise-making more difficult the understanding of processes after a discovery. The errors can be produced by inefficiencies in the placement of the RTLS beacons, lack of granularity in RTLS in short time stay areas, or proximity of the patients to the walls that produce confusions in the beacons detections, among others. These errors are usually repeated because the topology of the beacons has a direct effect on the quality of detection. Although these errors can be high in numbers, the time of errors usually is very short. That means that these errors have a low effect in the length of stay in areas, but a high effect in the number and kind of transitions. This has a big impact in techniques like process mining where the topology of the models discovered acquire more *spaghetti*. The correction of these common errors supported by the interaction with professionals can reduce the errors providing a cleaner view of the model that makes the model more usable.

For correcting the log, the expert should define a goodness model that could be used to correct the model according to the knowledge of the experts. On one hand, we need to define a Graph Model that define the restrictions of the process, and an Error Model, that describes the available edition operations and their cost. In the next subsections, the Graph Model and Error Model used for the experiments are described:

11.4.2   Physical Model as Graph Model

The easiest graph model that can be used for correcting an RTLS is the room's physical model. This model shows the distribution of the rooms of the RTLS deployed area. The Physical model is very easy to create. It is based on the physical map of the building and defines the transitions restrictions among physical rooms.

Figure 11.1 presents a graphic Physical model represented as a TPA. This model represents the possible transitions among the rooms. In that figure, circles represent the possible locations of patients, that are rooms or areas of the surgery department, and arrows represent the possible transitions that are possible to perform due to the disposition of the building. *Start* and *End* represents the starting and ending of a valid track. In that figure, you can see three kinds of areas. The *Wake Up* Area, the *Transfer* Area and the *Operating Rooms*. The *Operating Rooms* are the locations where the surgery take place. *Transfer* is the area of interchange among

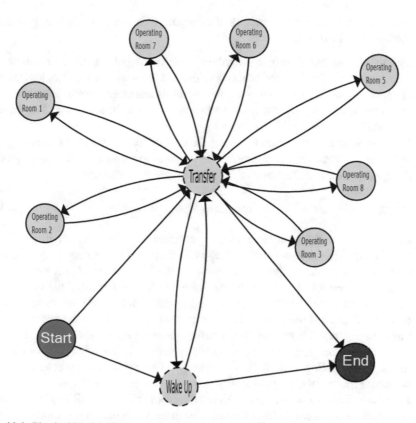

Fig. 11.1 Physical Model of the experiment expressed as a TPA

all the rooms*Wake Up* is the area where the patients can be placed before or after the surgery. However, if patients are admitted in the hospital they can avoid the stay in this room. For that, although is usual that patients spend some time in the *Wake Up* area, the tracking of the patients can start and finish directly on the *Transfer* area.

11.4.3 Interactive Error Model

The Error Model describes the possible adjustments that are compatible with the problem to solve. As the Graph model, the human expert can define the error model identifying all the available edition primitives that are desirable for the problem, as well as their cost, that can be used by the EC Algorithm for correct the input samples. For this experiment, we have defined three edition primitives that represent the three possible different kinds of corrections. The cost functions of each operation were defined using heuristics described in conjunction with process experts and depends on the semantic meaning of the locations on the process. The primitives defined are the following:

- **Delete**: This edition primitive is applied for correcting errors that are produced by signal reflections that insert locations in the RTLS sample that are not logical. For example, a user is in a room and a few seconds after that goes to the immediate upper room and then returns to the same room. This situation is a clear case of the localization error.

  The cost function is defined by using the cost of localization for correcting that situation, the algorithm can remove the illogical location from the sample using the *Delete* primitive. The cost of deleting a location is defined as:

$$D_{Location} = K + T^2 \tag{11.1}$$

  where T is the duration time of the permanence of the patient in a specific location, expressed in minutes and K is a constant that we have fixed to 10 for this experiment. According to the equation, the less duration has a location, the easier is to remove it and, on the contrary, the higher duration, the higher cost has. The rationale of this rule is that the longer duration of a location detected by a RTLS system the less probable is that this location is due to an error. For this experiment, This rule has been defined with an exception. If the location is unknown by the grammar, that it means is not in the list of possible locations, the cost of deleting is 0. This is because, if a location is not reachable by the structural model its error probability is the maximum.

- **Insertion**: This edition primitive solves the problems due to failures in a location that skips some areas in the samples. For example, when in a sample, the user has passed immediately from one area to another and, according to the structural model, these areas are not connected, the transition between this areas is a localization error. This error can be produced by reflections, signal inhibitions, beacons failure, etc. This primitive inserts a possible specific location in the middle of the illogical transition as a step of the search EC algorithm. The cost of deleting a location is a constant J, except if the location is an Operating Room that the constant is fixed to $10^4 J$. J is fixed to 100 for this experiment. The rationale of this exception is that the addition of an Operating Room has an important semantic charge. That means that this operation can easily change the meaning of the trace, producing more errors than corrections. For that, this operation should be avoided if possible. An important thing to take into account is that the locations added in a position of the trace are selected from the set of possible locations that are reachable from the previous node according to the Graph Model. This limits the number of operations available for the next iteration of the algorithm, making it more efficient in processing time and memory use.

- **Fusion**.The Fusion edition primitive fuse two consecutive locations that are referred to the same room. The cost associated with this operation is 0. The rationale of this is that, in RTLS, a continuous sequence of intervals of the same location is, usually, equivalent to a unique location which interval is the union of all of those intervals. RTLS systems do not provide consecutive locations. However, the inclusion of this edition primitive is important because in the middle of the process of search of the EC algorithm these situations are possible. In any case, the application of this edition primitive is not due to an error of the RTLS.

11.4.4 Results of the Algorithm Using the Physical Model

Figure 11.2 presents some real examples of corrected samples using the physical model. Figure 11.2a presents a simple insertion operation between Operating Room 5 and Wake Up locations. According to the structural model, is not possible a transition between these rooms, and the algorithm found that the most efficient change is to add a *Transfer* Location. This mistake can be produced for a quick transition between the *Operating Room 5* and *Wake Up* Areas. Figure 11.2b shows a more complex case, there is a not valid sequence formed by three Operating Rooms; that is corrected by removing the location with the lower time of stay and fusing the other two, referred to the same location. This mistake of the RTLS system probably was produced by reflections in Operating room 3 in the middle of the surgery process. Figure 11.2c sample presents a surgery in two Operating Rooms. The EC algorithm corrects the error removing the less probable location and adding the *Transfer* Area.

We have experimented with different Windows between −5 and +5. In Fig. 11.3 it is possible to see a graph representing the performance of the experiments. The blue line represents the time taken for the experiment in seconds by sample. The yellow line represents the percentual difference between the Correction trees of the windowed search in comparison to the Correction trees of the exhaustive search. The exhaustive search is equivalent to a − inf to inf Window and finds the

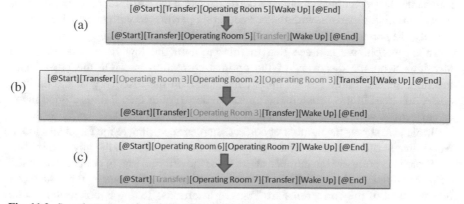

Fig. 11.2 Samples corrected according Physical Model

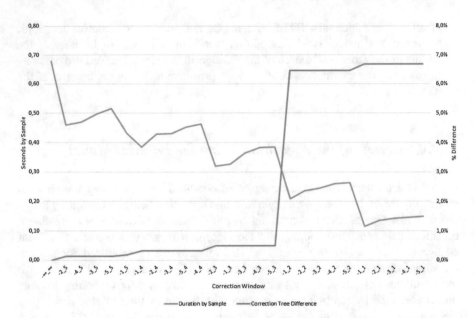

Fig. 11.3 Performance Comparison By Window in Physical Model Experiment

Table 11.2 Physical Model Sample Corrections

	Incorrect	Correct	Total
Samples	2244	1671	3915
%	57%	43%	100%

Table 11.3 Physical Model Events Statistics corrected

	# Events	# Events by Sample
Before correction	22.315	5,70
After correction	24.240	6,19

optimal correction tree for the selected Error Model. In other words, this difference represents the percentage of samples corrected that have a different correction set of operations in comparison with the correction set performed with exhaustive search, namely, the percentage of not optimal corrections tree inferred.

In the graph, we can see that in this problem the low limit window has a low impact on the discovery of the optimal correction tree. On the other hand, the high limit window has an important impact on the discovery of the optimal correction tree. In this problem, an upper window higher than 2 finds a good index of corrections with better performance.

Table 11.2 shows the number of correct samples according to the Physical Model. According to this data, 57% of the samples are not according to the physical model.

Table 11.3 compare the number of events of the original log, in comparison to the corrected log, and Table 11.4 shows the distribution of operations by type. As it can be seen most of the corrections are Transfer insertions. Taking a look at the results of the corrected sample, these corrections are due to the resolution of the RTLS

Table 11.4 Physical Model Events Statistics corrected by type

	OR	Transfer	WakeUp	Total
# Insertions	–	2.386	–	2.386
# Deletions	95	295	7	397
# Fusions	54	1	9	64

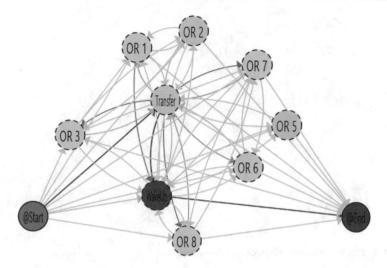

Fig. 11.4 TPA inferred without error Correcting

system in short-stay rooms like transfer. In these cases, the patient goes quickly from the *WakeUp* area to the *OR* area and the *Transfer* pass is not detected. In this case the algorithm corrects the system Inserting *Transfer* Locations in the middle (See Fig. 11.2a, c). Usually, Also, medium time reflection errors like the connection between different OR are solved adding Transfer states between the two operating rooms.

In the case of Process Mining inference, Fig. 11.4 shows the workflow inferred by PALIA algorithm using the Original Log. On the other hand, Fig. 11.5 shows the workflow inferred by PALIA using the log corrected using the Physical Model. It can be seen that the Corrected Model is easier to understand that original one.

Table 11.5 shows the Confusion Time computed aligning the original samples with the corrected samples. According to this, the total of confusion time is 0.05%. As expected, most confusions are produced between Transfer and rest of areas, as well as, consecutive Operating Rooms. This shows that although the correction has not a significant effect on the model because most of the problems are quick reflection errors, it has a clear effect on the human understanding of the flow.

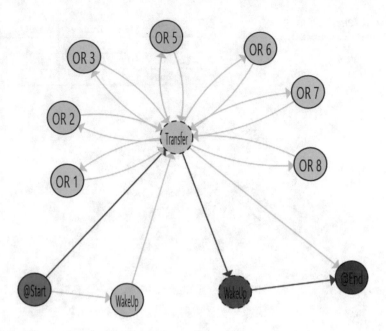

Fig. 11.5 TPA inferred with Physical Model experiment

11.4.5   Interactive Process Correction: Process Graph Model

Although the physical model can be used, as is, as a universal model for correcting errors of RTLS, it is possible to enrich the model with additional semantic restrictions to provide more precise indicators that can be provided by the expert interactively. In this line, we can take into account not only the physical model but also the process that patients follow, using heuristic information.

Figure 11.6 shows an example that, although is perfectly following the physical model, it seems illogical from the patient process point of view. In the example, the corrected sample shows that patient surgery takes place in two different Operating Rooms. Looking at the original trace, we can see that probably there was a long reflection error close to the end of the surgery. In this way, according to the process that the patients follow, it is logical to add a restriction limiting to one the valid number of Operating Rooms that can be occupied in the same trace.

Figure 11.7 shows a model that represents the process followed by the patient in the surgery department by applying this restriction. In this model, it is not allowed the presence of more than one operating room in the same patient flow. we have named this model *Process Model* because take into account the process restrictions in addition to the physical restrictions of the building rooms.

Figure 11.8 shows samples corrected using the process model that was not corrected using with the physical model. The Fig. 11.8a shows the new correction

Table 11.5 Confusion Time in Physical Model experiment

	OR 1	OR 2	OR 3	OR 5	OR 6	OR 7	OR 8	Transfer	WakeUp
OR 1	1,00000	0,00023	–	–	–	–	–	0,00007	0,00010
OR 2	–	0,99911	0,00075	–	–	–	–	0,00003	–
OR 3	–	0,00056	0,99925	–	–	–	–	0,00003	–
OR 5	–	–	–	1,00000	–	–	–	0,00001	–
OR 6	–	–	–	–	0,99874	0,00057	–	0,00001	–
OR 7	–	–	–	–	0,00126	0,99861	0,00060	0,00002	–
OR 8	–	–	–	–	–	0,00083	0,99940	0,00003	–
Transfer	–	–	–	–	–	–	–	0,99903	0,00010
WakeUp	–	0,00010	–	–	–	–	–	0,00075	0,99980

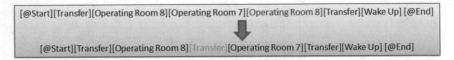

Fig. 11.6 Correcting limitations of Physical Model

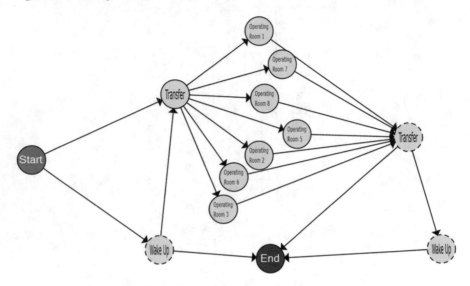

Fig. 11.7 Process Model of the Surgical Department

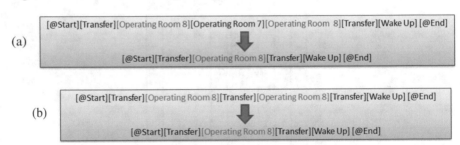

Fig. 11.8 Samples corrected according Process Model

of the sample of the previous Fig. 11.6. Also, Fig. 11.8b shows the elimination of a Transfer confusion in a surgery that was accepted by the physical model.

Comparing the performance of the algorithm in the Process Model Experiment (See Fig. 11.9) it is possible to see that this experiment requires more computation time than the previous one. Also, as in the Physical Model example, the higher window limit has more effect in the selection of optimal of the correction. In this case, it is needed a high limit window upper than 3 for achieving more optimal correction trees.

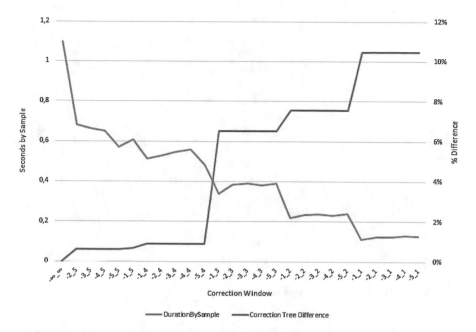

Fig. 11.9 Performance Comparison By Window in Process Model Experiment

Table 11.6 Process Model Sample Corrections

	Incorrect	Correct	Total
Samples	2.294	1.621	3915
%	59%	41%	100%

Table 11.7 Process Model Events Statistics corrected

	# Events	# Events by Sample
Before correction	22.315	5,70
After correction	23.902	6,11

Table 11.8 Process Model Events Statistics corrected by type

	OR	Transfer	WakeUp	Total
# Insertions	–	2.374	–	2.374
# Deletions	104	446	7	557
# Fusions	214	7	9	230

Table 11.6 shows the number of correct samples according to the Physical Model. According to this data, 59% of the samples are not according to the Process model. As expected, this index is higher than Physical Model example, because is more restrictive.

Seeing Tables 11.7 and 11.8, we can see that the corrections have decreased the number of events in comparison with the Physical Model experiment. Also, the number of deletions and fusions in OR and $Transfer$ have been significantly increased. This is because of the limitation of the new model in the acceptance of transitions among Operating Rooms, producing shorter sequences.

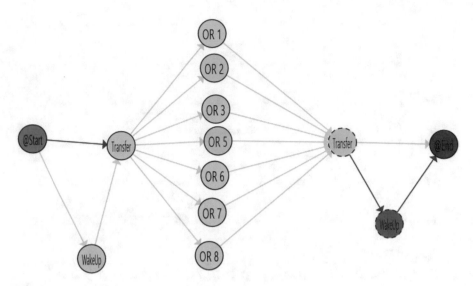

Fig. 11.10 TPA inferred with Process error model experiment

Figure 11.10 shows the final workflow inferred by PALIA. in a similar way to the Physical Model, the flow inferred is better understood than the not corrected model (Fig. 11.4).

Taking a look to Confusion Time of Process Model Correction Experiment (Table 11.9), it can be seen that in a similar way than Physical Model, there are confusions among $Transfer$ and the ORs as well as the contiguous ORs. However, the total of confusion time is, in this case, suppose a 0.4%. In comparison with Physical Model (0.05% of Confusion Time), Process Model Correction has discovered 8 times more RTLS detection problems. This supposes that the correction based on the Process Model is more accurate than the Physical Model one.

11.5 Discussion and Conclusions

The use of Interactive Trace Correction can be used for correcting RTLS models for providing better understandable IPIs. According to our experiments, the use of Error-Correcting techniques via the Edit Distance paradigm can correct the errors of RTLS systems conforming to the expected flows (Physical and Process Models), providing a much cleaner view in Process Mining solutions without other intrusive techniques that can affect the proper measure and without the manual correction of the corpus.

As we have seen in our experiments, although the RTLS System analyzed does not have a high percentage of error in terms of confusion time (0.05% and

Table 11.9 Confusion Time in Process Model experiment

	OR 1	OR 2	OR 3	OR 5	OR 6	OR 7	OR 8	Transfer	WakeUp
OR 1	0,99987	0,00023	–	–	–	–	–	0,00008	0,00010
OR 2	–	0,98524	0,00177	–	–	–	–	0,00003	–
OR 3	–	0,00107	0,98710	–	–	–	–	0,00006	–
OR 5	–	–	–	0,99183	–	–	–	0,00001	–
OR 6	–	–	–	–	0,99512	0,00059	–	0,00004	–
OR 7	–	–	–	–	0,00211	0,99191	0,00149	0,00024	–
OR 8	–	–	–	–	–	0,00082	0,98828	0,00026	–
Transfer	0,00013	0,01336	0,01113	0,00817	0,00277	0,00667	0,01023	0,99847	0,00010
WakeUp	–	0,00010	–	–	–	–	–	0,00081	0,99980

0.4% depending on the selected model), the impact in the view inferred by the Process Mining model is very high. This points out that without a big impact in the correction of the sample we can achieve much better Process Mining results.

Our experiments have demonstrated that it is important to select an adequate model for detecting and correcting more precisely the samples of the corpus. This technique applies a correction to a specific model, and if the model is not adequately selected, the perception of users about the real process might be erroneous. The Physical Model is a good starting point for defining this Model, being sure that the algorithm does not add more errors to the log and can be used for analyzing all the processes that take place in the same set of rooms, and to obtain more adequate corrections, the creation of richer models is required, like the Process Model. This interactive correction of traces combines the power of automatic correction with the heuristics provided by expert as heuristics incorporated to the error model. This not only allows a better correction, but also make the expert aware of the problem existing on the RTLS deployment. These kinds of Models help the correction of samples and provide more precise location results. In any case, this techniques can be used to objectively measure the difference between the real process deployed and the process perceived by the experts Using this information, Process experts, in our case, Medical Staff, can understand the errors in the processes and take decisions about their continuous improvement.

Another important issue to remark is the performance of the system. As the system follows an A^* search within a Windowed-Breadth First Search, the memory and the processing time can be compromised. In our experiments, we have analyzed the behaviour of the algorithm using different windows. We have compared the optimal solution discovering the better windows for each problem. Although in our example we have no performance problems, the length of the sequences can affect significantly the performance of the algorithm; in that case, the error model is crucial for having a better performance. The more precise the heuristics provided by the error model are, the quicker and more efficient the A^* search will be, improving the performance of the algorithm.

References

1. Álvarez García JA, Barsocchi P, Chessa S, Salvi D. Evaluation of localization and activity recognition systems for ambient assisted living: the experience of the 2012 EvAAL competition. J Ambient Intell Smart Environ 2013;5(1):119–32.
2. Amengual J-C, Sanchis A, Vidal E, Benedí J-M. Language simplification through error-correcting and grammatical inference techniques. Mach Learn. 2001;44(1–2):143–59.
3. Bendavid Y. RFID-enabled real-time location system (RTLS) to improve hospital's operations management: an up-to-date typology. Int J RF Technol Res Appl. 2013;5(3):137–58.
4. Botia JA, Villa A, Palma J. Ambient assisted living system for in-home monitoring of healthy independent elders. Exp Syst Appl. 2012;39(9):8136–48.
5. Buschmann T, Bystrykh LV. Levenshtein error-correcting barcodes for multiplexed dna sequencing. BMC Bioinform. 2013;14(1):272.

6. Chaaraoui AA, Climent-Pérez P, Flórez-Revuelta F. A review on vision techniques applied to human behaviour analysis for ambient-assisted living. Exp Syst Appl. 2012;39(12):10873–88.
7. Chang N, Rashidzadeh R, Ahmadi M. Robust indoor positioning using differential wi-fi access points. IEEE Trans Consum Electron. 2010;56(3):1860–67.
8. Chen M, Mao S, Liu Y. Big data: a survey. Mob Netw Appl. 2014;19(2):171–209.
9. Curran K, Furey E, Lunney T, Santos J, Woods D, McCaughey A. An evaluation of indoor location determination technologies. J Locat Based Serv. 2011;5(2):61–78.
10. Fernandez-Llatas C, Lizondo A, Monton E, Benedi J-M, Traver V. Process mining methodology for health process tracking using real-time indoor location systems. Sensors 2015;15(12):29821–40.
11. Fernandez-Llatas C, Martinez-Millana A, Martinez-Romero A, Benedi JM, Traver V. Diabetes care related process modelling using process mining techniques. lessons learned in the application of interactive pattern recognition: coping with the spaghetti effect. In: 2015 37th Annual International Conference of the IEEE Engineering in Medicine and Biology Society (EMBC); 2015. p. 2127–30.
12. Fernandez-Llatas C, Meneu T, Traver V, Benedi J-M. Applying evidence-based medicine in telehealth: an interactive pattern recognition approximation. Int J Environ Res Public Health. 2013;10(11):5671–82.
13. Fernández-Llatas C, Benedi J-M, García-Gómez JM, Traver V. Process mining for individualized behavior modeling using wireless tracking in nursing homes. Sensors. 2013;13(11):15434–51.
14. Gao X, Xiao B, Tao D, Li X. A survey of graph edit distance. Pattern Anal Appl. 2010;13(1):113–29.
15. Gu Y, Lo A, Niemegeers I. A survey of indoor positioning systems for wireless personal networks. IEEE Commun Surv Tutor. 2009;11(1):13–32.
16. Jameson JL, Longo DL. Precision medicine—personalized, problematic, and promising. Obstet Gynecol Surv. 2015;70(10):612–14.
17. Li N, Becerik-Gerber B. Performance-based evaluation of RFID-based indoor location sensing solutions for the built environment. Adv Eng Inform. 2011;25(3):535–46.
18. Liu H, Darabi H, Banerjee P, Liu J. Survey of wireless indoor positioning techniques and systems. IEEE Trans Syst Man Cybern Part C: Appl Rev. 2007;37(6):1067–80.
19. Martin N. Using indoor location system data to enhance the quality of healthcare event logs: opportunities and challenges. In: Daniel F, Sheng QZ, Motahari H, editors. Business process management workshops. Lecture Notes in Business Information Processing. Springer International Publishing; 2019. p. 226–38.
20. Marzal A, Vidal E. Computation of normalized edit distance and applications. IEEE Trans Pattern Anal Mach Intell. 1993;15(9):926–32.
21. Najera P, Lopez J, Roman R. Real-time location and inpatient care systems based on passive RFID. J Netw Comput Appl. 2011;34(3):980–89.
22. Navarro G. A guided tour to approximate string matching. ACM Comput Surv (CSUR). 2001;33(1):31–88.
23. Neuhaus M, Riesen K, Bunke H. Fast suboptimal algorithms for the computation of graph edit distance. In: Joint IAPR International Workshops on Statistical Techniques in Pattern Recognition (SPR) and Structural and Syntactic Pattern Recognition (SSPR). Springer; 2006. p. 163–72.
24. Shearer K, Bunke H, Venkatesh S. Video indexing and similarity retrieval by largest common subgraph detection using decision trees. Pattern Recognit. 2001;34(5):1075–91.
25. Stübig T, Zeckey C, Min W, Janzen L, Citak M, Krettek C, Hüfner T, Gaulke R. Effects of a WLAN-based real time location system on outpatient contentment in a level i trauma center. Int J Med Inf. 2014;83(1):19–26.
26. Sztyler T, Carmona J, Völker J, Stuckenschmidt H. Self-tracking reloaded: applying process mining to personalized health care from labeled sensor data. In: Transactions on Petri Nets and Other Models of Concurrency XI. Springer; 2016. p. 160–80.

27. Tan T-H, Gochoo M, Chen K-H, Jean F-R, Chen Y-F, Shih F-J, Ho CF. Indoor activity monitoring system for elderly using RFID and fitbit flex wristband. In: 2014 IEEE-EMBS International Conference on Biomedical and Health Informatics (BHI); 2014. p. 41–4.
28. Van Der Aalst W. Process mining: discovery, conformance and enhancement of business processes. Springer Nature Switzerland AG; 2011. https://link.springer.com/book/10.1007/978-3-642-19345-3
29. Van Der Aalst W. Process mining: data science in action. Springer Nature Switzerland AG; 2016. https://www.springer.com/gp/book/9783662498507.
30. Wichert R, Eberhardt B. Ambient assisted living. Springer Nature Switzerland AG; 2011. https://www.springer.com/gp/book/9783642181665.
31. Zeng Z, Tung AKH, Wang J, Feng J, Zhou L. Comparing stars: on approximating graph edit distance. Proc VLDB Endowment 2009;2(1):25–36.

Chapter 12
Interactive Process Mining in Type 2 Diabetes Mellitus

Antonio Martinez-Millana, Juan-Francisco Merino-Torres, Bernardo Valdivieso, and Carlos Fernandez-Llatas

12.1   Introduction

Type 2 Diabetes Mellitus (T2DM) is a chronic disease with a rapidly growing prevalence in the world [10]. Epidemiological studies estimate that there will be 693 million of people with T2DM by 2045 and that, almost half of all people will be living with an un-diagnosed diabetes [2, 4]. The disease is directly related to an increased morbidity and mortality [3], but several studies have shown that early diagnose and sustained life-style interventions reduced the incidence of complications and all-cause mortality, as well as an increased life expectancy [9, 18].

   Diabetes mellitus is a syndrome involving several factors which cause an impaired insulin secretion and/or action. This affection leads to a chronic hyper-

A. Martinez-Millana
Process Mining 4 Health Lab – SABIEN – ITACA Institute, Universitat Politècnica de València, Valencia, Spain
e-mail: anmarmil@itaca.upv.es

J.-F. Merino-Torres
Mixed Research Unit of Endocrinology, Nutrition and Dietetics, La Fe Health Research Institute, Valencia, Spain Department of Medicine, University of Valencia, Valencia, Spain

B. Valdivieso
Hospital at Home and Telemedicine Unit, The University and Polytechnic La Fe Hospital of Valencia, Valencia, Spain

The Joint Research Unit in ICT applied to the Reengineering of Socio-Sanitary Processes, The Medical Research Institute Hospital La Fe, Valencia, Spain

C. Fernandez-Llatas (✉)
Process Mining 4 Health Lab – SABIEN – ITACA Institute, Universitat Politècnica de València, Valencia, Spain

CLINTEC – Karolinska Institutet, Sweden
e-mail: cfllatas@itaca.upv.es

© Springer Nature Switzerland AG 2021
C. Fernandez-Llatas (ed.), *Interactive Process Mining in Healthcare*, Health Informatics, https://doi.org/10.1007/978-3-030-53993-1_12

glycemia (high blood glucose levels). Untreated diabetes leads to several micro- and macro- vascular injuries on several organs [11].

The normal process of glucose regulation starts when digestive system absorbs molecules of blood glucose from foods and drinks and transports them to the blood stream. Once in the blood, glucose molecules are used to fuel cells in their normal processes, but to get into the cell, there should be a mediator hormone produced by Langerhans islets β-cells in the pancreas. This hormone is the insulin. Among the several types of diabetes [17], T2DM is characterized by both an insulin action resistance and a progressive miss-function on the endogenous insulin release process. Different from other types of diabetes, like Type 1 Diabetes (related to an autoimmune reaction) or gestational diabetes (hormone-induced), T2DM is strongly linked with long-term defect originated by ageing and obesity [12]. T2DM accounts for the 90% of all diabetes cases and it has a prevalence in adult population that reaches 6% to 14%. The prevalence and incidence are region and cultural specific [16].

T2DM has no cure, but it can be controlled through a combination of lifestyle and pharmacological treatments. A good control of blood glucose levels decreases the risk of developing vascular and nervous complications. T2DM is commonly asymptomatic and is usually detected accidentally, as an abnormal blood glucose result in a routine laboratory test and confirmed with a Glycated Hemoglobgin (HbA1c) test . T2DM treatment consist on controlling blood glucose levels into normal thresholds to:

- Forewarn and delay macro-vascular complications and cardiovascular disease
- Forewarn microvascular and nervous complications

The American Diabetes Association (ADA) recommends a combination of interventions based on the risk of the patient. These interventions involve life-style, drugs and continuous follow-up ([1]):

- Changes on the food intake and nutritional habits. Adjusting the calories proportion of meals to the specific case and context of each subject and the overall strategy (weight loss or maintenance). Providing nutritional education is paramount to empower T2DM patients to design their own meal routines instead of following strict recipe compositions [14].
- Regular Physical Activity which increases insulin sensitivity and improves plas-matic parameters like blood glucose, fatty acids. Intensity should be moderate and prolonged during more than 30 min. Moderate intensity is calculated with several parameters, but a naäve approach is on the average beats per minute, that should be around 50% and 70% of the maximum peace (beats per minute) which is 220- Age. [18].
- Pharmacological treatment: There is no ideal pharmacological treatment for T2DM to help to control blood glucose levels (6%< HbA1c >7%) because all of them have side effects such as hypoglycemia, damage on B-cells and weight gain

- Diabetes self-management education to facilitate the knowledge, skills, and ability necessary for diabetes self-care and to manage the treatments.

The ultimate goal of the treatment is to individualize glycemic targets and perform interventions for the blood glucose lowering

12.2 Type 2 Diabetes as a Process

A process is defined as a series of actions or changes that happen either naturally or by the intervention of someone/something which ultimately leads to a result. Facing healthcare as a process is a difficult challenge. The number of actions and changes happening both naturally and by human intervention (or nonintervention) exceeds the current knowledge and understanding of T2DM processes, but decades of clinical research have leaded to a considerable body of agreement on the actions which lead to a correct management of the disease.

As a chronic disease, the clinical objectives of T2DM consist on maintaining the indicators of the disease into normality ranges and to delay or prevent the onset of complications. As we have seen, T2DM is a risk factor for co-morbidity and mortality but for the sake of clarity this chapter will focus solely on T2DM processes independently to other co-morbidities.

Variables related to T2DM evolution have been extensively studied. The standards of medical care defined by the American Diabetes Association (ADA) consider two main indicators for the glycemic control: Self-Monitored Blood Glucose (SMBG) and Glycated Heboglobine (HbA1c). Actually, these two indicators are elementary for a diagnosis of T2DM, and so, they are well-established indicators of the quality of care.

Besides, the (ADA) established goals for successful management of diabetes known as the ABCs of Diabetes: HbA1c <7.0 %, blood pressure <130/80 millimeters mercury , and low-density lipoprotein cholesterol (LDL-C) <100 mg/dL [20]. Another interesting indicator is the fasting blood glucose (the SMBG before having breakfast), which should be under 126mg/dL for people without the condition. The literature usually appeals to other indicators such as the Body Mass Index (BMI), cholesterol, creatinine and other indicators related to the life-style.

HbA1c reflects the blood glucose levels average during approximately three months and is the major tool to assess glycemic control and the evolution of the disease. ADA recommends to perform an HbA1c test two to four times year to evaluate the level of achievement of glycemic goals. A reasonable HbA1c level for T2DM adults is below 6.5–7%, but these tagets depend on several factors (duration of disease, lifestyle treated disease, life expectancy, sever hypoglycemia, etc..). Beyond HbA1c, ABCs recommends blood pressure below 130/80 millimeters mercury (Systolic/Diastolic) and low-density lipoprotein cholesterol (LDL-C) <100 mg/dL.

Despite the clinical and scientific evidence and the iterative release of guidelines, the management of T2DM is still not adequate. Prospective and observational studies reveal a significant distance between clinical guidelines and clinical practice [5, 19].

T2DM sails over different seas during its progression and regression. The regular follow-up of aforementioned indicators will produce changes in the therapy and recommendations of the diabetologists. But most specially, the sensitivity of glycemic values to changes in food intake habits, physical activity patterns and the normal evolution of the insulin resistance/production makes T2DM a dynamic process.

Previous studies have proposed risk prediction models to detect pre-diabetic and diabetic states by the use of Cox proportional hazards and logistic regression models [8, 15]. More recently, Nazari et al proposed the implementation of multi-state Markov model with continuous-time process to model T2DM [13]. In this work, authors proposed to consider time intervals between the changes in the disease states to provide a comprehensive view of pre-diabetes/diabetes states. Dagliati et al proposed careflow mining algorithm to detect the most frequent patterns of care in T2DM patients in a cohort of more than 1000 patients [7]. Authors concluded that progression of the disease is slow and the process of care is characterized by frequent modifications. Based on these findings, techniques that allow to handle high variability and noisy data have been suggested as more suitable, such as fuzzy models or Hierarchical Bayesian Logistic Regression [6, 21]. These models are based on probabilistic graphical models that allow to simplify complex networks of interactions and providing a better understanding of T2DM processes.

12.3   Process Mining Approach to Type 2 Diabetes

As we have seen in previous chapters, process mining is a technique that focuses on extracting knowledge from data stored in a warehouse or a corporate system which has the objective of providing analytics on the processes that produced that data. The management T2DM is based on the continuous adjustment of therapies and lifestyle counselling (e.g.: diet, physical activity, drugs) that aims to maintain and increase patients quality of life, by preventing, diagnosing and treating any type of episode, comorbidity or complication that may appear. This continuous process is supported by clinical and non-clinical activities that vary from one context to another and is highly influenced by the characteristics of the patient (which also change in the course of the disease).

Healthcare processes to manage T2DM are highly dynamic, complex, multidisciplinary and fitted-for-purpose, in the way that each endocrinology unit has its own interpretation to implement standard clinical guidelines. Understanding T2DM processes is not an easy task, even though it is clear that by its optimization patients' quality of life and use of clinical resources can be increased and optimized. The definition of Interactive Process Indicators (IPIs) for T2DM management would provide significant and meaningful information to analyze and understand the care process from both a single patient perspective or groups of patients.

The irruption and popularization of information and communication technologies has enables the collection and structured storage of any activity executed in a hospital. Any action or decision performed by a clinician, nurse, technician or manager is susceptible to be stored in a Hospital Information System (HIS) that compounds a huge number of databases, servers and components. Activities are stored as events, in a log format or as structured records in a database, containing information about when, who, what, to whom, and the result of that activity (among other relevant data). Process modelling techniques use this information to define how an entire process (composed by several activities) is being deployed using the data stored when the activity was held. Therefore it provides a high realistic view on how the process was implemented, helping the involved stakeholders to obtain information about the sequential order of the activities, the role of each actor, bottlenecks and unexpected paths. In this chapter we will analyze IPIs for the major indicator in T2DM management: HbA1c.

The types of data in which process mining is executed is crucial to determine which kind of techniques and approaches can be driven to obtain valuable information key indicators. Event logs (or records) are the most common way to organize data, nonetheless, it is important to discriminate which kind of data these records contain. In our experiments we analyze vital signs consisting of laboratory tests which are related to the therapies, the response of the patient (to the treatment and to the compliance) and his/her behaviours. Dealing with quantitative data and process mining needs to establish a level of abstraction to convert it into categorical data (temporal abstractions, categories consisting of ranges, rules, etc..)

Prior to apply the process mining models we need to perform some tasks to extract data, pre-process the data corpus, and finally to apply preliminary filters depending on the type of analysis. The extraction algorithms gathers and sorts all the recorded events using a temporal axis and then filtering for the type of observation (HbA1C). Thereafter, the corpus is built by connecting all the records. Finally the filtering algorithms extract only the activities matched to rules that have driven the analysis. After compiling all the relationships, discovering the nodes and the transitions, the model provides a set of workflows that reveal the pathways present into the analysed data set.

The workflows discovered using process mining are built up by nodes (activities) that are connected with arrows (transitions). According to the Business Process Theory, all the workflows must have a START and an END node, which will be represented by grey @Start and @End nodes that represent the first and the last record for a given patient in the data set considering a specific time range. In-between this nodes, a health process will be represented using the components shown in Fig. 12.1. Each node will contain the label defined in each type of analysis (in this example nodes are LOW, MED and HIGH) and will be connected through arrows to other nodes, indicating that a patient (or group of patients) has passed from one node (activity or status) to another.

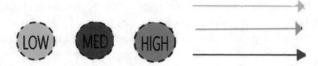

Fig. 12.1 Components of the workflows. Nodes are the states, in which the color reveals the time each patient remains in that state and the arrows are the transitions between the states, in which the color indicates the absolute frequency of the transition

Moreover, by applying an enhancement algorithm we are able to add a colour code to these components. This colour, which follows the traffic light approach, explains which is the absolute frequency of a given node or transition. A node will be red if it is a common activity or stage among patients and green if it is rare. The same will be applied to the transitions, an arrow will be red if there is a high flow of patients following that path or green if the flow is reduced. As mentioned the frequency is absolute, it represent the set of patients in each node/transition taking into account all the patients that accomplish the inferred workflow.

Figure 12.2 shows three illustrative cases of Interactive Process Indicators in the case of HbA1c in T2DM management. On the left side the Fig. 12.2 shows three examples of HbA1c trend and on the right side the corresponding process indicator. The first case (upper chart and workflow) shows the ideal case of therapy adjustment until the patient reaches the target value of 7%. In this case reflects that the measurements go up and down depending on the adjustment of pharmacological treatment and other supplemental interventions such diet and physical activity. The patient has HbA1c records every 2 months, which means is compliant with regular check recommendation. The inferred workflow has many indicators for this behaviour. The most significant is that there are only two transitions from start (S) and to end (E) nodes and these are in green. This characteristic reveals that the patient is compliant with the regular check-ups. Looking into the nodes, the workflow shows an intense transitions (in red) between HbA1c high (H) and low (L), which reveals the excursions of the tests up and down. This reveals that the patient has gone under an intense process of therapy adjustment or that the HbA1c was not successfully controlled. Finally there are two transitions for the medium (M) node, which is also connected to the end revealing that the patient was finally stabilized in a normal HbA1c value. The second case (middle chart and workflow) shows the case of a patient with high values of HbA1c during a long period. Even though the patient is compliant with the check ups (transition from S to H is in green), he expends most of the time with high values (node H in red), but finally is controlled and thus the transition to the end node comes from the medium node. The third case (lower chart and workflow) illustrate the paradigmatic case of a patient who has few tests. In this case the process is highlighted by a red transition from the start to the high node as the observations are considered as isolated events and not part of the same process due to the time distance between them, and this leads to assume that the patient has been in high state during this time. Moreover, the end

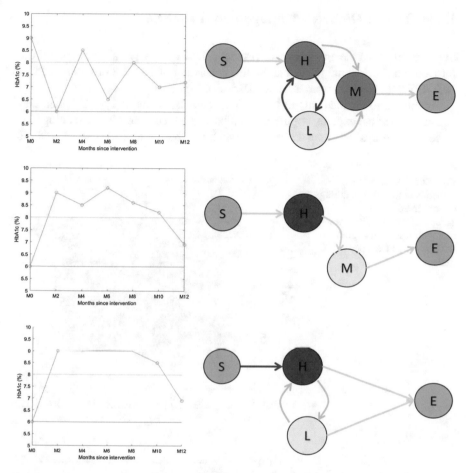

Fig. 12.2 Examples of Interactive Process Indicators for HbA1c management

transitions comes from the two nodes (H and L) showing that this patient has up and down episodes.

These three examples are useful to illustrate the Interactive Process Indicators which should be considered when analyzing real data, as they will be grouping data from several patients and a lot of information will be contained in the workflows.

Once data is defined and understood, process mining analysis should be driven to answer specific questions posed by endocrinologists and healthcare managers dealing with T2DM management:

- Which are the common paths followed by the majority of patients?
- Is there any recurrent exceptional or unexpected path?
- Does the care process comply with the clinical protocols?

12.4   Type 2 Diabetes Management Processes

In this example of the application of IPIs to T2DM we analyze an anonymized data set from La Fe Hospital (Valencia, Spain) consisting of 107,338 observations from 10,730 T2DM patients from 2010 to 2015 (See Fig. 12.3).

According to the medical guidelines for the management of Type 2 diabetes and consulted medical experts, population can be segmented according to their age into three main groups: less than 45 years old(45-), between 45 and 70 years old (45–70)

Fig. 12.3 Descriptive statistics of the HbA1c during the observed period. Temporal distribution of tests and their result. Histogram on the number of tests per patient

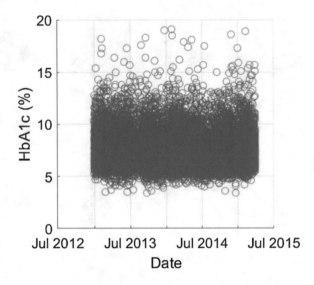

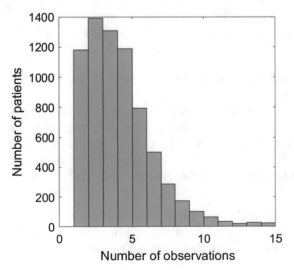

Fig. 12.4 Distribution of the
HbA1c levels for the three
age groups

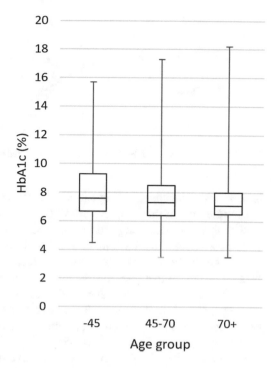

and over 70 years old (70+). Our analysis will be done based on these three groups
(See Fig. 12.4).

12.4.1   Analysis of HbA1C

HbA1c has been validated as a good estimator of the average blood glucose values
during the last 3 months, and despite it does not reflect some important events (e.g.:
blood glucose excursions), it is one of the main indicators for T2DM follow-up and
treatment decisions.

The main recommendations from standard guidelines can be synthesised into
two actions: to check up regularly through laboratory test and to keep the values
as closest as it is possible to 6.5–7%. For the first action patients are scheduled
to perform blood extractions and visits to endocrinologists in outpatient clinics
or general practitioners. For the second action, patients can have a wide range of
interventions, that depend upon several factors (life-style, diet or pharmacological
treatment). These interventions are primarily aimed to decrease HbA1c values, but
they should be balanced with patient's quality of life.

Based on the process oriented perspective of T2DM management, HbA1c should
be represented by three nodes, each of them standing for the category of the
measured value: LOW (HbA1c $\leq$ 6%), MED (6%<HbA1c$\leq$ 8%), HIGH (>8%). It

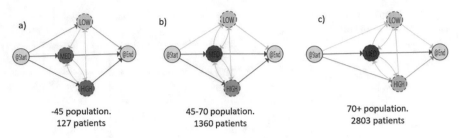

Fig. 12.5 Workflows for HbA1c in the three considered age groups

is clear that measurements beyond 8% should be categorized with more resolution, but for the sake of this chapter we will focus on the aforementioned targets.

The data set containing HbA1c observations is transformed into a event log in which each event has the following fields: Patient identification, timestamp of the observation, value of the observation. The process mining algorithm will process the data by assuming that two observations happening in a time range below 6 months are part of the same group of events (the second observation is a control of the effect of the proposed intervention), whereas a longer duration will lead to assume that the two observations are independent (regular follow-up).

The group of patients below 45 years old is composed by 127 patients. In the workflow (a) of Fig. 12.5 we can observe that the relative frequency of first observations are balanced between the three HbA1c levels (high, medium and low). The majority of the patients are more time in the Medium and High states than in the Low state and we can see that the transitions between these states are barely significant. This is an indicator of either a low compliance of the regular check ups or the inability to reduce the glycemic values during time.

The group of patients between 45 and 70 years old is composed by 1360 patients. In the workflow (b) of Fig. 12.5 we can observe a similar behaviour to the previous group but in this case patients are more time in the Medium state than in the High, which reveals a better performance of the interventions to keep patients in a normal range of glycemic values. However, the number of transitions and their absolute frequency could be indicating a low compliance to regular check ups.

The group of patients over 70 years old is composed by 2803 patients. In the workflow (c) of Fig. 12.5 we can observe that patients are more compliant with the regular check-ups, as denoted by the red transition to the medium node, and even more than in the previous group, patients stay more time in the medium range and less in the high state, which is also indicating the good response to the interventions in this group of age.

From a general perspective there are no clear paths in the management of HbA1c in T2DM patients, and the analysis must rely in the Interactive Process Indicators such as the strength of the transitions and the average time on each state. However, these analytics are useful to observe that the time between HbA1c tests is exceeding the ADA recommendations (transitions departing from start should be less populated) and as a consequence it is difficult to define the paths that each intervention and the patient response is reflected in the HbA1c behaviour.

Moreover, these analysis are also able to show exceptional or unexpected paths, as for example the transitions from High to Low in the three age groups. These transitions are revealing a significant decrease in the glycemic values, and thus a good response to the interventions. These patients could be analyzed more in detail to study the reasons underneath this good behaviour.

And finally, we can see that the group of patients showing a better behaviour is composed by patients over 70 years old, as the expend most of the time in normality (not healthy though) values. But also that the care process partially complies with the clinical protocols of regular follow-up of this crucial indicator in the T2DM management.

12.5 Conclusion

T2DM prevalence will increase in next decades, and will be proportionally linked to the ageing of population and increase in life-expectancy. Health institutions and healthcare professionals are currently highlighting the importance of reactive care in T2DM. HbA1c, as a reference parameter in the management of T2DM should be exploited to investigate the process of care and therapy and build processes which allow advancing in the understanding of both patient behaviour and individual responses to treatments.

In this chapter we have shown a first approximation of T2DM management to IPIs and process mining. The adjustment of process mining techniques enables the definition of IPIs revealing valuable information about the adherence to clinical guidelines and the ability of the interventions to meet their goals with respect to the blood glucose regulation. Besides, process mining methods for discovery and enhancement allowed to identify common and uncommon paths of patients by just loading HbA1c test in the form of an event log. The information contained in the workflows showed that some patient groups yield a better performance of the treatments in terms of HbA1c and that other patient groups need important interventions to normalize HbA1c values.

Flagship clinical trials such as the United Kingdom Prospective Diabetes Study (UKPDS) and the Kumamoto study confirmed the validity of this indicator to predict the development of complications. IPIs would be an interesting perspective to analyze temporal series of HbA1c and the onset of complications. Future work should look into the integration of other sources of data, such as the treatment recommendations and the complications development (using International Disease Codes for instance) to trace the care-paths that prevent/delay the worsening of T2DM patients and the effective therapies for patient's fenotypes.

References

1. American Diabetes Association. 4. Lifestyle management: Standards of medical care in diabetes—2018. Diabetes Care. 2018;41(Supplement 1):S38–50.
2. Beagley J, Guariguata L, Weil C, Motala AA. Global estimates of undiagnosed diabetes in adults. Diabetes Res Clin Pract. 2014;103(2):150–60.
3. Chatterjee S, Khunti K, Davies MJ. Type 2 diabetes. The Lancet. 2017;389(10085):2239–51.
4. Cho NH, Shaw JE, Karuranga S, Huang Y, da Rocha Fernandes JD, Ohlrogge AW, MalandaB. IDF diabetes atlas: Global estimates of diabetes prevalence for 2017 and projections for 2045. Diabetes Res Clin Pract. 2018;138:271–81.
5. Cooper JG, Claudi T, Jenum AK, Thue G, Hausken MF, Ingskog W, Sandberg S. Quality of care for patients with type 2 diabetes in primary care in Norway is improving. Diabetes Care. 2009;32(1):81–3.
6. Dagliati A, Malovini A, Decata P, Cogni G, Teliti M, Sacchi L, Cerra C, Chiovato L, Bellazzi R. Hierarchical bayesian logistic regression to forecast metabolic control in type 2 DM patients. In AMIA Annual Symposium Proceedings, vol. 2016. American Medical Informatics Association; 2016. p. 470.
7. Dagliati A, Tibollo V, Cogni G, Chiovato L, Bellazzi R, Sacchi L. Careflow mining techniques to explore type 2 diabetes evolution. J Diabetes Sci Technol. 2018;12(2):251–9. PMID: 29493360.
8. Goldstein BA, Navar AM, Pencina MJ, Ioannidis J. Opportunities and challenges in developing risk prediction models with electronic health records data: a systematic review. J Am Med Inf Assoc. 2017;24(1):198–208.
9. Gong Q, Zhang P, Wang J, Ma J, An Y, Chen Y, Zhang B, Feng X, Li H, Chen X, et al. Morbidity and mortality after lifestyle intervention for people with impaired glucose tolerance: 30-year results of the da qing diabetes prevention outcome study. Lancet Diabetes Endocrinol. 2019;7(6):452–61.
10. Guariguata L, Whiting DR, Hambleton I, Beagley J, Linnenkamp U, Shaw JE. Global estimates of diabetes prevalence for 2013 and projections for 2035. Diabetes Res Clin Pract. 2014;103(2):137–49.
11. Huxley R, Barzi F, Woodward M. Excess risk of fatal coronary heart disease associated with diabetes in men and women: meta-analysis of 37 prospective cohort studies. Bmj 2006;332(7533):73–8.
12. Kahn SE, Hull RL, Utzschneider KM. Mechanisms linking obesity to insulin resistance and type 2 diabetes. Nature 2006;444(7121):840–6.
13. Nazari M, Nazari SH, Zayeri F, Dehaki MG, Baghban AA. Estimating transition probability of different states of type 2 diabetes and its associated factors using Markov model. Prim Care Diabetes 2018;12(3):245–53.
14. Pan X-R, Li G-W, Hu Y-H, Wang J-X, Yang W-Y, An Z-X, Hu Z-X, Lin J, Xiao J-Z, Cao H-B, Liu P-A, Jiang X-G, Jiang Y-Y, Wang J-P, Zheng H, Zhang H, Bennett PH, Howard BV. Effects of diet and exercise in preventing NIDDM in people with impaired glucose tolerance: the da qing IGT and diabetes study. Diabetes Care 1997;20(4):537–44.
15. Shah ND, Steyerberg EW, Kent DM. Big data and predictive analytics: recalibrating expectations. JAMA 2018;320(1):27–8.
16. Talmud PJ, Hingorani AD, Cooper JA, Marmot MG, Brunner EJ, Kumari M, Kivimaki M, Humphries SE. Utility of genetic and non-genetic risk factors in prediction of type 2 diabetes: whitehall II prospective cohort study. BMJ. 2010;340(1):b4838–b4838.
17. Thomas LHP. Update on diabetes classification. Med Clin North Am 2015;99(1):1–16.
18. Tuomilehto J, Lindström J, Eriksson JG, Valle TT, Hämäläinen H, Ilanne-Parikka P, Keinänen-Kiukaanniemi S, Laakso M, Louheranta A, Rastas M, Salminen V, Aunola S, Cepaitis Z, Moltchanov V, Hakumäki M, Mannelin M, Martikkala V, Sundvall J, Uusitupa M. Prevention of type 2 diabetes mellitus by changes in lifestyle among subjects with impaired glucose tolerance. N Engl J Med. 2001;344(18):1343–50.

19. Vaghela P, Ashworth M, Schofield P, Gulliford MC. Population intermediate outcomes of diabetes under pay-for-performance incentives in England from 2004 to 2008. Diabetes Care 2009;32(3):427–29.
20. Vouri SM, Shaw RF, Waterbury NV, Egge JA, Alexander B. Prevalence of achievement of a1c, blood pressure, and cholesterol (abc) goal in veterans with diabetes. J Manag Care Pharm. 2011;17(4):304–12.
21. Yousefi L, Tucker A, Al-luhaybi M, Saachi L, Bellazzi R, Chiovato L. Predicting disease complications using a stepwise hidden variable approach for learning dynamic bayesian networks. In: 2018 IEEE 31st International Symposium on Computer-Based Medical Systems (CBMS). IEEE; 2018. pp. 106–11.

Chapter 13
Interactive Process Mining in IoT and Human Behaviour Modelling

Juan J. Lull, José L. Bayo, Mohsen Shirali, Mona Ghassemian, and Carlos Fernandez-Llatas

13.1 Introduction

The implementation of IoT means that sensors can be introduced in an area, enabling continuous human activity measurement and, through Wireless Sensor Networks, the output data may be sent to servers where information about the person may be processed and interpreted.

Ambient Intelligence (AmI), a concept that was proposed in 1990 by the European Commission Information Society and Technology Advisory Group (ISTAG) and Philips, consists on the creation of spaces where the technology serves the person in the most transparent way [12].

AmI lets the technology perform smart actions depending on the person's behaviour, such as switching lights on and off when the home resident moves from room to room [5].

J. J. Lull · J. L. Bayo
Process Mining 4 Health Lab – SABIEN – ITACA Institute, Universitat Politècnica de València, Valencia, Spain
e-mail: jualulno@itaca.upv.es; jobamon@itaca.upv.es

M. Shirali
Computer Science and Engineering, Shahid Beheshti University, Tehran, Iran

M. Ghassemian
BT Applied research labs, Adastral Park, Ipswich, UK

C. Fernandez-Llatas (✉)
Process Mining 4 Health Lab – SABIEN – ITACA Institute, Universitat Politècnica de València, Valencia, Spain

CLINTEC – Karolinska Institutet, Sweden
e-mail: cfllatas@itaca.upv.es

© Springer Nature Switzerland AG 2021
C. Fernandez-Llatas (ed.), *Interactive Process Mining in Healthcare*, Health Informatics, https://doi.org/10.1007/978-3-030-53993-1_13

In AmI, the *Ambient* side of the system includes sensors that provide the subject's context, i.e. a projection of the person as realistic as possible. The *Intelligence* side introduces the processing of the context so the environment around the subject may be enhanced. This enhancement depends heavily on the subject, since there are differences at the cultural level as well as gender, height, age, etc., so technology improvements in the environment are totally dependent on the specific person. Furthermore, the same person's behaviour changes in time, and the system should adapt accordingly. As an example, if the home or environment "knew" the person was feeling anxious or depressed, it could change lights or music accordingly. This would improve the life of a person invisibly.

One challenge for AmI is that IoT generates large amounts of data. For example, a simple heart rate measurement every second through a wearable, would account for around 90,000 measurement instances per day. If a person was monitored by a doctor every three months, around 8 million measurement instances would be available from visit to visit. This is something the doctor would not be able to interpret directly. The context would also be key here: heart rate could be high because of different possibilities, such as practicing sports, a stressful situation, a cardiovascular problem with no external manifestation, etc. GPS or other sensor data such as passive infrared sensors (PIR) or Bluetooth beacons, would add a context about the person. The situation in which we have a context as accurate as possible about the person is better than the nowadays usual way of following the person's health or wellness: A subjective survey based on what the person remembers about his health status during the previous months. As we can see, AmI may be of great help, by obtaining a more specific model of the person and ameliorating the subject's condition or dispatching the person to the doctor when necessary, than a visit to the doctor every three months with subjective data from what the subject remembers about his health condition.

By introducing IoT devices with sensors, the following aim could be achieved: the monitorization of the activity would generate and send the data through the IoT devices to a central server. The activity data would then be analysed and turned into meaningful behavioural data, e.g. the person is walking less than usual; heart rate is high and there is sleep deprivation; etc. *Systems with computing capabilities analye the assimilated data to recognize the activities of inhabitants or events. These can automate the domestic utilizations effectively and also can support the inhabitant by reducing the costs and improving the standard of living* [13].

It was stated earlier that the context of the subject is key. The correct analysis and integration of all the sensors may create an accurate context about the subject, so that real improvements could be introduced in the subject's life. Big data plays a key role here: Lots of information are available, and they must be interpreted correctly. The system that, based on the data, generates accurate human behaviour models, should be easily understood, since it is of vital importance that the models and decisions taken to help the person are correct. As seen in previous chapters, general pattern recognition models are prone to errors; those that act as black boxes, without information about how the models were generated, should be used with great care. Interactive pattern recognition models would be preferred, since they let us know and review the validity of the models. As [14] state, *at present, biology is*

the foremost field generating enormous amounts of data needing to be sorted. These
data also need to be analyzed for a better understanding of the research at hand.

Since we are trying to model behaviour, process mining techniques are suitable
for this study. A person's conduct is easily modelled as a series of steps or activities
with their corresponding timestamps. This has already been applied to different
fields, mainly the medical and elderly care one [7, 8], but also to education [1, 11],
consumer conduct [3, 10], etc. Examples include the successful differentiation and
modelling of male and female behaviours in shopping malls for customer experience
personalization [3], or the behaviour in a group of 25 in-house patients [4], amongst
others. In these cases, the interest is on how their behaviours are different, what is
unique e.g. in men's behaviour as opposed to women's behaviour, so that an added
value can be introduced in the consumers' experience.

In this chapter, an interactive process mining system is applied to data obtained
through IoT, specifically through PIR. The methodology lets us see different
behaviours in one single person and how this could be applied to intra-subject
studies with millions of measurement instances, discovering changes in individual
conduct and their specific characteristics.

13.2 Study Data and Procedure

The type of data that has been used here was described in [4]. Basically, data from
PIR sensors was acquired for 70 days. The sensors were at the person's home,
covering different areas:

- Kitchen
- Living room
- TV room
- Bathroom
- Bedroom
- Corridor
- Entrance
- Storage
- WC

The subject was a 28-year-old healthy male who was then studying and working
at the University.

Approximately 80,000 detection instances were recorded by the PIR sensors
(around 1,150 instances per day).

The process mining algorithm that was used is PALIA, implemented by the Institute of Information and Communication Technologies (ITACA) of the Universitat
Politècnica de València, Valencia, Spain [9].

We introduced the data for our model as: Whenever the sensor detected the
person, we classified that the person was in that area until he moved to another
area. In this way, we could assign times for each activity, in the following fashion:
One action is modelled as: **Location (Activity) + Start time + End time**.

Whenever the subject is detected in the entrance and until a new detection is performed, we assume the time in the entrance as outside the house.

An event log was created that included the different actions in time. Therefore, we had a single log that showed the actual position of the subject through time. The log was divided per day by separating the log into 24 h-days, that initiated at 0:00. Each 24 h-day is stored as a trace inside the log.

Since PIR data is usually contaminated, we discarded data that could have been generated because of problems with the sensors, inside a noise removal process.

The correction algorithm, based on the heuristic topological distance, has been formally defined elsewhere [8]. Informally, it consists on the comparison and edition of two different Timed Parallel Automata (TPA), one of them representing the possible transitions inside the house, the base Interactive Process Indicator (base IPI), and the other one representing the trace that we want to correct. The edition of each trace TPA minimizes the differences between the evolved IPI corresponding to a trace, and the base IPI, deleting, adding or fusing nodes.

Specifically:

- Consecutive events in the same place were fused into one event (fusion weight was set to 0).
- Consecutive events between areas that were not connected, were discarded (e.g. the entrance and the bathroom are not directly connected so two consecutive events with entrance and bathroom were discarded; this was achieved by assigning a weight of 0 to the deletion of nodes).
- The creation of nodes was not permitted (weight of node addition: −200).

The possible movements inside the house are represented in the graph that shows the base IPI, depicted at Fig. 13.1.

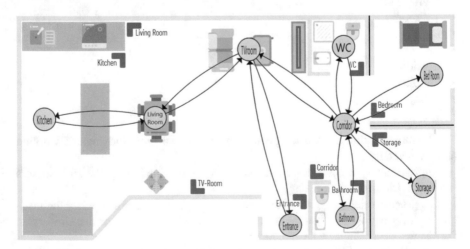

Fig. 13.1 Base IPI graph representing possible connections between areas in the house (Start and End nodes have been omitted in the Figure)

According to the structure of the house, the subject could move from the kitchen to the living room and vice versa. From the corridor, he could move to the bedroom, the WC, the bathroom or the storage, etc. However, places such as the corridor and the kitchen are not directly connected in the house, so two consecutive events with a corridor and a kitchen events do not appear as connected in the base IPI and this kind of connection would be discarded as an outlier when comparing a trace TPA against it.

Each corrected TPA is defined as an evolution IPI. Those indicators represent different behaviours in the subject.

13.2.1 Clustering Behaviour Models

Finally, a Quality Threshold Clustering algorithm based on heuristic distance (see [8]) was applied, in order to group similar behaviours. The algorithm has two parameters, similarity and minimum density.

The first parameter, similarity percentage, indicates that individual traces in a cluster cannot be differentiated by more than the parameter value, according to their distance.

The second parameter, minimum density percentage, indicates that in order to consider a group as a valid one, the density of members should account at least for a minimum density size. In practice, this means that groups will need a minimum number of trace TPAs that constitute them. Otherwise, it would be considered as an outlier TPA and would not be introduced in any group.

Both parameters were optimized, by testing with different levels of similarity and density. In the end, 20% similarity and 5% minimum density were selected. Lower levels of similarity generated groups with similar behaviour but subtle changes, while 5% minimum density lead to classify groups with less than four elements as outliers. The parameters should be changed depending on the study. If subtler changes should be detected (i.e. in the case of an elderly person that we need to study because she or he has changed their behaviour as of late), the parameter values would be different (in that case, a lower similarity ratio would be chosen). The user needs to interact with the model, so it is perfected.

The applied clustering method discovers the number of groups (i.e. there is no previous definition of the number of groups that must be achieved, [4]).

The days classified as outliers were reviewed and two days were detected that did not have data from parts of the day and were discarded. The two days were removed from the data.

13.3 Results

Four groups, showing different behaviour through the day, were detected. Apart from them, 3 outliers were found that did not fulfil the conditions of distances

Table 13.1 Groups obtained
through heuristic distance
clustering

Group	Days	Calendar colour
0	35	Red
1	22	Navy blue
2	4	Green
3	4	Yellow
Outliers	3	Light blue
Total	68	

and density. The groups were formed by 35, 22, 4 and 4 days. These are shown in Table 13.1.

The groups show several differences among them. A table with average duration and standard deviation per activity per day, along with a workflow, are presented for each group.

In each workflow, the colour of the nodes reflects the average time per day dedicated in each area via a heat map: The redder a node representing a location, the longer the subject stayed at that location. The greener, the less time the subject spent there. The same colour scale is shared across the different day groups. This means that green represents 0 h while red represents the maximum amount of time spent at a single location, around 13 h.

The arrow colours represent the number of times the subject moved from one place to another. The colours range from green to red (few movements up to highest number of movements). This scale has been adjusted for each group, so opposite to the node duration colours, this one does not represent the same number of executions at every workflow.

The different classified days can be seen in the calendar represented in Fig. 13.2, with the colour codes that appear at Table 13.1.

13.3.1   Group 0

The group 0, consisting of 35 days/traces (1 trace per day) out of 68 day, has the characteristics shown in Fig. 13.3 and in Table 13.2.

The subject spent most of the time outside the house (as stated previously, it is assumed that detection instances in the entrance correspond to either entering or leaving the house). The second place the resident stayed most was the bedroom and then the tv room. We can see this in Fig. 13.3 (reddest colour is associated to the entrance and then the next ones are the bedroom and the tv room) and in Table 13.2. Specifically, the subject was outside for approximately 14,5 h and 4 h in the kitchen.

When using PALIA, the user may hover the cursor over the node and see specific data, such as the information shown in Table 13.2.

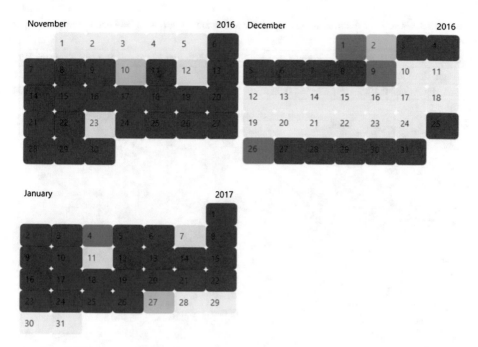

Fig. 13.2 Distribution of classified days in a calendar view

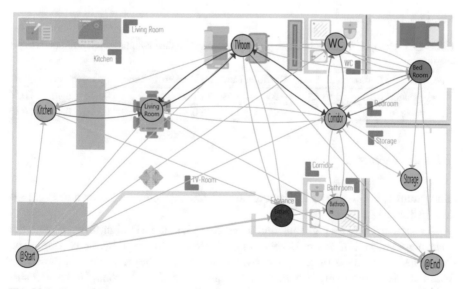

Fig. 13.3 Group 0 Flow

Table 13.2 Group 0, duration in hours per day and standard deviation between different days per location

Location	Bathroom	Bedroom	Corridor	Entrance	Kitchen	Liv. room	Storage	TVroom	WC
Avge. duration	0,22	7,05	0,18	11,41	0,57	0,28	0,03	3,90	0,31
Std. deviation	0,13	1,67	0,03	5,37	0,09	0,06	0,05	0,39	0,04

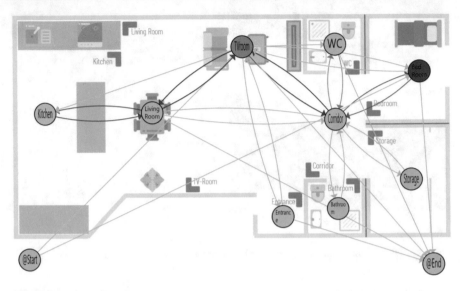

Fig. 13.4 Group 1 Flow

Table 13.3 Group 1, duration in hours per day and standard deviation between different days per location

Location	Bathroom	Bedroom	Corridor	Entrance	Kitchen	Liv. room	Storage	TVroom	WC
Avge duration	0,26	13,13	0,35	0,68	1,67	0,39	0,07	6,90	0,50
Std. deviation	0,16	1,40	0,05	0,91	0,14	0,02	0,11	0,44	0,05

13.3.2 Group 1

The group 1, consisting of 22 days/traces has the characteristics shown in Fig. 13.4 and in Table 13.3.

As shown both in Fig. 13.4 and in Table 13.3, it is straightforward that the maximum amount of time was spent in the bedroom, followed by the tv room. The home resident moved frequently between the corridor, the tv room and the living room and less frequently between the living room and the kitchen. He moved still less frequently between the corridor and the bedroom. In this second cluster of days, the subject did not practically leave the house, less than 3/4 h per day. In the rest of the groups, the subject left the house for longer periods.

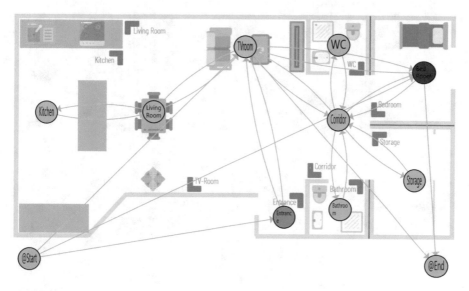

Fig. 13.5 Group 2 Flow

Table 13.4 Group 2, duration in hours per day and standard deviation between different days per location

Location	Bathroom	Bedroom	Corridor	Entrance	Kitchen	Liv. room	Storage	TVroom	WC
Avge duration	0,12	11,95	0,22	6,52	0,83	0,31	0,03	3,54	0,43
Std. deviation	0,05	1,45	0,01	2,61	0,06	0,01	0,03	0,26	0,04

13.3.3   Group 2

The group 2, consisting of 4 days/traces (1 trace per day) has the characteristics shown in Fig. 13.5 and in Table 13.4.

As Table 13.4 and Fig. 13.5 show, the subject stayed most of the time in the bedroom, but it was less than the time spent there on days from Group 1. The second place was the entrance, i.e. outside home, and then the tv room. This group represented four days.

13.3.4   Group 3

The group 3, consisting of 4 days/traces (1 trace per day) has the characteristics shown in Fig. 13.6 and in Table 13.5.

During the four days in group 3, the subject stayed most of the time in the tv room. In the second place was the bedroom and in the third place was the entrance.

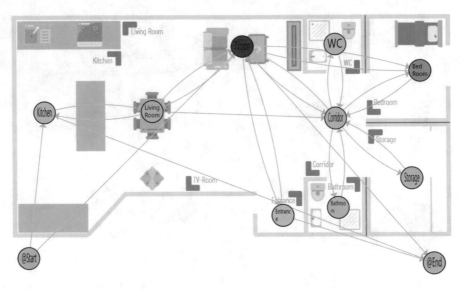

Fig. 13.6 Group 3 Flow

Table 13.5 Group 3, duration in hours per day and standard deviation between different days per location

Location	Bathroom	Bedroom	Corridor	Entrance	Kitchen	Liv. room	Storage	TVroom	WC
Avge duration	0,53	6,29	0,24	2,15	1,21	0,36	0,07	12,68	0,40
Std. deviation	0,19	1,47	0,01	1,38	0,08	0,01	0,02	0,56	0,04

13.4 Interpreting Group IPIs

As can be seen in the results, the automatic clustering identified two main cluster evolution IPIs that accounted for most of the days, groups 0 and 1. The reason behind the classification can be easily seen by visual inspection of the aggregated workflow.

The results may be interpreted as shown in Table 13.6. This understanding of what the relation is between the data and the real person, needs the expert that can add critical meta-information to the context. In this case, there was information about the subject that was available: he studied and worked at the same time, at the University, with a flexible timetable. So, it is feasible he was mainly studying some days, while on other days (most of them) he was working.

Individual days can be seen (in PALIA, the calendar view lets the user enter into any of the days and see the workflow corresponding to that day). Thus, it is easy to inspect the individual TPA corresponding to a day in a group.

As an example, we can see the individual traces for some of the days that were classified differently. Figure 13.7 shows one of the days classified as group 0.

Table 13.6 Interpretation of group IPIs

Group	Main characteristics	Interpretation
0	High time in entrance; kitchen: around half hour; around 7 h sleep; less than 4 h in the living room	Working outside
1	High time in bedroom, then tv room; nearly no time outside	Studying for an exam
2	High time in bedroom; less than 8 h outside; less than 1 h in the kitchen	Leisure: Going out
3	High time in the tv room; more than 1 h in the kitchen	Leisure: At home

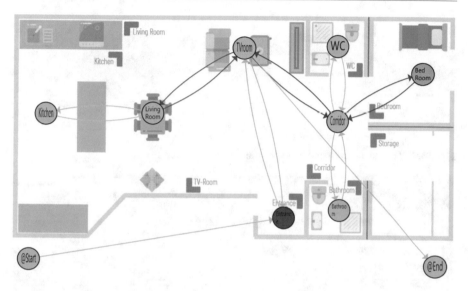

Fig. 13.7 Workflow corresponding to the resident's behaviour on January 14 2017, group 0

Figure 13.8 shows the workflow for a day in group 1. Another workflow for group 1 is shown at Fig. 13.9. They can be compared to the cluster TPA and between them and see their similarities. Figure 13.10 shows the workflow for a day that was not classified in any group, and was thus considered an outlier.

The comparison between days inside a group, or between one day and the TPA representing the group, visually shows the differences between data. In Fig. 13.11, the workflow representing the subtraction of 7 November from 19 January, both in the same group, shows the following differences: time spent at the tv room was higher (5 h 48 min. vs 3 h 43 min.) while time spent at the bedroom was lower (14 h 40 min. vs 15 h 55 min.). A higher number of transitions between the kitchen and living room was also detected in day 7 Nov. compared to 19 Jan. (32 and 16 transitions, respectively). However, in general terms both workflows are very similar between them.

The comparison between days in different groups clearly shows the distinction in behaviour that motivated the different classification. In Fig. 13.12, big changes can be observed both between the duration in the locations of the house and the transition between the locations. The most significant changes between days were

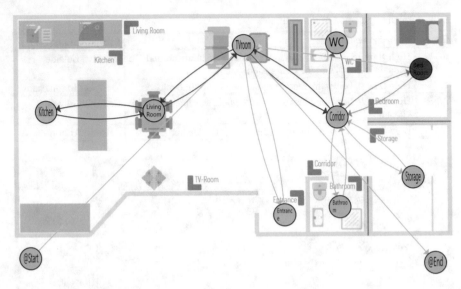

Fig. 13.8 Workflow corresponding to November 7 2016, group 1

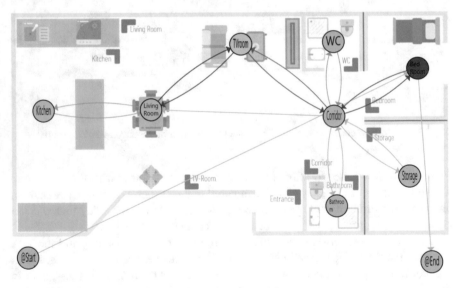

Fig. 13.9 Workflow corresponding to January 19 2017, group 1

the time spent in the bedroom (7 h 34 min vs 15 h 55 min.) and in the entrance - outside the house- (14 h 7 min. vs 1 h 22 min.). Areas that make nearly no difference at all can also be seen, such as the living room, the WC or the corridor, and are thus painted white. The transitions between areas in the house was also lower in 14 Jan.

As can be seen, automatic detection of different behaviours is straightforward. Different patterns in the resident behaviour can be visually detected. Also, outliers are easy to detect and inspect in order to classify them as data that must either be discarded, or that correspond to very different behaviour to the other days.

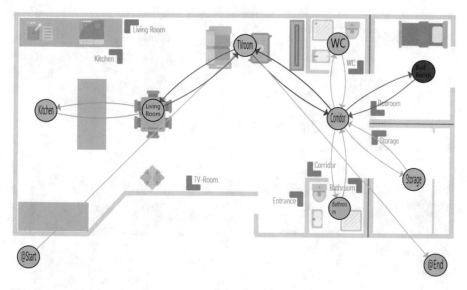

Fig. 13.10 Workflow corresponding to November 10, 2016, outlier

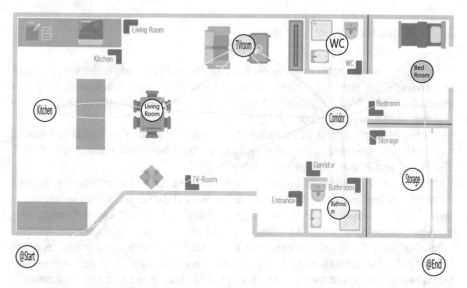

Fig. 13.11 Resulting workflow after subtracting 19 January from 7 November TPAs, both corresponding to the same group 1

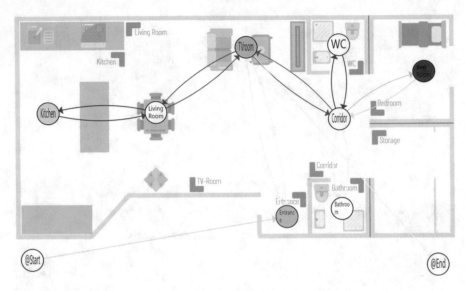

Fig. 13.12 Resulting workflow after subtracting 14 January TPAs from 7 November, corresponding to group 0 and group 1, respectively

13.5 Conclusion

IoT can improve our lives in many aspects, in case we can analyse the vast amounts
of information it provides. The more sensors and smart devices we have, the better
the context we can create around the subject, and the more accurate the information
and decisions about the subject we can take.

As Farahni et al. stated, in the terms of IoT and health, timely big data processing
and analytics are needed to have actionable data on multi-scale, multi-modal,
distributed and heterogeneous large datasets [6].

Behaviour modelling is an inherently complex task, since there is a great
inter-subject and intra-subject heterogeneity. Modelling the individual behaviour is
most complicated since the same subject changes his or her conduct every day,
in subtle or obvious ways. Creating a model that correctly displays the average
behaviour in a group of subjects is a task that has been accomplished in many
studies and with techniques different to IPM. However, modelling the intra-subject
behaviour without sacrificing the concept drift (i.e. processes are continuously
changing in time) may be a titanic task. As [2] state, *Concept drift has been
shown to be important in many applications (...). However, existing work tends
to focus on simple structures such as changing variables rather than changes to
complex artifacts such as process models describing concurrency, choices, loops,
cancellation, etc.*

In this chapter, we have shown how different process models can be inducted
from a subject's behaviour. We have shown how modelling differences in conduct

in a subject, with IoT data that calls for big data, can be achieved through IPM. The techniques applied in this chapter could easily be applied to different fields, because of the exploratory and visual characteristics of interactive process mining.

References

1. Bogarín A, Romero C, Cerezo R, Sánchez-Santillán M. Clustering for improving Educational process mining. In: ACM international conference proceeding series, New York, Association for Computing Machinery; 2014. p. 11–5.
2. Bose RPJC, Van Der Aalst WMP, Žliobaite I, Pechenizkiy M. Handling concept drift in process mining. In: Lecture notes in computer science (including subseries lecture notes in artificial intelligence and lecture notes in bioinformatics). LNCS, vol. 6741. Berlin/Heidelberg: Springer; 2011. p. 391–405.
3. Dogan O, Bayo-Monton J-L, Fernandez-Llatas C, Oztaysi B. Analyzing of gender behaviors from paths using process mining: a shopping mall application. Sensors. 2019;19(3):557.
4. Dogan O, Martinez-Millana A, Rojas E, Sepúlveda M, Munoz-Gama J, Traver V, Fernandez-Llatas C. Individual behavior modeling with sensors using process mining. Electronics. 2019;8(7):766.
5. Eisenhauer M, Rosengren P, Antolin P. A development platform for integrating wireless devices and sensors into Ambient Intelligence systems. In: 2009 6th IEEE annual communications society conference on sensor, mesh and ad hoc communications and networks workshops, SECON workshops 2009. 2009.
6. Farahani B, Firouzi F, Chang V, Badaroglu M, Constant N, Mankodiya K. Towards fog-driven IoT ehealth: promises and challenges of iot in medicine and healthcare. Futur Gener Comput Syst. 2018;78:659–76.
7. Farid N, De Kamps M, Johnson O. Process mining in frail elderly care: a literature review. In: Proceedings of the 12th international joint conference on biomedical engineering systems and technologies. SCITEPRESS – Science and Technology Publications; 2019. p. 332–9.
8. Fernández-Llatas C, Benedi J-M, García-Gómez J, Traver V. Process mining for individualized behavior modeling using wireless tracking in nursing homes. Sensors. 2013;13(11):15434–51.
9. Fernandez-Llatas C, Valdivieso B, Traver V, Benedi JM. Using process mining for automatic support of clinical pathways design. In: Methods in molecular biology, vol. 1246. Humana Press, New York, NY; 2015. p. 79–88. https://link.springer.com/protocol/10.1007%2F978-1-4939-1985-7_5
10. Gou Z, Tsugawa S, Korkaew A, Yamaguchi S, Khamket T, Manaskasemsak B, Rungsawang A. An interest-based tour planning tool by process mining from Twitter. In: 2016 IEEE 5th global conference on consumer electronics, GCCE 2016. Institute of Electrical and Electronics Engineers Inc.; 2016.
11. Mukala P, Buijs JCAM, Van Der Aalst WMP. Exploring students' learning behaviour in moocs using process mining techniques. Eindhoven: Department of Mathematics and Computer Science, University of Technology; 2015. p. 179–196
12. Riva G, Vatalaro F, Davide F, editors. Ambient intelligence: the evolution of technology, communication and cognition towards the future of human-computer interaction. Amsterdam/Fairfax: IOSS Press; 2005.
13. Saralegui U, Ángel Antón M, Ordieres-Meré J. An IoT-based system that aids learning from human behavior: a potential application for the care of the elderly. MATEC Web Conf. 2017;125:05010.
14. Sen S, Datta L, Mitra S. Machine learning and IoT a biological perspective. Boca Raton: CRC Press; 2019.

Chapter 14
Interactive Process Mining for Medical Training

Jorge Munoz-Gama, Victor Galvez, Rene de la Fuente, Marcos Sepúlveda, and Ricardo Fuentes

14.1 Process Mining in Medical Training

Process Mining has been widely used in healthcare in different medical areas [18], and recently some applications in the medical training field has been developed. In particular, the use of Process Mining in the training of procedural skills has opened a branch of opportunities to fill gaps in this field.

Procedural skills are essential to perform surgical procedures and to obtain good clinical outcomes [4]. Literature suggests that surgical procedures can be seen as a process [16], so it is possible to analyze surgical procedures with Process Mining. This perspective allows focusing on the sequence of steps of a surgical procedure, an aspect rarely considered in the medical training research and practice. Also, this view enables the development of different applications that can be useful in the medical training context for tasks like teaching, assessment, giving feedback, among others.

In this chapter, we will use the Central Venous Catheter insertion as a running case to illustrate the POME (Process-Oriented Medical Education) methodology. This surgical procedure has six main steps: first, to prepare implements and patient for the procedure; then, a vein is punctured using a trocar (a needle with a hole to introduce a guidewire); next, the guidewire is passed through the trocar; later, the trocar is removed, and the catheter advanced through the guidewire; finally, the guidewire is removed and the catheter installed.

J. Munoz-Gama (✉) · V. Galvez · M. Sepúlveda
School of Engineering, Pontificia Universidad Católica de Chile, Santiago, Chile
e-mail: jmun@uc.cl; vagalvez@uc.cl; marcos@ing.puc.cl

R. de la Fuente · R. Fuentes
School of Medicine, Pontificia Universidad Católica de Chile, Santiago, Chile
e-mail: rdelafue@med.puc.cl; rfuente@med.puc.cl

© Springer Nature Switzerland AG 2021
C. Fernandez-Llatas (ed.), *Interactive Process Mining in Healthcare*, Health
Informatics, https://doi.org/10.1007/978-3-030-53993-1_14

14.2   POME Methodology

Figure 14.1 shows the POME (Process-Oriented Medical Education) methodology overview. This methodology facilitates the analysis of surgical procedures as a sequence of steps and uses the results for medical training tasks. It is composed of three stages: first "Model Stage", second "Data Stage" and third "Analysis Stage". Each stage has its components and relations between them, which we explain below.

"Model Stage" consists of developing a graphical representation (i.e. a model) of the surgical procedure as a process. In "Process Modeling" step, a first draft of the model is designed and then is assessed the model experts agreement level through a "Delphi Panel" step. Experts should be doctors who have experience performing the procedure. Both steps are iterative: depending on the level of agreement reached in the "Delphi Panel" the model is modified, to then assess the expert's agreement level with the model again. This stage ends when the level of agreement reached is the desired.

"Data Stage" focus on generating data to analyze surgical procedures as processes. That means creating Event Logs. In order to do so, executions of the procedure are needed, which are commonly captured through video recordings ("Execution and Recording" step). These videos are used for different tasks in medical education, but still is not clear their effectiveness and how to use them [6]. We tag the videos with the activities defined in the model developed in "Model Stage". Tagging videos allow getting the entire sequence of steps of an execution, and therefore an Event Log with all the executions.

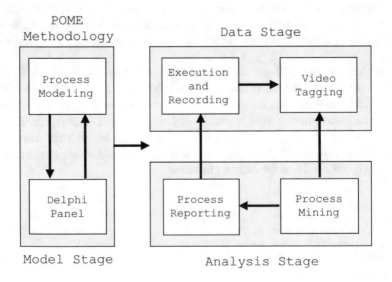

Fig. 14.1 POME methodology overview

In "Analysis Stage" the Event Log generated in "Data Stage" and the model generated in "Model Stage" are used to perform the analysis with Process Mining algorithms. With the information obtained after treating the data, it is possible to create a report ("Process Reporting" step). Designing the report will depend on the goal of the application. However, the main requirement is to create an easy-to-interpret report for doctors.

14.3 Model Stage

14.3.1 Process Modeling

The first step in our methodology is to have a Generic Surgical Process Model of the procedure in analysis. This model has been defined as "a simplified pattern of a medical procedure in a formal or semi-formal representation" [16]. This generic model will not only be useful to have a reference standard to compare the executions made; rather, it is a representation in which the procedure is broken down into sequential steps, decision points and alternative pathways. This breakdown of the procedure has been defined as an input that all procedural training must have [5, 10, 24].

The development of this model is not trivial due to the inherent difficulties of generating process models for the healthcare and medical education domains:

1. Surgical processes show a lot of variability among executions due to the experiences, skills and preferences of the health personnel, the patient's characteristics, and the availability of resources and technology [15, 16].
2. When consulted how they perform a procedure, experts tend to omit relevant information [25]. This omission can reach up to 70% of the steps necessary for a correct execution [21], and it has been attributed to the automation of high levels of expertise [9].
3. An adequate representation of a procedure requires a holistic approach to procedural competence. Whoever performs a procedure must have not only the necessary technical skills but also the skills that ensure the patient's physical and psychological comfort, such as the care necessary to avoid mechanical and infectious complications. Thus, McKinley et al. have defined the following dimensions as necessary components of any representation of a procedure: preparation; infection control; communication and work with the patient; teamwork; security; procedural competence; post-procedure care [13].

In this context, the objective when developing a model for Process-Oriented Medical Education (POME) is to have a model without local or speciality biases, versatile to be applied to different settings and centres, complete from the point of view of having all the technical information necessary for the execution and complete because it includes those steps necessary to obtain a holistic representation of the competencies required for adequate health care.

Thus, the generic process model is obtained in two stages: one is the generation of a first model of the procedure, and second is the validation of the model using the Delphi Methodology. For the first stage, we rely on published checklists for the chosen procedure. A checklist is a list of observable activities or behaviours, organized consistently, that allows an observer to record the performance dichotomously (i.e. done or not) in an assessment context [7]. All published checklists are analyzed in terms of their psychometric validity, their completeness of activities and the presence of the seven dimensions of competence, defined by McKinley [13]. Using the list of activities defined in the checklists as a reference, a representation of the procedure is constructed in BPMN notation, a notation that, in addition to being a de facto standard, has proven to be easily understood by users in the healthcare area [19, 20]. The result of this first stage is a first generic process model, which will be subjected to a validation process that avoids biases of speciality or local practices that make the model little applicable to other health centres or realities. The process is explained below.

14.3.2   Delphi Panel

Delphi methodology has proven to be an effective tool in many disciplines to achieve consensus among experts on a given topic [3, 8]. It is characterized by the anonymous interaction of experts, who in successive and controlled rounds can modify their answers after knowing the answers of the rest of the participants. This interaction concludes when the consolidated responses represent the majority of the group [14]. The realization of the Delphi panel requires a structured characterization and selection of experts. For this purpose, we used the recommendations of Okoli and Pawloski [17]. In our case we define a minimum time of experience in the procedure, a minimum number of monthly executions and additionally meet one of the following characteristics: be the local manager of the procedure, be an accredited instructor, be the head of a service where the procedure is performed frequently or have participated in guides or publications regarding the performance of the procedure.

Once the experts from different specialities and health institutions have been selected, they are invited to participate in an online survey. In the survey, the activities defined in the first model are ordered sequentially, asking the experts to express their agreement with the inclusion of this activity in the final model, through a 5-point Likert scale: (1) under no circumstances should be included, (2) should not be included, (3) may or may not be included, (4) should be included, (5) must be included. Also, they are asked to propose new activities, modify proposed activities, and propose changes to the place they should occupy in the sequence. Once the experts complete the survey, the results obtained for each activity are presented in a second survey, showing them as the percentage obtained by each item on the Likert scale. Also, the new proposed activities are added, and they are asked to express themselves regarding the suggested modifications for any activity. In this

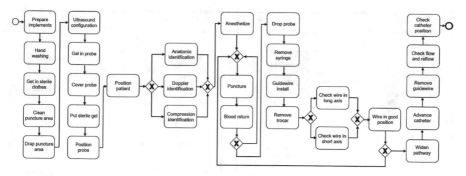

Fig. 14.2 BPMN model of the Central Venous Catheter installation. (Adapted from [2])

second survey, they are again invited to weight the inclusion of each activity in the final model of the procedure based on the same 5-point Likert scale. This sequence is repeated up to a third time if the previously defined agreement criterion is not reached. To ensure the adequate methodological quality, planning and execution of the Delphi panel, it should follow the recommendations of Diamond et al.: a reproducible selection of participants, the definition of a stopping criterion, a maximum number of rounds, and an exclusion criterion for each item [3].

The proposed modelling methodology allows obtaining a representation of the procedure in BPMN notation, based on the information available in publications and subsequently enriched through the consensus of experts from different centres. This mixture of information allows us to have a process model without local or speciality biases that can be applied to analyze. Figure 14.2 shows the model obtained for the running case.

14.4   Data Stage

14.4.1   Execution and Recording

Processes analyzed with Process Mining commonly have an information system behind them, recording all the data generated during their execution. Even when its database is not recording the data with an Event Log shape, it is possible to build them using this data. In [11], these type of processes are called *plugged* processes (left image in Fig. 14.3).

However, some processes are not supported by information systems, because in some parts its execution is not recorded in common databases, is based on hands-on work or involves the mixture of other data sources than common database systems (e.g. paper data or logs, spoken decisions). Process Mining can help to analyze these processes, but creating the Event Log needs a different treatment than *plugged* processes. In [11], these type of processes are called *unplugged* processes (right image in Fig. 14.3).

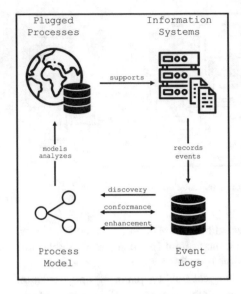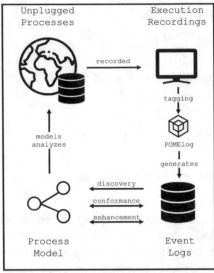

Icons made by Freepik, Pixel perfect, ultimatearm and srip from www.flaticon.com

Fig. 14.3 Process Mining for plugged processes (left) and unplugged processes (right)

How to collect data to analyze *unplugged* processes is the question, and the answer will depend on the context. In the medical training field, execution of surgical procedures commonly are video recorded, so the primary source of data cames from them. In our running case, we uploaded the executions recorded to a platform called POMElog [11], where it is possible to watch the executions and tag the videos with the sequence of activities defined in the "Model Stage" of POME methodology. With POMElog, data is created as Event Logs, and this platform delivers it ready to analyze the data using Process Mining.

14.4.2 Video Tagging

POME methodology involves video tagging as a way to obtain data from videos, which should be done by experts in the surgical procedure in analysis. Because of that, the lack of surgeons experienced and the little available time they have [22] is a challenge that needs to be addressed. In this step, experienced doctors are needed or, at least, doctors well trained in how to execute the procedure. This is crucial to ensure data quality and no-biased results.

Methods to control the bias generation during data collection, as well as methods to generate the Event Logs will depend on the data resource type used. To avoid bias, in our running case, we use the Levenstein distance [1] to decide how different are the tags between different taggers. To generate the Event Logs, we developed

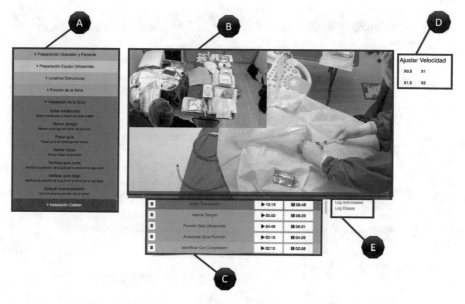

Fig. 14.4 POMElog and features [11]

POMElog, a web-based platform where videos can be tagged and doing so generate the data.

POMElog [11] allow doctors to tag videos in a user-friendly way, because of the features it has. Following Fig. 14.4, POMElog contains all the activities of the model designed in the Model Stage (section A), different views to help the tagger precisely decide which activity is being executed (section B), give the option to select the starting and ending point of time an activity is executed (section C), adjust the speed of the video (section D) and finally export the event log (section E).

14.5   Analysis Stage

Once created the Event Logs, it is time for the "Process Mining" step. Process Mining algorithms receive as input the data, and the chosen algorithm depends on the task of interest. If the objective is to know the common pathway followed by executions of a surgical procedure, Discovery algorithms can be used to see it and its deviations. If the objective is to compare the model generated in the "Model Stage" of POME methodology with data obtained in "Data Stage", Conformance Checking algorithms can help to accomplish this task.

After "Process Mining" step ends, it is necessary to design an easy-to-understand report for doctors. "Process reporting" step consists of showing the results of the last step in a way doctors can understand and use in medical training tasks. The report will vary depending on the objective for what it was generated. Figure 14.5 shows

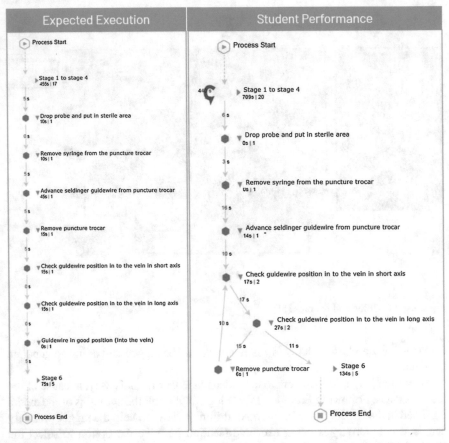

Fig. 14.5 Diagram of the Guidewire Install surgical procedure stage included in the feedback report. The expected execution is shown on the left side and the student's performance is shown on the right side [12]

an example. It was generated using Process Mining as a way to give feedback to students about the sequence mistakes they did during their training [12].

Designing the reports should consider doctors are not expert in Process Mining but healthcare. It is essential to establish requirements for the report, and then test with them if the report accomplishes them. Also, it is crucial to evaluate their understanding and ease of interpretation of the report. With this, the likelihood of use of the application designed will increase. Validation techniques [23] can help on this task (expert opinion, effects analysis, among others).

14.6   Conclusion

This chapter describes the POME methodology, which allows considering the sequence of steps as a point in medical training applications. This methodology proposes a novel strategy to analyze surgical procedures as processes, creating all the elements needed to run a Process Mining project. "Model stage" allows to obtain an abstraction of a surgical procedure, "Data stage" proposes a new way to use videos and obtain data from them, and "Analysis Stage" take in consideration context variables as bias and ease-of-understanding of the information given to doctors. We use the Central Venous Catheter insertion procedure as a running case, showing a successful case of using this methodology. This example encourages the use of Process Mining with other surgical procedures, enabling the development of new tools to the medical training field.

References

1. Cohen WW, Ravikumar P, Fienberg SE. A comparison of string distance metrics for name-matching tasks. In: Proceedings of the 2003 international conference on information integration on the web, IIWEB'03. AAAI Press; Palo Alto, California, USA. 2003; p. 73–8.
2. De La Fuente R, Fuentes R, Munoz-Gama J, Dagnino J, Sepúlveda M. Delphi method to achieve clinical consensus for a BPMN representation of the central venous access placement for training purposes. Int J Environ Res Public Health. 2020;17(11):3889
3. Diamond IR, Grant RC, Feldman BM, Pencharz PB, Ling SC, Moore AM, Wales PW. Defining consensus: a systematic review recommends methodologic criteria for reporting of Delphi studies. J Clin Epidemiol. 2014;67(4):401–9.
4. Fecso AB, Szasz P, Kerezov G, Grantcharov TP. The effect of technical performance on patient outcomes in surgery: a systematic review. Ann Surgery 2017;265(3):492–501.
5. Grantcharov TP, Reznick RK. Teaching procedural skills. BMJ. 2008;336(7653):1129–31.
6. Green JL, Suresh V, Bittar P, Ledbetter L, Mithani S, Allori A. The utilization of video technology in surgical education: a systematic review. J Surg Res. 2019;235:171–80.
7. Hales B, Terblanche M, Fowler R, Sibbald W. Development of medical checklists for improved quality of patient care. Int J Qual Health Care J Int Soc Qual Health Care 2008;20(1):22–30.
8. Hasson F, Keeney S, McKenna H. Research guidelines for the Delphi survey technique. J Adv Nurs. 2000;32(4):1008–15.
9. Hoffman RR.   Human factors contributions to knowledge elicitation.   Hum Factors. 2008;50(3):481–8.
10. Huang GC, McSparron JI, Balk EM, Richards JB, Smith CC, Whelan JS, Newman LR, Smetana GW Procedural instruction in invasive bedside procedures: a systematic review and meta-analysis of effective teaching approaches. BMJ Qual Saf. 2016;25(4):281–94.
11. Leiva L, Munoz-Gama J, Salas-Morales J, Galvez V, Lam Jonathan Lee W, de la Fuente R, Fuentes R, Sepúlveda M. Pomelog: generating event logs from unplugged processes. In: Proceedings of the Dissertation Award, Doctoral Consortium, and Demonstration Track at BPM 2019 co-located with 17th International Conference on Business Process Management (BPM 2019). 2019;2420:189–93.
12. Lira R, Salas-Morales J, Leiva L, de la Fuente R, Fuentes R, Delfino A, Nazal CH, Sepúlveda M, Arias M, Herskovic V, Munoz-Gama J. Process-oriented feedback through process mining for surgical procedures in medical training: The ultrasound-guided central venous catheter placement case. Int J Environ Res Public Health. 2019;16(11):1–21.

13. McKinley RK, Strand J, Ward L, Gray T, Alun-Jones T, Miller H. Checklists for assessment and certification of clinical procedural skills omit essential competencies: a systematic review. Med Educ. 2008;42(4):338–49.

14. Mead D, Moseley L. The use of the Delphi as a research approach. Nurse Res. 2001;8(4):4–23.

15. Müller R, Rogge-Solti A. BPMN for healthcare processes. In: Proceedings of the 3rd central-European workshop on services and their composition (ZEUS 2011); Feb 2011.

16. Neumuth D, Loebe F, Herre H, Neumuth T. Modeling surgical processes: a four-level translational approach. Artif Intell Med. 2011;51(3):147–61.

17. Okoli C, Pawlowski SD. The Delphi method as a research tool: an example, design considerations and applications. Inform Manag. 2004;42(1):15–29.

18. Rojas E, Munoz-Gama J, Sepúlveda M, Capurro D. Process mining in healthcare: a literature review. J Biomed Inform. 2016;61:224–36.

19. Rolón E, Chavira G, Orozco J, Soto JP. Towards a framework for evaluating usability of business process models with BPMN in health sector. Proc Manuf. 2015;3:5603–10.

20. Scheuerlein H, Rauchfuss F, Dittmar Y, Molle R, Lehmann T, Pienkos N, Settmacher U. New methods for clinical pathways-Business Process Modeling Notation (BPMN) and Tangible Business Process Modeling (t.BPM). Langenbeck's Arch Surg. 2012;397(5):755–61.

21. Sullivan ME, Yates KA, Inaba K, Lam L, Clark RE. The use of cognitive task analysis to reveal the instructional limitations of experts in the teaching of procedural skills. Acad Med. 2014;89(5):811–6.

22. Walter AJ. Surgical education for the twenty-first century: beyond the apprentice model. Obstet Gynecol Clin. 2006;33(2):233–6.

23. Wieringa RJ. Design science methodology for information systems and software engineering. Berlin/Heidelberg: Springer; 2014.

24. Wingfield LR, Kulendran M, Chow A, Nehme J, Purkayastha S. Cognitive task analysis: bringing olympic athlete style training to surgical education. Surg Innov. 2015;22(4):406–17.

25. Yates K, Sullivan M, Clark R. Integrated studies on the use of cognitive task analysis to capture surgical expertise for central venous catheter placement and open cricothyrotomy. Am J Surg. 2012;203(1):76–80.

Chapter 15
Interactive Process Mining for Discovering Dynamic Risk Models in Chronic Diseases

Zoe Valero-Ramon and Carlos Fernandez-Llatas

15.1 Introduction

An enormous amount of data is nowadays available thanks to the massive introduction of Electronic Health Records (EHR) in medical systems. This data supposes the witnesses of the patients' journey along the health care pathway. This data by itself does not suppose any significant progress, but it provides a great opportunity for creating new awareness, and allowing more effective and precise treatments. However, data analysis is needed to gain the knowledge to improve, not only the quality of the provided care but also to improve the experience of the patient. Data analytic gives value and meaning to collected data and facilitates personalised decisions enabling a full circle of care around an individual in the personalised medicine paradigm [9]. All these data have been also used to develop health risk models in the preventive medicine approach. Risk Models are statistical tools intended to offer *an individual probability for developing a future adverse outcome in a given time period* [33]. Risk Models are computed in a moment and have validity over time. Risk values of an individual patient, play an important role in the decision taken by health professionals, who decide treatments delivered to patient depending on them. Predictive models and decision support systems, including risk

Z. Valero-Ramon (✉)
Process Mining 4 Health Lab – SABIEN – ITACA Institute, Universitat Politècnica de València, Valencia, Spain
e-mail: zoevara@itaca.upv.es

C. Fernandez-Llatas
Process Mining 4 Health Lab – SABIEN – ITACA Institute, Universitat Politècnica de València, Valencia, Spain

CLINTEC – Karolinska Institutet, Sweden
e-mail: cfllatas@itaca.upv.es

© Springer Nature Switzerland AG 2021
C. Fernandez-Llatas (ed.), *Interactive Process Mining in Healthcare*, Health Informatics, https://doi.org/10.1007/978-3-030-53993-1_15

models for clinical use or diagnostic tools, support health professionals addressing the management of patients with chronic diseases.

There are several definitions for chronic conditions, the World Health Organization (WHO) defines them as diseases of long duration and generally slow progression [35] and other author [6] as having one or more of the following characteristics: they are permanent, leave residual disability, are caused by non-reversible pathological alteration, require special training of the patient for rehabilitation, or may be expected to require a long period of supervision, observation or care. Both definitions agreed in the fact of being of long duration. Some of the chronic diseases with greater impact are coronary heart disease, stroke, many varieties of cancer, depression, diabetes, asthma, chronic obstructive pulmonary disease or hypertension among others. Over 50 million people in Europe have more than one chronic disease, due to either random co-occurrence, possible shared underlying risk profile, or synergies in disease development [29]. Chronic conditions require ongoing management over a period of years or decades, so individuals' behaviour should be taken into consideration.

Personalised medicine approach lays on treatment strategy based on individuals' unique behaviour, moving away from the *one size fits all* approach. Consequently, behind the idea of precision and personalised medicine, there is a need to discover concrete patients' behaviour and individualised models. The adequacy of treatments to categorised patients in a more precise way, not only increases the effectiveness of care pathways but also improves patients' experience of care. Precision medicine cannot only be based on genetic sequencing, or simple stratification founded on collected variables or risk models [10]. This scenario is even more important in the case of chronic diseases, were the continuum of healthcare for patients and population, focused on prevention and management of patients with chronic conditions and/or multiple morbidities is crucial.

While current understanding of risk models relies on models that consider static snapshots of variables or measures, rather than ongoing, dynamic feedback loops of behaviour considering changes and different states. Moreover, diseases are not static, they evolve towards different destinations, especially when talking about chronic health problems. In the same way, the human being is not static, an individual evolves throughout her/his biography in age, lifestyle, socioeconomic status, or intercurrent diseases, and all these aspects affect the patient's evolution. Conventionally, individuals' health modelling, assessment, and management, have been done from a static and time-invariant set of concepts, definitions, and propositions, assuming linear relationships among variables. However, the temporal perspective of the clinical information is crucial for a complete understanding.

Although the main benefits of using risk and prediction models in the healthcare domain are clear, since they are now implemented, do not respond well to unexpected changes in patient's conditions, as they suit standard conditions rather than unusual or unpredictable ones [7]. Individual differences cause great variances in the execution of risk models. In consequence, risk models of chronic conditions should be dynamic, including disease variability and dependencies with other conditions (such as comorbidities, social conditions or age). In this line, Process Mining

Technologies can construct individualised behaviour models [14]. Moreover, there is a rising interest in discovering more accurate stratification groups, that may allow a better care delivery and maximise the process value based on each group conditions [25]. There is a necessity to include health behaviour, mental health, social determinants, and individual preferences to achieve a full precision medicine-based care [17]. Accordingly, there is a concern to stratify individuals built on their behaviour rather than in their disease [2]. Process Mining could also help with this concern.

In this chapter, the authors propose a method for discovering different dynamic risk models for chronic diseases, based on the stratification of individuals' behaviour using the Interactive Process Mining paradigm. As explained in previous chapters, Interactive Process Indicators (IPIs) are Process Indicators produced as a result of the application of interactive paradigm with professionals, therefore, disease dynamic modelling is possible creating the corresponding IPIs, as explained through this chapter. Using this method, we are not also able to discover better models, but also to analyse and study them through Process Mining techniques and tools. These IPIs could be used for a better understanding of medical processes.

15.2   Chronic Conditions

Obesity is nowadays considered a chronic disease which worldwide prevalence has reached a pandemic dimension. The worldwide predominance of overweight and obesity has doubled since 1980 to an extent that nearly a third of the world population is now classified as overweight or obese [1]. WHO defines overweight and obesity as abnormal or excessive fat accumulation that may impair health. Body mass index (BMI) is a simple index of weight-for-height that is commonly used to classify overweight and obesity in adults. It is calculated by dividing a person's weight in kilograms by the square of his/her height in meters (kg/m^2) [36]. WHO also establishes a normal BMI range as 18.5 to 24.9, while a BMI greater than or equal to $25\,kg/m^2$ and below $30\,kg/m^2$ is considered to be overweight, and similarly, a BMI greater than or equal to $30\,kg/m^2$ is classified as obese. However, obesity and overweight are more than a simple excess weight, they are a major risk factor for noncommunicable diseases. Based on literature research, comorbidities known for their association with overweight and obesity are cardiometabolic factors, including risk factors (hypertension, hyperlipidemia and type II Diabetes Mellitus) and cardiovascular diseases (ischemic heart disease, cerebrovascular disease, and peripheral vascular disease), asthma, and musculoskeletal disorders (osteoarthritis of the lower limbs and sciatica) [4, 22, 26]. When a patient is classified as obese, the risk of comorbidities is considered as severe [22]. However, this is not only a question of patient's current state but it is also indeed more important to consider obesity onset, obesity evolution, weight fluctuations, duration of obesity (known as the time since BMI was first known to be at least $30\,kg/m^2$), or even parental BMI to see comorbidities association and treatment [13, 32]. Nevertheless, in real practise, if a patient decreases his/her weight, and, after a re-computation, achieves a normal BMI, automatically all these risks disappear from the actual static care approach.

In summary, the evolution of the risk model is not taken into account. The changes in the individual risk values are usually connected to the behaviours, attitudes, and beliefs of patients. That means, people with the same disease and treated with the same treatment respond in different ways. Knowing the patient as an individual is key to select the best treatment for him or her [37].

Hypertension is another of the well-known chronic conditions. Hypertension, also known as high or raised blood pressure (BP), is a condition in which the blood vessels have persistently raised pressure. Based on WHO information, hypertension is a serious medical condition and can increase the risk of heart, brain, kidney and other diseases. It is a major cause of premature death worldwide, and an estimated 1.13 billion people worldwide have hypertension [34]. Blood pressure is based in two numbers, systolic blood pressure representing the pressure in blood vessels when the heart contracts or beats. And the diastolic blood pressure representing the pressure in the vessels when the heart rests between beats. Hypertension is diagnosed if, when it is measured on two different days, the systolic blood pressure (SBP) readings on both days is 140 mmHg or more, and/or the diastolic blood pressure (DBP) readings on both days is 90 mmHg or more or taking antihypertensive medication [20].

On the other hand, blood pressure shows noticeable oscillations over the short and long term [18]. Short-term fluctuations are these occurring within a 24 h, whereas long-term fluctuations occurring over more-prolonged periods (days, weeks, months, seasons, and even years). These variations are the result of complex interactions between environmental and behavioural factors and cardiovascular mechanisms [24]. It means, these variations over time are important and should be taken into account.

Hypertension is a lifelong disease that is manageable but generally not curable. New technologies now enable patients to generate accurate home-based BP readings that could be stored directly into the electronic medical record. Using more frequent BP measurements in conjunction with assessment of social health determinants and data analytics can be generated more personalised interventions that can improve BP control [21].

15.3 Assessing Chronic Conditions with Risk Models

In the literature, there are several approaches to standardise risk models in medicine using time-stamped data. Knowledge-Based Temporal Abstractions (KBTA or TA) is one of them [27]. TA are mainly methods to achieve a switch from a qualitative time-stamped description of raw data, to a qualitative interval-based representation of time series, intending to abstract high-level concepts from time-stamped data. TA has been used to approach health processes in some areas such as prognosis of the risk for coronary heart disease [23], for defining typical medial abstraction patterns

[5], and for the assessment of costs related to Diabetes Mellitus [11]. Previous works tried to generate an automatic summarising of the patient's current based on his/her data through temporal abstraction. However, the great majority of clinical variables, such as weight, blood pressure or temperature, have numerical results, but TA techniques are based on discrete labels, and in consequence, it is excluding important information from the analysis. Other work in the literature performed a dual approach, using TA in combination with Process Mining for blood pressure and temperature [15].

In this line, other authors suggested the importance of taking into account the full set of behaviours through real-time measurements to create models over time and, in consequence, infer patterns, context, and states of patients, with the ultimate objective of developing personalised interventions [28]. Nonetheless, modelling methodologies rely on predictive strategies rather than the evolution of patient measurements or pathways. Going a step forward, it is needed to implement a data-driven approach capable of discovering patients' behavioural models as temporal and dynamic flows succeeding precision medicine paradigm [10]. With this objective, Data-Driven Models are key for supporting the discovery of individuals' behaviour process [8].

15.4 Interactive Data Rodeo for Creating Dynamic Risk Models

In this section, a complete use case of an Interactive Data Rodeo is described as a proof of concept of the Interactive Process Mining methodology. The main objective of the Interactive Data Rodeo was to obtain dynamic models associated with chronic diseases, concretely to obesity and hypertension. And the ultimate goal was to use these models as IPIs for the understanding, measurement, and optimisation of the processes associated with obesity and hypertension diseases and related interventions, allowing health professionals to navigate behind the models and to discover the specificity of the processes associated with individuals. A complete Data Rode was implemented to obtain a set of IPIs that can be used as indicators for understanding and measuring the behaviour of individuals within obesity and hypertension processes, that can support health professionals in their daily practice regarding these chronic diseases. This was carried out following the flow described in Chap. 9 and which different steps are highlighted in Fig. 15.1.

The implementation of the methodology was performed in a real scenario with real data, using retrospective data of a tertiary hospital in Spain. The corpus considered was collected from real patients. Data were extracted from the EHR of the hospital between 2012 and 2017, from primary care, hospital admissions, emergency, outpatient and morbidity diagnosis services, as described in Table 15.1. All data were anonymised previous to the extraction. In the following sections, there are explained all steps performed within the Data Rodeo flow.

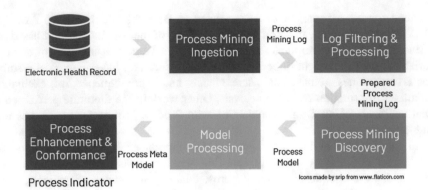

Fig. 15.1 General Data Rodeo Flow

Table 15.1 Data description

Table	Description	Unique patients/observation	Period
Patients Anonymize	General information about patients: age, identifier, some diagnoses	50,196	–
Primary Care	Data collected in primary consultations: variables and annotations	17,853/215,523	2017
Hospital Admissions	Type of admission, ICD9[a], Diagnostics, DRG[b], date	10,403/180,797	2012–2016
Emergency	Severity description, Admission service code, destination service, date	34,054/180,797	2010–2017
Outpatient	Provision type, date	36,667/706,888	2012–2017
Morbidity Diagnoses	ICD9[a] code, diagnose date	48,080/1,048,575	1993–2017

[a]International Statistical Classification and Related Health Problems
[b]Diagnosis-Related Group

As explained in Chap. 9, the process of ingestion is the first step in a Data Rodeo and is in charge of providing the Data Log to start the Process Mining flow. In this concrete case, the hospital experts provided the data in several Comma-Separated Values (CSV) files, concretely one CSV file per table included in Table 15.1, where values were represented in a set of rows and columns. At this point, it was performed the selection of the relevant data for the creation of the corresponding IPIs. As there were established two main chronic diseases under the study, obesity and high blood pressure or hypertension, information was extracted from *Patients Anonymize* and *Primary Care*, which description is included in Tables 15.2 and 15.3 respectively.

At this stage, data were processed to compute the variables that were used for creating events and trace data during the following stage. There were also completed two actions: format corrections and adding new semantic values. Format corrections

Table 15.2 Patients Anonymize description

Column name	Data type	Example
ID_ANON	Global unique identifier	000269d4-b40a-df4f-a1c0-56db3f989ad2
Age Group	Integer – group of age by 5 years	40
Overweight	Integer: 1/0, overweight diagnose	0
Obesity	Integer: 1/0, obesity diagnose	1
Unspecified Overweight or Obesity	Integer: 1/0	1

Table 15.3 Primary Care description

Column name	Data type	Example
ID_ANON	Global unique identifier	000269d4-b40a-df4f-a1c0-56db3f989ad2
Measure Date	String	20170830
Code Measurement	String – type of observation	BMI, Weight, Height, SBP, DBP,. . .
Numerical Result	Floar – result of the measurement	87.5
Text Result	String – indicates void numerical result	Yes/No
Age Group	Integer – group of age by 5 years	45

were applied to *Measure Date* and *Numerical Results*, whereas a new semantic variable for the result was added. The semantic result provides a semantic vision that facilitates the understanding of the chronic condition process semantically. In the case of obesity, it was introduced the BMI semantic result as follows: *Underweight* for BMI numerical result <18.5; *Normal* for BMI between 18.5 and 24.9; *Overweight* or *Pre-Obese* for BMI between 25.0 and 29.9; and *Obese* for BMI greater than 30.

Cut-off points considered for BP were those specified by the American Heart Association (AHA) for the classification of Hypertension [3]. So BP semantic result was introduced as follows: *Normal* for SBP numerical result <120 mmHg and DBP numerical result <80 mmHg; *Elevated* for SBP between 120 and 129 mmHg and DBP <80 mmHg; *Hypertension stage 1* for SBP between 130 and 139 mmHg or DBP 80–89 mmHg; and *Hypertension stage 2* for SBP ≥140 mmHg or DBP ≥90 mmHg.

Event data was composed by the start corresponding to *Measure Date*; the completion time or end adding a second to the start; the name of the node, the identification of the trace, and metadata correlated with the event. The name of the node was based on the BMI and BP semantic results as Named events, defined by the clinicians according to the mapping of the process. The identification of the trace corresponded with the *ID_ANON* and finally, the metadata associated with the event store overweight and obesity diagnoses, *Obesity*, and *Overweight* columns respectively. Whereas the trace data, considered as the set of metadata related to the same case, included the *Age Group*. At this point the Process Mining Log was created and ready for the next stage, Log filtering, and processing.

After creating the Log, the next stage is filtering and processing the data to select the adequate Log for constructing the IPI. At this point, we have applied a different filtering strategy for the two different IPIs, Obesity and Hypertension. In the case of obesity, we have implemented five different filters in the following order. First, void traces were deleted, second, there were selected patients with more than four observations during the period, then traces were sequenced assuming ending of the current trace was the beginning of the next one, fourth a fuse filter was applied to fuse equal traces. At this point, from the 17,853 initial unique patients, there were obtained the flows for 2,260 patients after implementing previous filters. Finally, a clustering filter was used for stratification. The objective was to extract sub-logs from the main log representing a set of subpopulations based on BMI characteristics. We have selected Topological Distance as it maximises the similarity between two traces, concretely *Weighted Topological Distance (WTD)* [14] augments similarity in the topology structures of the inferred workflow. This distance was used with Quality Threshold Cluster (QTC) [12] as the Clustering algorithm. QTC algorithm requires a *quality threshold* to decide the maximum distance among traces in the cluster. At this point, better results arose with a quality threshold of 0.12 for the clustering algorithm and 0.01 of similarity.

A similar strategy was applied in the case of Hypertension, implementing six different filters in the following order. First void traces were deleted, second patients with both SBP and DBP measures at the same moment were selected, third patients with more than four measures during the period were chosen. Fourth, traces were sequenced assuming the ending of the current trace was the beginning of the next one, fifth equal traces were fused. At this time, trace clustering using WTD and QTC was used to obtain sub-populations based on BP behaviour. Better results were achieved for the quality threshold of 0.12 and 0.02 similarity.

Process Mining Discovery phase objective is to obtain the Process Model representing the given model using the appropriate discovery algorithm. PM Discovery algorithm used in this work was PALIA (Parallel Activity Log Inference Algorithm) [16]. PALIA has been widely tested in real healthcare scenarios, such as follow up protocols of patients with diabetes [11], for discovering surgery department flow [16], malnutrition assessment [30], for the characterisation of emergency flows, measuring organisational change effects [19] or obesity modelling [31]. For the experimentation of this work, we have used the implementation of the PALIA algorithm provided by the PMApp tool [19]. After applying the Process Mining Discovery algorithm we obtained the Process Model ready to be processed in the next step.

Model Processing stage's main purpose is to process logs to compute the metadata associated with the model. To create useful dynamic models of chronic conditions is needed to compute the metadata related to the model, for example, two patients could have the same BMI events, but their timing and frequency are completely different. It is the analysis of these differences the key point in the understanding of the dynamical characteristics of the model. PALIA support metadata associated to models in several ways, concretely in this work we have used metadata computed to nodes and edges with statistical information, so we can comprehend how the executions of the models have been performed. This statistical information includes the execution number, the duration average, the duration median, the duration aggregation, the case number and the duration by case. PALIA also supports storing the relationship between the topological structures of the model with the log events, so it is possible to navigate from the model to the individual. This feature helps in the understandability of the model and the trust of the professional in the model. The result of this step was a Process Meta-Model ready for the next stage of the Data Rodeo.

Until this stage, we had been accessing, collecting and processing data, but the interactive paradigm implies not only to extract information but also to present this information to the human experts, in this case to the health professional. This phase supposes the last one in the Data Rodeo flow and its result is the IPI presented to the user. PMApp tool provides a visualisation area joint with enhancement capabilities. Thanks to heat maps we were able to highlight statistical data of the model with colours in nodes and edges. At the end of this stage, two IPIs were produced: the Dynamic Obesity Risk Model and the Dynamic Hypertension Risk Model.

15.4.1   Interactive Process Indicators for BMI and BP

Once all steps of the interactive Data Rodeo were applied, two interactive Process Indicators were obtained: the *Dynamic Obesity Risk Model* and the *Hypertension Dynamic Risk Model*. These two models represent the BMI and BP behaviour of the population considered respectively. The Strategy previously explained for BMI has, as a result, nine different groups plus a set of outliers representing the stratified population in nine well-defined sub-populations with the same BMI behaviour. These nine groups are included in Figs. 15.2–15.10 from the most prevalent dynamic behaviour to the less prevalent.

Figures represent models where, the nodes, have been colored with a gradient that means the median time of stay, and edges have been painted with a gradient symbolizing the number of patients, that, proportionally follow this transition, where gradient scale goes from green (minimum value) to red (maximum value).

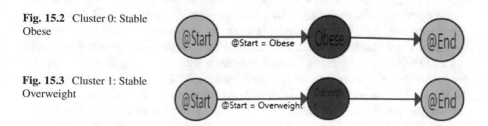

Fig. 15.2 Cluster 0: Stable Obese

Fig. 15.3 Cluster 1: Stable Overweight

Fig. 15.4 Cluster 2:
Increasing Risk

Fig. 15.5 Cluster 3:
Increasing Obesity

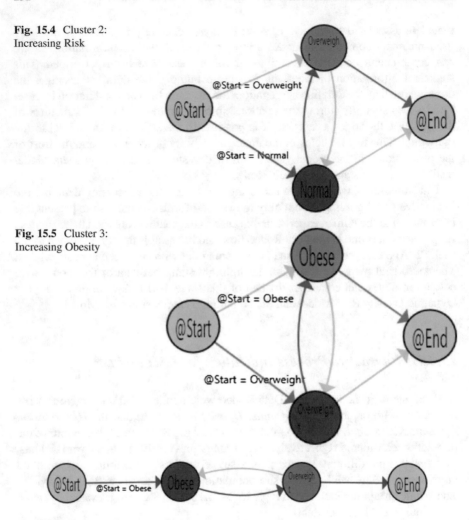

Fig. 15.6 Cluster 4: Decreasing Risk

Within this IPI a two-stratification level is observed, where the first level corresponds with the behaviour in the period, it is increasing, decreasing or stable BMI, since the second level models weight itself. An example of this two-stratification could be seen in cluster 3 (Fig. 15.4), which represents increasing BMI behaviour from normal to the overweight stage, it means an increasing pattern over time.

Following this schema, the most numerous group is the *Stable Obese Risk Model* with 742 patients representing the 32.8% of the population in Fig. 15.2, it is pursued by *Stable Overweight risk model* with 683 patients, 30.2% of the population showed in Fig. 15.3. It means 63% of the considered population was obese or overweight during the period with no changes. The third cluster displays *Increasing Risk Model* (Fig. 15.4), including 269 patients gaining weight during the period from

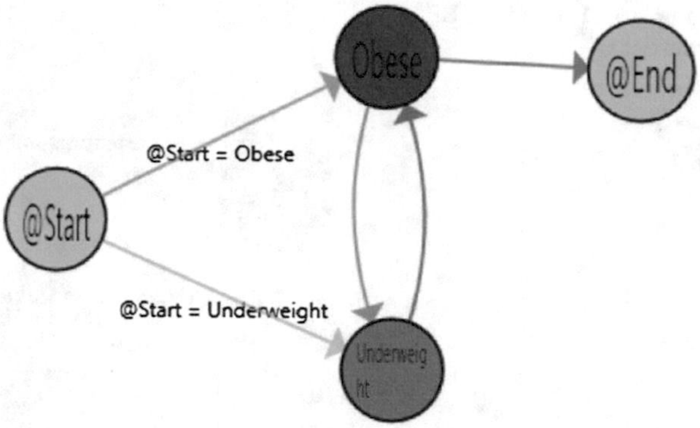

Fig. 15.7 Cluster 5: Possible
errors

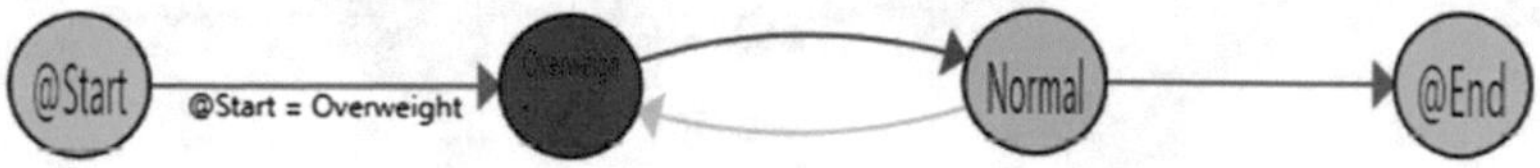

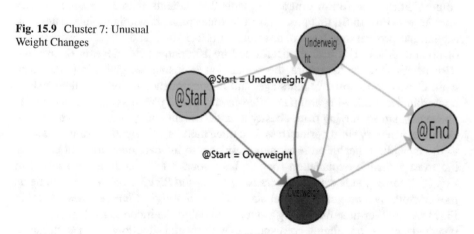

Fig. 15.8 Cluster 6: Decreasing to normal

Fig. 15.9 Cluster 7: Unusual
Weight Changes

Fig. 15.10 Cluster 8: Stable
Normal

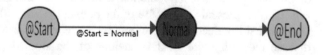

Fig. 15.11 Dynamic BP:
cluster 0

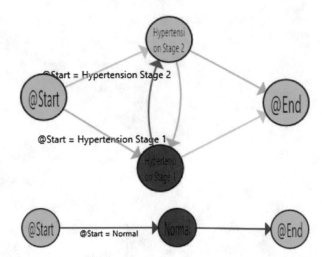

Fig. 15.12 Dynamic BP:
cluster 1

normal to the overweight stage, and consequently also increasing their risk of comorbidities. The fourth group represents 204 patients with *Increasing Obesity Risk Model* (Fig. 15.5), this group also illustrates patients within an increasing risk model, but progressing from overweight to obese stage and worsening their risk of comorbidities. The fifth group formed by 105 patients, represents *Decreasing Risk Model* (Fig. 15.6), where the population is losing weight, slimming down from obesity to the overweight stage, and in consequence decreasing their risk of comorbidities. Following group *Possible errors* with 57 patients (Fig. 15.7), includes obese population moving from obesity to underweight and going back to the initial situation, in a very short period (less than three months). Navigating from the model to the individual, health professionals were able to indicate measurement errors as the most plausible explanation for this behaviour. The seventh group showed in Fig. 15.8, corresponds with the *Decreasing to Normal Risk Model*, where all patients moved from overweight to normal stage. *Unusual Weight Changes Risk Model* in Fig. 15.9, another time navigating from the model to the individuals, health experts detected that this population corresponded with special situations, such as surgeries or pregnancy. Finally, a population with a *Stable Normal Risk Model* included in Fig. 15.10, represents only 1.8% of the population with 40 patients.

This first obtained IPI represents the Dynamic Risk Model for obesity chronic disease modelling the BMI behaviour of the studied population, this means a dynamic obesity stratification based not only on BMI stage in a concrete moment but also and more importantly, on individuals' behaviour over time.

Likewise, the strategy applied for BP generated sixteen groups plus a set of outliers representing the stratified population in sixteen sub-populations with the same BP behaviour. These groups are included in Figs. 15.11–15.26 from the most prevalent dynamic behaviour to the less prevalent.

Figures from 15.11–15.26 also represent models where the nodes have been coloured with a gradient using the median time of stay and edges by the number

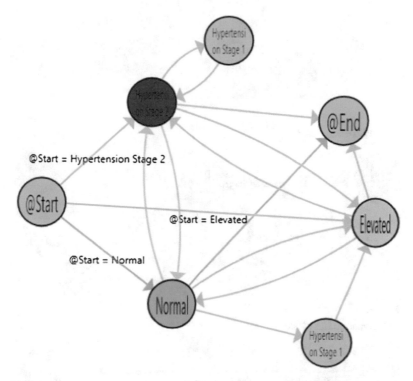

Fig. 15.13 Dynamic BP: cluster 2

of patients, that, proportionally follow this transition, where gradient scale goes from green (minimum value) to red (maximum value). These 16 groups show intrinsic variability of BP, as a continuous variable that fluctuates in response to various physical and mental changes. Nevertheless, obtained groups represent patients' BP behaviour in two-level as in the obesity case. The first level includes the conduct within the period, it is increasing, decreasing, stable and irregular risk models. Whereas the second level includes the different BP stages. With this two-stratification level, we obtained *Stable Risk Models* for normal BP with 335 patients representing only the 9.3% of the studied population (Fig. 15.12) in cluster 1, for hypertension stage 1 with 185 patients (Fig. 15.15) in cluster 4, and hypertension stage 2 with 118 patients (Fig. 15.19) in cluster 8.

Increasing BP Risk Models include cluster 0 (Fig. 15.11) with 655 patients increasing their BP from hypertension stage 1 to stage 2. Cluster 3 (Fig. 15.14) also includes an increasing pattern, with 223 patients moving from elevated and hypertension 1 to hypertension stage 2; cluster 11 (Fig. 15.22) represents a similar behaviour, with 103 patients mainly moving from normal BP to elevated BP or hypertension stage 2. Last, cluster 15 (Fig. 15.26) also includes patients with an increasing risk model, from normal BP to hypertension stage 2. Increasing BP Risk Model represents 29.7% of the population.

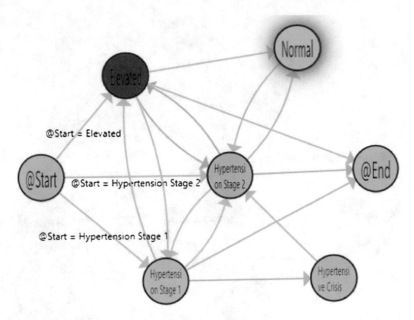

Fig. 15.14 Dynamic BP: cluster 3

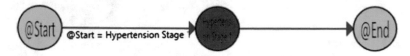

Fig. 15.15 Dynamic BP: cluster 4

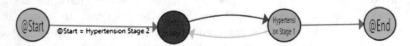

Fig. 15.16 Dynamic BP: cluster 5

Irregular BP Risk Models include patients with constant changes in their BP values, showing they have not well controlled their BP. These groups are: cluster 2 shows 239 patients mainly finalising with normal BP but with long episodes of different hypertension stages illustrating how important is to consider the whole process (Fig. 15.13). Similarly, cluster 13 shows patients the majority of the time with normal BP, but with several episodes of elevated and hypertension stage 2 (Fig. 15.24). The rest of clusters, cluster 7 with 122 patients (Fig. 15.18), cluster 12 with 102 patients (Fig. 15.23) and cluster 14 with 88 patients (Fig. 15.25) are clear examples of patients with decompensated BP with several episodes of different hypertension stages.

Decreasing BP Risk Models are represented by cluster 5 with 146 patients decreasing from hypertension stage 2 to stage 1 (Fig. 15.16). Cluster 6 with 132

Fig. 15.17 Dynamic BP:
cluster 6

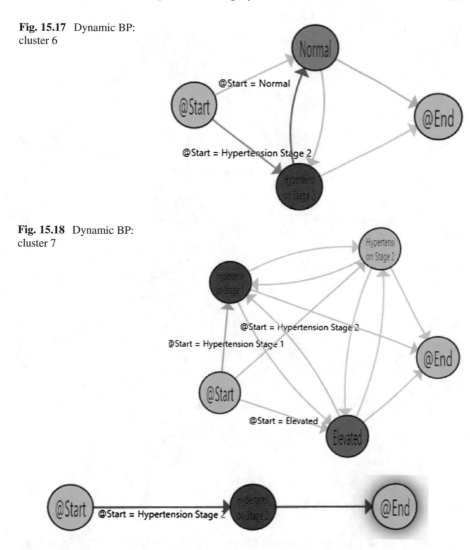

Fig. 15.18 Dynamic BP:
cluster 7

Fig. 15.19 Dynamic BP: cluster 8

patients diminishing their BP from hypertension stage 2 to normal (Fig. 15.17). In cluster 9, there are included 118 patients moving from hypertension stage 2 to elevated BP (Fig. 15.20), whereas in cluster 10 106 patients finalised the period with normal BP although they came from elevated BP (Fig. 15.21).

Once again, this second IPI, the Dynamic Risk Model for Hypertension chronic disease, has allowed the characterisation of the population into sub-groups based on their dynamic BP behaviour, rather than a static classification based on a BP static measure.

Fig. 15.20 Dynamic BP:
cluster 9

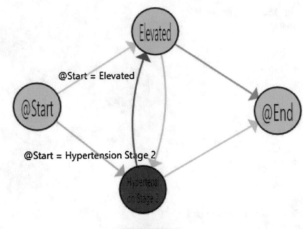

Fig. 15.21 Dynamic BP:
cluster 10

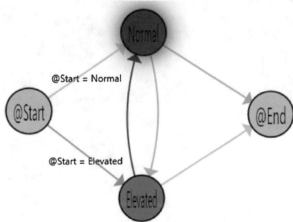

15.5   Discussion and Conclusions

The utilisation of Interactive Process Mining in a concrete health scenario, chronic
disease, through a concrete methodology implementing a Data Rodeo has permitted
to obtain two valuable and innovative Process Indicators that could be used for
understanding and measuring chronic underlying processes. Interactive Process
Mining has the potentiality of presenting findings over data in an understandable
view to health experts so they could find new medical evidence. Moreover, it can
be self-adapted to the population is applied and ca be automated over an emerging
cloud of personal devices, allowing health professionals to analyse individualised
behaviour and to compare current status with past inferred workflows, and to
measure changes in treatments or adherence. The formalisation of the application
of Interactive Process Mining through the Data Rodeos methodology has eased
the generation of the interactive Process Indicators interactively. Thanks to data
analysis interactions between health professionals and Data Rodeo experts, we have

Fig. 15.22 Dynamic BP: cluster 11

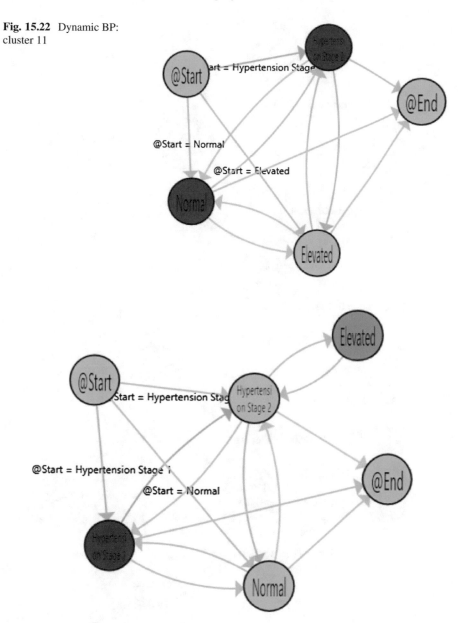

Fig. 15.23 Dynamic BP: cluster 12

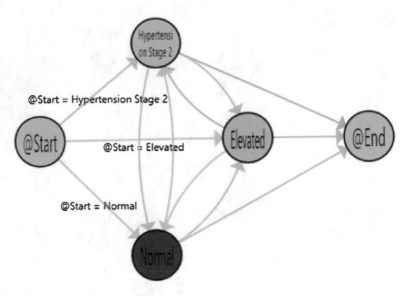

Fig. 15.24 Dynamic BP: cluster 13

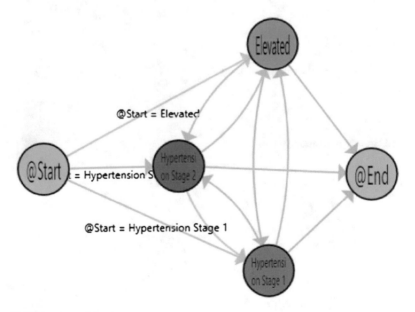

Fig. 15.25 Dynamic BP: cluster 14

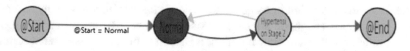

Fig. 15.26 Dynamic BP: cluster 15

transformed raw data coming from a real HER from a tertiary hospital in Spain, in understandable information. As a result, two Dynamic Risk Models have been generated for obesity and hypertension chronic diseases.

On one hand, the Interactive Data Rodeo has permitted to characterise the population dynamically into nine sub-groups with the same BMI behaviour, building the first IPI, the Dynamic Obesity Risk Model. Three behaviour patterns were discovered within this IPI, one for patients with a stable BMI pattern, but two other models for population changing their BMI during the studied period, showing increasing and decreasing models. This finding could be very relevant for health professionals as it shows how the population could by stratify based on their weight evolution rather than in an isolated BMI data, and treat them in consequence. If we consider two patients from two different sub-groups of the Dynamic Obesity Risk Models, the first one from Stable Overweight (Fig. 15.3) and the second one from Decreasing Risk (Fig. 15.6) groups; they have the same BMI at the end of the period, it is Overweight, but their behaviours are different. In a classic and static approach, the only insight is the BMI result, nevertheless, this IPI let us consider other dimensions of the problem. The first patient has not made any improvement in her/his health status at any moment, consequently, the patient is probably not well-engaged with diet counselling or not properly motivated. On the other hand, the second patient is losing weight, she or he is doing things well and treatment is working. Therefore, interventions should not be the same for these two patients to succeed in their weight loss. In the first case, health professionals should influence general health behavioural changes or deep in what other things could be influencing the patient so weight loss is not happening. Whereas in the second case, they should continue to motivate the patient and maximise correct attitudes. This IPI has allowed the classification of the population regarding dynamic weight behaviour and has shown insights in an understandable way. With this information, health professionals could put in practice concrete and personalised interventions in specific groups trying to influence in particular behaviours.

On the other hand, we were even capable, working in close collaboration with health professionals, to discover measure errors and unusual weight changes sub-groups. Health professionals were able to navigate from the model to the individuals of these clusters to analyse the population characteristics of these groups to avoid errors that will continue occurring or what kid population is suffering from this unusual weight changes. These facts showed the potentiality of the interactive paradigm.

In the case of blood pressure, following the Data Rodeo methodology a second IPI was obtained, the Dynamic Hypertension Risk Model. This IPI reflects BP variability and fluctuation in response to various changes, this is why hypertension flows have more spaghetti effect than obesity flows. By analysing IPI groups health professionals could infer if common BP behaviours have associated common population characteristics or patterns. The Dynamic Hypertension Risk Model has presented sixteen different sub-groups with population BP continuum and evolution. Once again, health professionals could compare different groups' BP evolution, personalise interventions for the different groups and test their efficacy and effectiveness over time.

Even more, at that point the application of a Data Rodeo allowed us to combine both chronic conditions analysis, obesity and hypertension. We considered the IPI for the Dynamic Obesity Risk Models, and we implemented a new Data Rodeo to obtain BP flows for each group, intended to discover differences in BP flows among the different BMI behaviours. This second round for the Data Rodeo run very fast, as we started from the knowledge acquired in the first data analysis.

Figures 15.27–15.30 represent four insights of BP' dynamic evolution for four different groups of the Dynamic Obesity Risk Model. Figure 15.27 shows how normal BMI population is within a normal BP stage, both in duration and path, although with some hypertension episodes. Whereas the population with a Stable Obese Risk Model clearly shows different dynamic behaviour for BP (Fig. 15.28). Within this group, patients followed a hypertension flow, spending most of the time in the elevated BP stage. Following the example, we can look at BP evolution for an increasing weight group, concretely the Increasing Overweight Risk Model. This model includes the population increasing their obesity risk, moving from normal weight to overweight. Figure 15.29 illustrates BP flow for this population, highlighting that although the most common path is normal BP, the population included in this risk model is experimenting long episodes of hypertension stage 1, applying median to duration time spent per node. This situation endorses the fact that excess weight is translated into a higher risk of hypertension. Looking into a decreasing weight group, in Fig. 15.30 is presented the dynamic BP flow for Decreasing Risk Model. The flow shows that patients spent most of the time in Hypertension stage 1, followed by stage 2. Although patients are losing weight, the effects of this improvement on their health status have not yet been noticed on BP. This could mean weight loss benefits might be visible when this deficit is maintained over time or with a more drastic weight reduction.

Chronic conditions should be approached following personalised medicine considering several and complementary dimensions, social determinants, inter-relationships between diseases and health behaviours among others, to achieve the best treatment strategy for each patient, therefore patient's unique behaviour should be considered. This relies on a concern of stratification groups and risk models established on behaviours and dynamic evolution rather than in static measures or predictions. Indeed, health variables are dynamic by themselves, and diseases not only vary over time but also are dependent on previous stages, behaviours, and conditions. However, current risk models for chronic diseases are far from dynamic flows, they have been approached by a static and time-invariant set of concepts inferring linear relationships among variables. Moreover, the massive data available

Fig. 15.27 Dynamic BP flow for Stable Normal BMI Risk Model

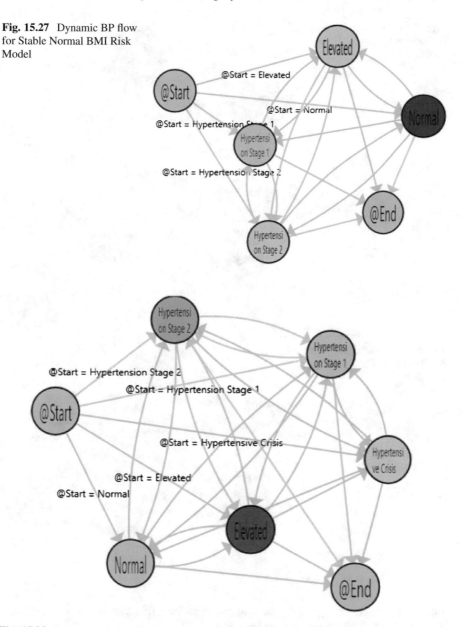

Fig. 15.28 Dynamic BP flow for Stable Obese BMI Risk Model

Fig. 15.29 Dynamic BP flow
for Increasing Risk BMI Risk
Model

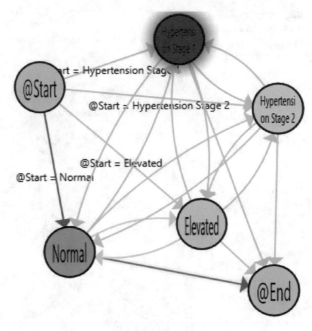

Fig. 15.30 Dynamic BP flow
for Decreasing Risk BMI
Risk Model

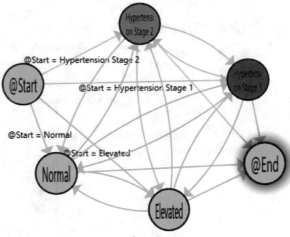

nowadays supposes a great opportunity to transform this data into understandable information for health professionals.

In this chapter, we have implemented a complete Data Rodeo following Interactive Process Mining methodology to build two different IPIs for two chronic conditions, obesity and hypertension, with the ultimate goal of understanding, quantifying and qualifying obesity and hypertension processes. These two IPIs represent the Dynamic Obesity Risk Model and the Dynamic Hypertension Risk

Model respectively and let us go a step ahead in the area of risk modelling inferring real processes behind data.

References

1. Afshin A, Sur PJ, Fay KA, Cornaby L, Ferrara G, Salama JS, Mullany EC, Abate KH, Abbafati C, Abebe Z, et al. Health effects of dietary risks in 195 countries, 1990–2017: a systematic analysis for the global burden of disease study 2017. The Lancet. 2019;393(10184):1958–72.
2. Alvarez C, Rojas E, Arias M, Munoz-Gama J, Sepúlveda M, Herskovic V, Capurro D. Discovering role interaction models in the emergency room using process mining. J Biomed Inform. 2018;78:60–77.
3. American Heart Association. Understanding blood pressure readings, May 2020.
4. Audureau E, Pouchot J, Coste J. Gender-related differential effects of obesity on health-related quality of life via obesity-related comorbidities: a mediation analysis of a French nationwide survey. Circ Cardiovasc Qual Outcomes. 2016;9(3):246–56.
5. Balaban M, Boaz D, Shahar Y. Applying temporal abstraction in medical information systems. Ann Math Comput Teleinform. 2003;1(1):56–64.
6. Bernstein AB. Health care in America: trends in utilization. Center for Disease Control and Prevention, National Center for Health Statistics, 2004.
7. Campbell H, Hotchkiss R, Bradshaw N, Porteous M. Integrated care pathways. BMJ. 1998;316(7125):133–7.
8. Chambers DA, Feero WG, Khoury MJ. Convergence of implementation science, precision medicine, and the learning health care system: a new model for biomedical research. JAMA 2016;315(18):1941–2.
9. Chouvarda IG, Goulis DG, Lambrinoudaki I, Maglaveras N. Connected health and integrated care: toward new models for chronic disease management. Maturitas. 2015;82(1):22–7.
10. Collins FS, Varmus H. A new initiative on precision medicine. N Engl J Med. 2015;372(9):793–5.
11. Concaro S, Sacchi L, Cerra C, Stefanelli M, Fratino P, Bellazzi R. Temporal data mining for the assessment of the costs related to diabetes mellitus pharmacological treatment. In: AMIA annual symposium proceedings. vol. 2009. American Medical Informatics Association; 2009. p. 119.
12. Danalis A, McCurdy C, Vetter JS. Efficient quality threshold clustering for parallel architectures. In: 2012 IEEE 26th international parallel and distributed processing symposium. IEEE; 2012. p. 1068–79.
13. Everhart JE, Pettitt DJ, Bennett PH, Knowler WC. Duration of obesity increases the incidence of NIDDM. Diabetes. 1992;41(2):235–40.
14. Fernández-Llatas C, Benedi J-M, García-Gómez JM, Traver V. Process mining for individualized behavior modeling using wireless tracking in nursing homes. Sensors. 2013;13(11):15434–51.
15. Fernandez-Llatas C, Sacchi L, Benedi JM, Dagliati A, Traver V, Bellazzi R. Temporal abstractions to enrich activity-based process mining corpus with clinical time series. In: IEEE-EMBS international conference on biomedical and health informatics (BHI). IEEE; 2014. p. 785–8.
16. Fernandez-Llatas C, Valdivieso B, Traver V, Benedi JM. Using process mining for automatic support of clinical pathways design. In: Data mining in clinical medicine. New York: Springer; 2015. p. 79–88.
17. Glasgow RE, Kwan BM, Matlock DD. Realizing the full potential of precision health: the need to include patient-reported health behavior, mental health, social determinants, and patient preferences data. J Clin Transl Sci. 2018;2(3):183–5.

18. Grassi G, Bombelli M, Brambilla G, Trevano FQ, Dell'Oro R, Mancia G. Total cardiovascular risk, blood pressure variability and adrenergic overdrive in hypertension: evidence, mechanisms and clinical implications. Curr Hypertens Rep. 2012;14(4):333–8.
19. Ibanez-Sanchez G, Fernandez-Llatas C, Martinez-Millana A, Celda A, Mandingorra J, Aparici-Tortajada L, Valero-Ramon Z, Munoz-Gama J, Sepúlveda M, Rojas E, et al. Toward value-based healthcare through interactive process mining in emergency rooms: the stroke case. Int J Environ Res Public Health. 2019;16(10):1783.
20. Joint National Committee on Detection, Treatment of High Blood Pressure, and National High Blood Pressure Education Program. Coordinating Committee. Report of the joint national committee on detection, evaluation, and treatment of high blood pressure. National Heart, Lung, and Blood Institute, National High Blood Pressure . . . ; 1995.
21. Milani RV, Bober RM, Milani AR. Hypertension management in the digital era. Curr Opin Cardiol. 2017;32(4):373–80.
22. Must A, Spadano J, Coakley EH, Field AE, Colditz G, Dietz WH. The disease burden associated with overweight and obesity. JAMA. 1999;282(16):1523–9.
23. Orphanou K, Stassopoulou A, Keravnou E. DBN-extended: a dynamic Bayesian network model extended with temporal abstractions for coronary heart disease prognosis. IEEE J Biomed Health Inform. 2015;20(3):944–52.
24. Parati G, Ochoa GE, Lombardi C, Bilo G. Assessment and management of blood-pressure variability. Nat Rev Cardiol. 2013;10(3):143.
25. Porter ME, Teisberg EO. Redefining health care: creating value-based competition on results. Boston: Harvard Business Press; 2006.
26. Schienkiewitz A, Mensink GBM, Scheidt-Nave C. Comorbidity of overweight and obesity in a nationally representative sample of German adults aged 18–79 years. BMC Public Health 2012;12(1):658.
27. Shahar Y. A framework for knowledge-based temporal abstraction. Artif Intell. 1997;90(1):79–133.
28. Spruijt-Metz D, Hekler E, Saranummi N, Intille S, Korhonen I, Nilsen W, Rivera DE, Spring B, Michie S, Asch DA, et al. Building new computational models to support health behavior change and maintenance: new opportunities in behavioral research. Transl Behav Med. 2015;5(3):335–46.
29. Struckmann V, Snoeijs S, Melchiorre MG, Hujala A, Rijken M, Quentin W, van Ginneken E. Caring for people with multiple chronic conditions in Europe. EuroHealth. 2014;20(3):35–40.
30. Valero-Ramon Z, Fernandez-Llatas C, Martinez-Millana A, Traver V. A dynamic behavioral approach to nutritional assessment using process mining. In: 2019 IEEE 32nd international symposium on computer-based medical systems (CBMS). IEEE; 2019. p. 398–404.
31. Valero-Ramon Z, Fernandez-Llatas C, Martinez-Millana A, Traver V. Interactive process indicators for obesity modelling using process mining. In: Advanced Computational Intelligence in Healthcare-7. Berlin/Heidelberg: Springer; 2020. p. 45–64.
32. Wannamethee SG, Shaper AG, Walker M. Overweight and obesity and weight change in middle aged men: impact on cardiovascular disease and diabetes. J Epidemiol Community Health. 2005;59(2):134–9.
33. Whittemore AS. Evaluating health risk models. Stat Med. 2010;29(23):2438–52.
34. World Health Organization. Hypertension; Mar 2020.
35. World Health Organization. Noncommunicable diseases; May 2020.
36. World Health Organization. Obesity and overweight; Mar 2020.
37. Ziegelstein RC. Perspectives in primary care: knowing the patient as a person in the precision medicine era. Ann Fam Med. 2018;16(1):4–5.

Chapter 16
Interactive Process Mining-Induced Change Management Methodology for Healthcare

Gema Ibanez-Sanchez and Martin R. Wolf

16.1 Towards an Interactive Change Management Model in Value-Based Healthcare

The life expectancy of world's population is increasing vertiginously. This is accompanied by a growth of chronical diseases, especially among older adults, which has a direct impact on the health systems around the world. In consequence, every major economy struggles with rising healthcare costs, and the necessity of finding ways to assure sustainability of the healthcare systems.

A widely known paradigm is the approach of Value-Based Health Care [43]. Its main objective is to provide value to the patient through better care, at lower costs, resulting in better health. This is generally possible by means of an optimization of existing resources, which implies a global change in healthcare organizations at all levels – not only organizationally but also individually.

The Digital Transformation of healthcare is one of the options to facilitate this shift. In a world with many data sources (mobile, HIS, IoT, wearables...), Big Data technologies [36, 45] might help to interpret this data to analyse the current situation and to find ways to move forward. However, these techniques, in some cases, can act as *black boxes*, where an health expert is not able to understand how a result was obtained, or which criteria were used to achieve the results. These are critical questions that cannot be answered by those traditional *black box* approaches,

G. Ibanez-Sanchez (✉)
Process Mining 4 Health Lab – SABIEN – ITACA Institute, Universitat Politècnica de València, Valencia, Spain
e-mail: geibsan@itaca.upv.es

M. R. Wolf
Faculty of Electrical Engineering and Information Technology FH, Aachen University of Applied Sciences, Aachen, Germany
e-mail: m.wolf@fh-aachen.de

© Springer Nature Switzerland AG 2021
C. Fernandez-Llatas (ed.), *Interactive Process Mining in Healthcare*, Health Informatics, https://doi.org/10.1007/978-3-030-53993-1_16

which is one of the reasons, why these approaches have not been well accepted by the medical community. In particular, health experts need to trust information technology which can be ensured by transparency in all aspects of the technology usage, especially when it might have any negative impact on the patients' health. In consequence, adequate visual tools and methodologies are needed to support healthcare professionals to understand the results of Big Data applications and to transfer this newly generated knowledge into practical activities. Nonetheless, this implies not only a radical change for the used tools and technologies, but also for the mindset of healthcare professionals and its culture *data value* (most medical professionals see the logging of data as a waste of time that distracts them from the care of their patients) [36], and the coordination among teams that are usually hardly able to adopt new approaches in a timely manner [22, 32].

There are methodologies and/or paradigms that try to help on identifying improvements in health organizations and driving changes, such as Lean Six Sigma [54]. Such methods have been successfully applied in other fields and are now being adopted to the healthcare environment [8, 17]. One of these approaches is a combination of Lean Thinking and Six Sigma, where the first part is a dynamic, knowledge-driven and patient-centred process (flow focused) through which all people in a defined organization continuously eliminate waste and create value, being more effective by doing many small improvements. The second one is a more data and process-based approach (problem-focused) resulting in dramatic improvements in service quality and patient satisfaction, by refining system's output if variations in all processes inputs can be reduced. Then, the common purpose of both is to reduce variability and waste through the identification of issues, their prioritization and the proposition of changes to fix them. Nevertheless, changes usually result in resistance [58]. Typical comments associated with resistance are *"Why should we change if we already have a solution in place?"*, *"I don't have time"*, or *"I won't be able to understand it"*, being one of the main barriers contributing to its low penetration. Concretely, Lean Six Sigma has a failure rate between 60% and 70% [56], being very hard to implement and sustain. Researches highlight several barriers and possible obstacles to change [12, 34]. One of its reasons is that multiple stakeholders with different perspectives and priorities are involved which makes collaboration more difficult and results in resistance, even if it is obvious that proposed tools and techniques could provide improvements. Other barriers in the adoption of Lean Six Sigma in healthcare are the lack of leadership, engagement of senior leaders, the understanding of what it is and how it may benefit organizations, and appropriate culture [1, 16, 35]. These barriers can only be reduced at the level of individuals' behaviour because they are the basis of each organization and of the Lean approach. Lean Six Sigma also supports the coordination of individual's relation, supported by effective communication, which is needed to deal with these pitfalls. Furthermore, shared goals and knowledge enable visibility of the overall work process and the linkages between different jobs, facilitating employees' alignment. Whereas, it arises other concerns related to the dilemma between personal feelings, attitude and perceptions against team views (experience).

There are several more aspects that need to be taken into account at the time of leading a change. Although Lean Six Sigma provides insights to deal with, it is more focused on reducing waste and variability and there are other concepts, like Change Management, heavily focused on driving organizations through changes. Nonetheless, Change Management, firstly, is based on exploring organization's effectiveness and on examining the process of organization development [57]. Furthermore, Change Management contributes specific models, tools and techniques to prepare and support individuals and organisations to successfully adopt changes in order to drive organizational success, and to work on reducing resistance to carry out this change process shortly and smoothly [23, 41]. Change of individual behaviour is the centre of every change achievement in organizations. The behaviour of a person is influenced by her/his personality and context, having concrete expectancies related to change, and affecting their performance and effort into the adoption of it. Once individuals are motivated to do something, the organization is ready to embrace any change. But somehow, individuals are ruled by the norms of the groups they belong to, and in many cases, those groups are interconnected composing a whole system – so, this effort is not trivial at all.

Learning processes of acquiring knowledge that lead to behavioural changes are part of individual changes, in which the performance of the person will be reduced in certain phases. There are several models about the phases of a change process from a psychodynamic point of view that usually run from a first shock or denial phase up to a final phase of acceptance. The best known model [31] on these phases, where most of other models are based on, is presented in the Fig. 16.1. In general, people facing as change run through these phases successively.

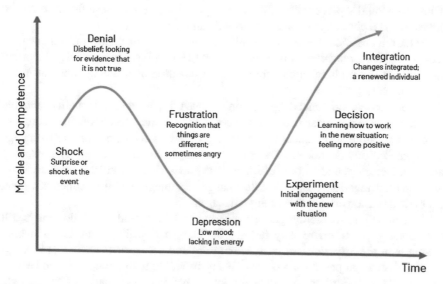

Fig. 16.1 The process of change and adjustment based on [31]

In this transition, individuals can feel learning or survival anxieties that, in a professional environment, could take the form of fear to temporary incompetence, punishment for incompetence, loss of personal identity or loss of group membership. Survival anxiety must be greater than learning anxiety but learning anxiety must be reduced rather than increasing survival anxiety. So, how to reduce learning anxiety? For example, the individual could be smoothly introduced to the change, then might agree with it, get trained, feel more involved in the process, follow positive role models, or even have a coach. Albeit, these are actions need to be guided by an expert.

The emphasis is on a healthy development, authentic relationships and healthy organizations, believing that people want to continue learning, which leads us to a set of guidelines and techniques for this purpose. Starting at the individual level, literature [13] proposes five areas to pay attention to achieve a positive response to change. These are (1) nature of the change (2) persons who benefit in the change (3) organizations that handle the change (culture) [50]; (4) types of personality of each individual, and (5) previous individual experience.

Teams are also a key pillar in organizational life to accomplish complex tasks. There are different types of organizational teams, each with significant benefits and downsides. Additionally, when a team is working in uncertainty, greater teamwork is needed. But not only this is a matter of managing a team, the team must also be effective. Here five elements have been identified that contribute to team's effectiveness, which are: define a team goal and a plan for it, identify roles, procedures, interpersonal relationships and inter-team relations at the organizational level. At that point, resistance can be faced in different ways, like feeling insecure and worried, feeling of loss of prestige, or not feeling involved in the change process. Thus, individual's personality [38] might also influence and be influenced by the team, so it is a challenge balance teams with all these aspects.

At the organizational level, it is highly significant to identify how the organization works, e.g. like a machine, or like an organism [21, 42], but it is especially important to point out the political map behind the organization as a crucial element in the change process [49].

Acceptance is influenced by person's behaviour, her/his personality, and the context in which it is located, and it is necessary to facilitate its conditions in order to gain best possible acceptance. However, if people lack the right mindset to change and organizations do not set strategies to manage and embrace the change, they are even though bound to fail (readiness level for a change) [59]. Here individual, team and organizational aspects of the changes are integrated into a coherent whole, enabling a framework for this change management.

Although these methodologies are diverse and widespread, their adoption is still low. Some aspects where they fail are the lack of objective data, being mainly obstacles in the *situation analysis*, *monitoring* and *assessment* phases. It is a key aspect of being prepared for a change, being critical to assess the nature and extent of its effects [2]. Furthermore, data are not always ready for analysis, which might lead to more time, extra costs and efforts, being translated into a slow and frustrating process [14]. Usually classical models (surveys, questionnaires, interviews...) are used [20] to measure the evolution of changes, which are based on subjective data coming from end-users (patients) resulting in a tremendous effort when trying to synthesize the information gathered to evaluate the effectiveness of the changes applied. It entails a considerable investment of energy and resources, resulting in evaluations that need more time than expected. In consequence responsible persons do not know if the change is going to be effective enough or not, and cannot react in time, which leads in many cases to the failure of the project.

With that purpose, Interactive Process Mining (IPM) is proposed as an instrument to alleviate this crucial aspect of data analysis as it has been demonstrated that Interactive Pattern Recognition models converge better and quicker than other do [19]. From available computerized data, Interactive Process Mining enables process discovery automation, which reduces considerably the invested effort in the identification of the processes. It offers medical experts a direct understanding of it by allowing them to navigate into the different levels of data, offering a high granularity, until to figure out the root cause of issues, being possible to apply their experience and knowledge and modify the processes accordingly in an interactive and iterative way. Interactive Process Mining is able to measure objectively changes, before, during and after any optimization, to identify an initial starting point, its evolution, its (in) effectivity and reasons for that, from top to bottom and from bottom to up.

IPM appears to offer a completely pragmatic approach, which does not mean that it does not take advantage of the benefits that others have. In this chapter, we propose a knowledge-based change management methodology (Fig. 16.2) to improve healthcare organizations based on Interactive Process Mining as the tool and, with this, are going promote the real digital health transformation in health organizations.

The proposed methodology has the objective of creating a team-based problem-solving culture, encouraging digital health transformation in healthcare organizations to elevate the value chain. In this system health professionals become 'Augmented Intelligence' through practical solutions that are provided by Interactive Process Mining.

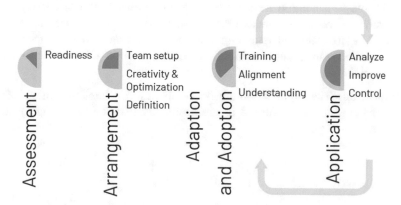

Fig. 16.2 Interactive Process Mining-informed change management methodology for healthcare

16.2 Interactive Process Mining-Informed Change Management Methodology for Healthcare

The proposed methodology is thought to support health organizations to develop change culture mindset, while introducing IPM in its daily practice. Existing clinical evidences indicate which could be a better practices, but IPM allows investigating organization reality and providing evidences in a fast and agile way (who, how, when, why, where...). Following a painless process, where health professionals pass from the learning to hands-on phase in a transparent way, so that the methodology is presented in following four phases:

- **Assessment**. The Assessment phase comprises the first contact with the health organization, where professionals driving the change need to know how the organisation is really working and which barriers could exist that might obstruct the change.
- **Arrangement**. When the main stakeholder who are driving the change know all ins and outs of the organization, it is time to present the rules and frames in which the change need to be implemented. The Arrangement phase is a flexible phase that takes into account the complexity and necessities of the organization and provides a general overview of the scope of the project and steps to follow. This phase should introduce IPM to make health professionals get familiar with the new working philosophy.
- **Adaptation and Adoption**. Having identified key success factors of the change in the previous phase, the Adaption and Adoption phase takes them into account, facilitating the entry of IPM in the organization gradually. The guidelines established in the previous phase, help everyone involved in the change process, to be clear about the role and how to act, reducing the risk of abandonment. At the same time, IPM initiates an adaptation process divided into shakedown, research, and production stages, and which results in:

  - training health experts in the use of the solution proposed by IPM,
  - adapting IPM to special use cases and the corresponding domain until obtaining meaningful information in a format that health professionals can easily understand (Interactive Process Indicators) to make decisions, and
  - reaching a deeper understanding of medical data through IPM, which then can be applied at the point of care and/or the identification of improvements in the organization.

- **Application**. The Application phase comprises the implementation of any new change process identified in the health organization to provide value to patients.

16.3 The Team

The team behind the methodology (Fig. 16.3) is lead by a switch manager, who initiates and leads the change into the organization. As it has been introduced in the previous chapter about Data Rodeos, IT professionals work closely together with the Interactive Process Miner to make available the data needed. The Interactive Process Miner is in charge of forming a multidisciplinary team with medical experts to generate a symbiosis wherein the Interactive Process Miner is able to comprehend the data coming from the hospital. Then, (s)he can connect data with the PM tool and turn it into information, which is interpreted by health team, enabling decision making. Health experts can be managers, directors, heads of unit, clinicians, which can be doctors, and nurses and IT professionals. Albeit every stakeholder has her/his concerns, there should be a common understanding of the general objective followed by the organization, in which a combination of different interests could coexist. I.e. managers, directors, and/or heads are more focused on measuring Quality of Service, crossing services, or doctors that have medical knowledge that can apply in their daily practice to change treatments and improve patients' health, without forgetting nurses that have know-how about real operations in hospitals.

16.4 Assessment Phase

This phase is essential to set foundations of a propitious environment for the transformation. The main objective of this phase is to state the readiness level of the health organization for the change, utilizing stakeholder maps, where to identify people that can resist or foster the change.

The first step is to have informal meetings, starting with the person who leads the change and the management of the organization that in some cases might be

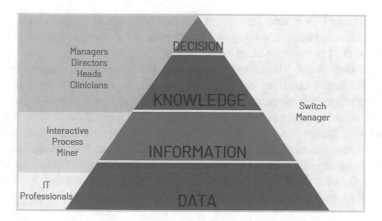

Fig. 16.3 The team behind the interactive model

the same person, being of paramount importance to get management support. For that purpose, the premises in which the transformation is done is introduced to the management team, how it is going to be implemented in the health organization, presenting the methodology, tools, techniques and structure of the plan to be executed. Furthermore, it is appropriate to agree on an additional time that health team should dedicate to the current change process and if a reward strategy is needed.

The switch manager carries it out, asking key questions, thus being able to identify medical staff that should participate. The meetings should be done one by one, maybe taking coffee in a relaxed environment, to figure out the real functioning and dynamics of what happens in the health organization, experiencing the environment. These are the actual day-to-day activities carried out by individuals, processes followed, pressures, expectations and concerns. Likewise, structure, systems and policies in place, basically how things are formally organized, but most important are all unwritten activities that emerge over time such as power, influence, culture or norms. This information allows aligning driving forces towards change as well as outputs as the target, policies, procedures, rules, communication, team, or resources (not only at the human level but also at the monetary and time).

16.4.1 Readiness Assessment

The *readiness assessment* is supposed to be done for internal use only. Gathered information should not be shared with the organization. For this reason, information inquiry should not take place with the use of any questionnaire or with provided assessment overview (because otherwise the results of the inquiry would be requested by the customer). However, the assessment criteria should be used to ask the right questions during preparing meetings, to structure the answers and to generate summarizing results. Areas that should be covered during the assessment phase are the following:

- **Management Support.** The extent management agrees to and (actively) supports the new changes. Management Support is the most important driver (or preventer) of any change in an organization.
- **Target Definition.** The extent targets are clearly defined, communicated and accepted in the organization. Optimally targets are defined in the scope of an aligned strategy. Well-defined strategy and targets ensure that health professionals are used to aligning and following changes and innovations.
- **Processes Definition.** The extent processes and standardized proceedings are defined and followed in the organization. Well-defined processes ensure – on the one hand – that medical experts are used to aligning proceedings (i.e. at changes) and follow these defined standards. On the other hand, permanently defined processes may increase the resistance to change these processes.

- **Communication Level.** The extent relevant information is shared within the health organization. A good level of internal communication ensures that changes are discussed and aligned with personal work processes. Fast communication structures help to rapidly adopt innovations within an organization – *Exception.* In some organizations, the focus is on negative communication (e.g. gossip). In these cases, communication may slow down and hinder innovation.
- **People Involvement.** The extent medical teams are (voluntarily or with pleasure) involved in (organizational) decisions of the health organization. If health professionals can participate in decisions of an organization, they feel involved and are more willing to accept the decisions. This affects also the acceptance of a change, any driving forces of a change and, thus, the speed of introducing innovations.
- **Overall Performance.** The overall performance of the health organization, not just financially but also considering all relevant Performance Indicators. A good overall performance is an indicator of effective organizational structures, processes, communication and employees. Thus, it is a summary of the above-mentioned criteria. It also displays a certain level of satisfaction (unless the pressure to perform is insanely high), but also a certain extent of resisting forces (*why should we change?*). That is the reason why a high overall performance impacts the introduction of any change negatively.
- **Dissatisfaction.** The extent medical staff is not satisfied with the actual situation and wishes to change. Dissatisfaction is – analogously to performance – an indicator of ineffective organizational structures. It comprises driving forces that may support any change in the situation.

The Fig. 16.4 may be used to continuously assess the readiness of the organization. Any actual status that has been queried in the scope of any meetings or interviews can be depicted as 'X' in the sheet.

(*) *Displayed 'Minimally Required Values' (MRV) required values are only an estimation and may differ between organizations. Furthermore, not sufficiently fulfilled criteria may be compensated by high fulfilment of other criteria.*

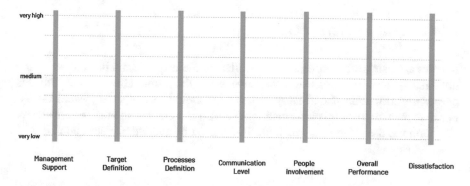

Fig. 16.4   Tool to assess the Readiness of an organization (*)

Table 16.1 Assessment criteria

Area	Questions
Management support	Does the management actively support the introduction of (1) innovations generally (2) IPM particularly? Who is supporting? How does the support look like?
Target definition	Are there (1) any strategy (2) any concrete targets that aim to introduce new and innovative technologies? Are these targets (or strategies) (1) documented, (2) broadly communicated, (3) accepted and followed in the health organization?
Processes definition	To what extent does the health organization uses processes to ensure standardized proceeding and high-quality results? Are the processes in the health organization (1) defined and documented (2) accepted and followed by the medical staff, (3) frequently controlled? Are processes in the health organization often changed and adopted to innovations?
Communication level	Do health professionals feel informed about the actual situation of the organization and with sufficient details? Do health professionals share relevant information to colleagues? What is the speed of communication in the health organization? Do they complain about not being informed (or involved) into certain situations?
People involvement	Are health team usually involved in organizational decisions (i.e. introduction of new technologies)? Are health team ready to get involved in organizational decisions? Do they like it?
Overall performance	What is the overall performance of the health organization considering all relevant performance indicators (i.e. finance, quality of care, patient satisfaction, health experts' satisfaction, process compliance, organizational effectiveness...)? How satisfied are health experts with the overall performance of the organization? What is the performance of the health organization considering (1) the ability, (2) the willingness to change?
Dissatisfaction	Are health experts dissatisfied with the actual situation? Why? What do health experts wish to change?

In order to fulfil the tool to assess the readiness of the health organization, the following questions (Table 16.1) to interrogate assessment criteria are presented.

16.4.2 Stakeholders' Map

Besides assessing the readiness it is important to identify relevant persons who may influence – either in a positive or negative way – the introduction of IPM. For this purpose, information about every stakeholder should be gathered systematically. For documentation of this information, GDPR requirements should be considered. Furthermore, the information in Table 16.2 should be queried in a structured way.

Table 16.2 Stakeholders information

| Stakeholder (SH) | Impact of the project to SH | Gap in support | | Concerns/ issues/resistance of SH | Interest/wins of SH | Who can influence stakeholder | Strategy to influence/involve SH (what, how, when, who) |
		Current mindset(*) of SH	Support needed(*) of SH				
<Name>	*<Description>*	*<R/N/A/S/C>*	*<R/N/A/S/C>*	*<List>*	*<List>*	*<Name>*	*<Description>*
...	...	...	...	...	...	...	...

16.5 Arrangement Phase

In order to prepare the participants to new working procedures, a dedicated preparation workshop should be conducted. This workshop not just aims to inform (and train) the medical staff about the change process, but also to introduce IPM, presenting its potential to solve problems and to generate ideas on how (and in which areas) it could be applied in the own hospital, as well as, to create a comfortable atmosphere to work.

The workshop preparation is divided into 5 stages (Fig. 16.5). It is organized as a whole morning workshop, where all the health professionals take part, optimally voluntarily.

16.5.1 Stage 1: Team Setup

The workshop starts welcoming participants with coffee, cookies and drinks. The idea is to make participants feel save and welcomed. Then, each participant presents themselves, introducing their name, function and experience with technology (data science, process mining), with the purpose to know each other and that moderators know expectations from them, too. It should continue with a brief introduction of the conductors, who they are, what they do, and why they are there. At this point, participants can ask questions. Then, there should be an overview to the agenda of the workshop.

16.5.2 Stage 2: Orientation and Creativity

It continues with a creativity session to figure out processes and main issues, for which several creativity and consolidation techniques have been selected. Even though these techniques are considered to be appropriate in change processes, by helping on the development of empathy in the pursuit the value through human-centred research [27, 46, 48], they should be considered as proposals; they can be easily replaced by more appropriate ones [33]. Anyhow, the first part of the session is dedicated to the identification of processes, forcing participants to envision current

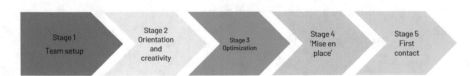

Fig. 16.5 Five stages of the Arrangement phase

issues in the organization to make them aware of worries, to, secondly, prioritize these concerns. Some proposed methods are:

- **Persona.** Each persona card tries to focus on capturing different behaviours, i.e. 'the teamworker', 'the shaper'. The more the needs, desires, habits and cultural backgrounds of a specific group of people in the organization are fully expressed, the more realistic it becomes. Participants are divided into groups with 3–4 people each. Every group has to fill in one, partially prefilled, persona sheet, and the role of the persona-sheet should be different from the roles of its group members.
- **A day in the life.** Proceeding of this exercise is to list activities of a normal day and/or any important situations/concerns that come to participants, as well as ideas of solving them or potential improvements. There could be crossed interactions among stakeholders and identified processes and game characters could be used as a source of inspiration.
- **Journey patient.** It is a synthetic representation that describes step-by-step how a patient interacts with a service. The service is mapped from the patient perspective, describing what happens at each stage, and what obstacles and barriers patients may encounter. This map should also represent emotions (positive/negative) experienced during the interactions, even when it is with other services or processes.
- **Empathy map.** Depending on the type of target that the organization wants to resolve, there are methods such as the empathy map that are more focused on the patient's experience. It is a patient's centred canvas split into four quadrants (says, thinks, does, and feels). It is used by putting all the existing knowledge on the table, identifying missing information. It should follow the rule of 'one person per map', producing an overview of who the patient is, and to identify inconsistencies in the perception of the same patient from various team members (and so intervene to mitigate the conflict) that might affect to the process.
- **Experience principles.** These are inspiring values that help to create a shared experience vision within the organization, by applying it consistently across several processes and initiatives. They might incorporate insights about what patients expect from the organization or specific service. It should be used to guide multiple teams or work-streams to pursue the same goals in terms of the patient experience. Contrary to the previous one that wants to state the experience of the patient, this method might contribute to defining values that offer a concrete service.
- **Offering map.** It is also a very interesting method to clarify what a service provides to the patients, detailing the value proposition into specific groups of features. It could be depicted by words, pictures, diagrams, or a combination of them, being more detailed in specific areas or functions.
- **Service blueprint.** It is a diagram that displays the entire process, by listing all the activities that happen at each stage, performed by the different stakeholders. The service blueprint is built by first listing all the roles involved on a vertical axis, and all the steps required to deliver the process on the horizontal axis.

The resulting matrix allows representing the flow of actions that each role needs to perform along the process, highlighting the actions that the patient can see and the ones that happen in the back-office. The difference with other methods presented is that the service blueprint analyses an existing service or specifies a well-defined concept, but is not used as an ideation tool.

Once, issues have been identified and prioritized, these are shared with the rest of medical team.

This is an example of techniques that are helpful in inviting health professionals to reflect, raise issues, and prioritize them. Although these techniques share some similarities, they have characteristics that make them more appropriate in some cases than others.

16.5.3   Stage 3: Optimization

Evidence highlights that agile methodologies are ideal for projects with high variability due to constantly changing requirements and those where the value of the product delivered is a priority [18, 39]. Thus, it does an especial emphasis on agile methodologies requirements prioritization to be more efficient at the time to prioritize tasks to be implemented taking into account project constraints, the complexity around requirements, and available resources (time, costs, and employees) [15]. Reflecting on what is known from agile requirement literature, and knowledge related to change transformation, these agile practices could be extended and applied in the proposed methodology to nurture the optimization development, helping in the prioritization of the questions detected in the previous step. Techniques [4] such as the 100-dollar test, or MoSCoW, among others are contextualized in the proposed methodology and presented as follows:

- **The iron triangle** takes into account the triangle between (1) time, (2) cost, and (3) scope, so if needed resources are not in place to solve a problem arisen by a question, maybe it is necessary to make sure that it is possible to meet them by reducing scope, or prioritizing adequately before being selected.
- **MoSCoW** term comes from Must-have, Should-have, Could-have and Won't-have and is related to user stories, although in this case should be considered as questions or issues to be solved that directly affects the value offered to the patients.

  - Must-have user stories are critical, failing the whole project if one must-have story is not implemented.
  - Should-have user stories need to be implemented too, but are usually less critical and can be implemented later.
  - Could-have user stories improve User Xperience, not being critical.
  - Won't-have user stories are less important.

- **Kano Analysis** involves features, but instead, improvements or changes should be classified into four categories having in mind patients' benefit:

  - Delighters. are new, or of high value to the patient
  - Satisfiers. offer value to the patient
  - Dissatisfiers. do not affect the level of satisfaction if they are not present
  - Indifferent. will not affect the patient in any way and should be eliminated

- **The 100-Dollar test** is a method where each person gets 100 units to distribute among the given matters. If they are too many, it is recommended to use more units. After distributing the units, it is calculated the total for each one and rank them accordingly.

16.5.4   Stage 4: Mise en place

It is a crucial phase when a plan to drive the culture change in the health organization is presented, because it clearly states the why, what, who, how and when to achieve this transformation. Opening with the presentation of a short-term plan, which should enclose the following points.

- **Vision and mission [7].** The purpose of this first step is to give health experts a reason to desire to be involved in the change process of adopting digital health transformation. Linking goals to motivations facilitates their involvement in the change, and the clearer the objectives are, the greater the benefit to the individual, the team and the health organization is. This linkage generates an awareness of the necessity of change and what it is needed for. Here it is important to discuss and clarify any aspects to be sure that all people are on board in accordance with main goals and purposes.
- **Team.** As introduced in Sect. 16.3 there is a list of relevant stakeholders for the change. According to results from the Arrangement phase health professionals could be divided into the following groups [25], specifying their roles and duties for each one:

  - **Sponsors** of the change. Who pays for it? Are they involved??
  - **Participants** in the change. Anyone who is participating in the change process.
  - **Authorities** approving the change. They are usually managers and directors inside the health organization, although it could be further as in the case of the sponsors.
  - **Core team** managing the change. It is usually composed by the change manager and the interactive process miner, although as later is introduced, other roles may be needed like a communicator or a training manager, that are introduced later.
  - **Experts** supporting the change. The interactive process miner is a crucial role to strengthen the understanding of the rationale behind IPM and to emphasize

its benefits for the incoming adopters. Furthermore, at this point, the role of **champions** is introduced. They facilitate the change by assessing how things are going on and by identifying what needs to be done. They are in a triangle among sponsors, implementers and the core team. They recognize resistance and propose ideas to work around, helping in the preparation of training materials if needed. They are fascinated by transmitting their enthusiasm, using their own words. Champions [24] have extensive knowledge of the ground level, being considered as one of the most successful factors in the process of change. As Everett Rogers suggested in his theory [47], champions act as social influencers, persuading individuals to adopt an innovation, which leads to that the critical mass that adopts the change when enough other individuals have done it before. At this point, the adoption becomes self-sustaining, and it should be taken special care of having an appropriated number of champions on board, having clear tasks and being, of course, well prepared (trained). Besides, managers must be aware of the additional work that champions are doing and, if possible, there should be a kind of reward. Any other specific role identified as being essential is also welcome to this group.

- **Communication.** An effective communication is fundamental [29] for proper implementation of the change. Findings suggest that change generates uncertainties that need to be addressed [3, 44]. For that, it is needed to define clear rules about how communications are performed in both directions from the core team towards the rest of the group, and vice versa [52] to tackle queries of employees, generate community spirit, and build trust until having a commitment. Aspects that should be covered are mainly a communication plan, which entails activities for coordinating, motivating, and managing conflicts. It might consist of periodic updates, meetings with individuals, or in-group, as well as consultation schedule (normal business hours, weekends, 24×7...), and defining clear contact persons for each topic (suggestions, issues...), i.e. from the core team, the experts or the champions. The plan should be agreed among all involved persons, taking into account their agendas. Another aspect is the type of messages in terms of content and used code (verbal or non-verbal); and methods and modalities of communications where channels, media and technologies of communication have to be considered. It is important to emphasis feedback as it can help to identify not only resistance but also to diagnose gaps on why a change may fail, as well as, to enrich significant key performance indicators, contributing to the adoption of the change. Last but not least, from empirical researchers [30], several recommendations may be suggested:

  - Redundancy helps to keep the message.
  - It is more effective to use different channels than just one.
  - People prefer face-to-face communication.
  - Line hierarchy is the most effective communication channel.
  - Opinion leaders are effective changers of attitudes, especially to remind that management supports any action during the change process.

- **Training.** A variety of factors, besides ability, can influence training effectiveness, e.g. management actions, but mainly employee motivation, attitude, and expectations. Individuals who lack motivation prior to training are less likely to succeed and may require some preparation in advance. To provide clear guidelines could contribute significantly to training effectiveness [55]. Therefore, employees should be informed about training content at this stage, and a minimum set of rules should be established related to the training e.g. supervisory and peer support (champions), the kind and amount of available resources (in time and equipment), training sessions and follow-ups. Furthermore, other actions contributing to employees' involvement in the training process are e.g. participation in the requirement assessment, choice of degree of attendance, or preferences for training methods. Additionally, elements like rewards (which are explained more in detail in the next point) might encourage persons taking advantage of the new skills and knowledge on the job. It is best to pick a method that encourages active participation of employees and provides adequate feedback. Interactive methods that allow more individualized instruction and increased employees control over learning, like with IPM with its interactive and iterative nature, facilitate this active participation in the learning process. At the same time, this is incrementally incorporated to the daily practice of the organization, assuring the length of time that employees are using acquired skills and behaviours on the job. The final phase of the training process, and probably the most important in terms of increasing effectiveness, is evaluation. Since IPM is normally used by the employees, this evaluation could be translated into performance indicators, where the benefits of the training are reflected as e.g. in increased productivity.
- **Rewards.** Reinforcement strategies are one of the most effective contributions to change [53]. As it is mentioned in the Assessment phase, it is one of the elements that should be agreed with the management team from the beginning [6] in case it was identified as a facilitator. In scope of the Reward strategy it should be identified which behaviour impacts the performance of the change, and how it can be measured, and who interventions involved in each case can be identified. When speaking about rewards, there are two main classes [5, 37], (a) financial reinforcement, which is one of the most used mechanisms in practice, and (b) non-financial reinforcement. Sometimes this might be given in form of feedback, positive or negative, social reinforcement in terms of compliments, general recognition etc. or even in other ways such as recognizing the effort by giving more responsibility, or more autonomy to the employee.
- **Indicators.** It is well known that Key Performance Indicators (KPI) are a powerful tool to measure performance in organizations. KPI are usually measured after a process is finished, postponing results that did not provide the opportunity to react in time [9]. By cons, KPIs should be established from the beginning to state the current status of the organization and to monitor the progress over time, helping on identifying which priorities should be set. But, what is an indicator? And, what is it for? There seems to be an obvious answer to these questions, but there is none. Many organizations are working with wrong measures, clinging

to indicators that reflect past performance and do not contemplate the ones that really measure states that the organization wants to achieve in the future. Even though this is clear, the process of identifying such truly beneficial indicators is not a trivial path. The scientific evidence [40] proposes dedicating full-time teams for monitoring them, in order to make modifications necessary to adapt the indicators to the changes that the organization may undergo to increase its performance, which is costly in terms of both, downtime and money. Furthermore, cascading down of performance measures, breaking one measure down into parts as it goes down to different teams is not a good practice. While this looks logical, it leads to chaos, helping the organization go nowhere quickly. Instead, it is going in the right direction to determine which root causes hinder the performance increase and which success factors contribute to it. With that purpose, it is necessary to have the possibility not only to recognize the necessary indicators to show a good summary, but also to generate more complex views. These views should comprise information of the organization from different perspectives, e.g. an objective could be to reduce the length of stay in the emergency service. In this example, the patient goes through admission, triage and the waiting room, until is called for his/her first visit with the doctor, who can order several tests. It is a blood test that is analysed by the laboratory, a hospital transversal service and an RX test, done in external consultations, being both independent units of the emergency room. Meanwhile, the patient awaits the results of the tests in the waiting room, until (s)he is called and meets the doctor again that discharges her/him. The process followed by patients carries valuable information that would help employees to understand what the real pathway at the emergency service is. It may help to identify bottlenecks that directly affects the performance. Thus, many questions need to be answered to find those success factors that help improving the performance of the emergency service, e.g. the laboratory takes a long time until it delivers the results, but a lot of questions arose while waiting for an answer. As discussed in previous chapters, IPM enters the scene to shed light on these and other questions through the definition of Interactive Process Indicators.

16.5.5 Stage 5: First Contact

The final stage of the workshop is aimed to introduce formally IPM to the health experts in order to make them aware of the added-value of using new technologies and the direct benefits to their daily practice.

This phase has the aim of presenting the grounds to embrace IPM in the health organization, and to make all involved medical staff aware of the new processes.

16.6 Adaptation and Adoption Phase

After the two previous phases that concentrate on getting into the health organization, the Adaptation and Adoption phase is focused on entering directly to the work with IPM. In the first steps of the methodology, the weakest and most relevant points of the health organization should be underlined. It is the starting point where the organization begins to embrace the culture of change while experiencing a digital health transformation through the adoption of IPM. From here, first indicators could be considered as complementary information to what IPM finds out. This technology enables process discovery iteratively by involving health experts from the very first minute. Based on sessions known as 'Data Rodeos', IPM facilitates the measuring, understanding and assessing of health process through Interactive Process Indicators, from more abstract top overview to low-level detailed medical information, endowing health professionals with well-rounded knowledge to the decision making. As explained in previous chapters, the team, made of at least one interactive process miner and a health expert, performs a series of meetings (Data Rodeos) following the stages of shakedown, research and production. This allows them, to find the best Interactive Process Indicators to present the medical data until the medical team reaches a deep understanding of the reality of the health organization. The health expert could carry out sessions on its own, where support materials is available, as well as a communication channel with the interactive process miner to get support. These sessions, both group and individual, allow them to investigate new evidence.

It should be taken care to try to avoid overproduction, if different people asking the same questions or requesting similar information with multiple forms. For that reason, it is important to guide Data Rodeos with questions that might help in the ongoing research:

- What is the standard case?
- How much does it differ from the real case?
- Are clinical outcomes as expected?
- Is the operational throughput good enough?
- Could be mortality numbers reduced?

The drivers within IPM are clinical processes or pathways, which are represented as workflows, where all events could be recognized as either value-added or non-value added. In here, it could highlight the critical path where more effort is necessary for looking into details to identify e.g. bottlenecks. In some cases, these workflows could become a 'spaghetti' diagram, which is an easy way to see the wasted time. The more 'spaghetti'-like the diagram is, the clearer the need for redesigned work becomes visible, in which case clustering might shed some light. In general, workflows could be used:

- To understand each step of the process
- To orient new staff to the process
- To clearly describe the process to other departments
- To identify where there are problems

Looking at the three first bullets, it is clear that visual representations combined with other techniques, as are introduced below, are primordial to let clinical staff understand the performance of the health organization under different viewpoints. This is what in this book is called as Interactive Process Indicator. Starting with the Shakedown phase, Data Rodeos are conducted according to the plan defined in the Arrangement stage. During the Research phase, several iterations are carried out, where health experts and interactive process miners validate visual representation to assure that the results are comprehensive, objective and explorative. These iterations are done until figuring out the best-fitting Interactive Process Indicator. Then IPM solution goes through the Production phase to generate a version for health experts, with which they can continue to work more autonomously.

A deep understanding of how work currently happens is essential before trying to fix it. Workflows are visual descriptions that improve comprehension and that emphasize the level of variability in the process, where events can depict total end-to-end time, e.g. length of stay, time for a specific job without waiting times (e.g. an urgent operation), or an incident where a task must be reworked (e.g. a medical error). It also provides a common language to talk about the process among all stakeholders. Moreover, it could include information related to resources, e.g. number of people to reflect the utilization and capacity of the service in terms of available time, work time, utilization of that time and capacity of resolution per patient's episode.

There are cases where corresponding data is available to conduct a Data Rodeo, but it is not like this in all cases. In a hypothetical case that the health organization wants to reduce the number of lost medical devices, they might use a check sheet. It is structured to collect data, keeping instances of quality problems in a specific problem. This tool helps to know what kind of data is needed to be collected, to be able to monitor the quality of the process and to understand where the health organization might want to make some improvements, and then incorporate this information to the data model.

There is no 'one-size-fits-all' solution in healthcare, although there are widespread indicators that might be interesting to assess the status of the health organization under financial (costs), patient (experience), internal (health experts) or performance (quality of care) perspectives. For example, in the case of the experience of a patient, it could be possible to measure PROMs and PREMs. PROM's (Patient Reported Outcomes Measurement) objective is to capture patients' perception of their health, being some measures of distress/anxiety or unmet needs. Instead, PREM's (Patient Reported Experiences measurement) objective is to capture patients' perception of their experience with health care or service, e.g. length of stay. Furthermore, ICHOM Standard Sets [28] are of valuable relevance since it defines outcomes that matter to most patients having a certain health condition e.g. stroke, opening up new possibilities to compare performance globally and allowing clinicians to learn from each other. As it is introduced, the Quadruple Aim [10, 11, 51], add the importance of the patient and practitioner experience to these compelling goals, which is key for the good performance of any health organization. Additionally, a manager might be interested in knowing the workload of each service (e.g. emergency room, laboratory. . .), or teamwork among others.

Other representations might complement the information offered by the mentioned workflows. Some histograms show the frequency of occurrence of a particular event (e.g. duration in the waiting room at the emergency service). With this information the frequency distribution, if it is a normally or randomly distributed event or if it is spread or very concentrated distribution (e.g. there are more patients in the morning) can be understood a little bit better. This can be either looking at inputs and outputs in a quantitative way, and also helps to compare what needs to be done which patient and what is required by the health organization. Control charts are another representation, which provides information about the stability of the process, specifically with regard to its target value and/or variation. Averages and ranges with acceptable numbers related to the mean in the central line. When the value is outside of the limits, it is time to figure out the root cause. Scatter diagrams are plots of XY pairs of numerical data. It can be seen whether there is any kind of correlation or pattern because correlation and pattern are not the same. Considered a useful tool to root cause analysis.

Apart from workflows and some of the proposed tools to represent additional information in the form of indicators, there are other approaches to identify when it is needed to do a change. Process Quality measures the capability of a process to produce to its expected capability (trying to eliminate "defects"), considered a defect as any process output that does not meet patients' expectations. Hence, when an IPM solution is delivered in the Production phase, health professionals continue monitoring the organization to detect the need for a change. At that moment, the Application stage starts to identify root causes and applies the necessary modifications in the organization.

Last but not least, this phase measures the technology acceptance of IPM solution. The study of success factors for the adoption of technology is something that has been measured for a long time. It establishes that teaching and providing support is essential, as well as social influence in the perceived usefulness factor. However, the one that mostly impacts is the lack of management support. The engagement depends on health experts' interest, expectative and effort to adopt new technologies [26]. It is of special interest to define a plan that mitigates this sort of issues. Medical team should trust, use and accept the new technology, which should improve the efficiency and quality of care, which should be easy to use, and needs the minimum effort of learning. Some relevant questions that might arise:

- How well does the system perform?
- How relevant is it to health expert's job?
- How useful is it?
- How much does it make performance easier and satisfying?
- How does it facilitate more informed and accurate decisions?

Technology acceptance should be measured during the whole adaptation process to be sure that improvements are welcome.

16.7 Application Phase

This phase is where new changes happen, after improvement is identified in the Adaptation and Adoption phase, here is necessary to go through the following steps that frame them orderly to reduce resistance and assure a smooth transition.

16.7.1 Analysing Change

The aim of this stage is to analyse and figure out a solution. Understanding change complexity determines an uncertain context that needs additional team work. Any change implies time, and people, being primordial to know the availability level of personal capability and capacity to implement the change, so that, firstly, a team where each representative has to be familiar with the topic that is going to be investigated need to be clearly define. Secondly, one or more preparatory meeting(s) should be carried out.

With the information coming from IPM and proposed root cause analysis tools (5 why's, cause & effect...), a definition of a proper solution can be elaborated. This includes the identification of the non-value added activities, delays, rework, bottlenecks and other forms of waste.

- What is the desired end-result? Is it to reduce waiting times in emergency service?
- Is there clinical evidence that helps in solving the problem?
- How quickly is change needed?
- What are the teams affected by the change? Are they from the laboratory, radiology, or dietary?
- How do you know to do your work? Do you ask your line supervisor?
- Do all health experts do a task in the same way?
- Does information arrive on time?
- Can any paperwork be eliminated?
- Is information available, reliable and up-to-date?
- Are there any immediate improvements without significant investments?

It should take special care to countermeasures and implementation plans in terms of (what, who, when, expected outcome) and the definition of a follow-up plan. Starting from the current state and keeping in mind the future process, it is possible to make quick modifications in an editor available in IPM, to depict the new process that is to be achieved. Most of the time root causes can be attributed to something not being specified. Likewise, during a change process, there may be organizational assets that should be preserved or practices that need to be maintained.

16.7.2 Norming Change

As in the Arrangement phase, and after having analysed the proposed change, it is needed to present how it is going to be performed, including:

- Scope definition to let medical staff know what the change is aimed for.
- Team involved in the change, taking new measures for better coordination. It is required to find out current concerns about new changes and needs to be covered. At this level, it is important to define how tasks are accomplished, by dividing and scheduling work, defining roles in terms of what people do and what they do together. In the case that more than one service (e.g. radiology or nursing) are working together, a new profile that acts as a link with other parts of the organization may be needed (**link manager**).
- An effective communication helps on the alignment between health professionals, enabling visibility of the overall work process, and linkages between different positions, reducing resistance and contributing to that all clinical staff understand which corrective actions are required.
- In specific cases, training will be required to teach about new ways of working.
- A reinforcement strategy may help on the motivation of the medical team involved to accomplish with their assigned tasks.
- New indicators derived from forthcoming change should be offered in IPM.

16.7.3 Performing Change

All change should firstly be tested in scope of an experiment, starting small. The challenge is to develop critical short-term priorities that keep health experts' operations functioning while laying the groundwork for broader, longer-term transformational change.

16.7.4 Monitoring Change

IPM has proper indicators to monitor change. It implies to establish a baseline performance to compare the results during and after applying the solution into the health organization, being possible to compare the results to the baseline performance. To assure that no unexpected change occurs the process is monitored. This helps to know if the actions have the expected impact, and letting us know what actions have been successful, also confirming if the understanding of the problem was right. Health experts should be informed about if progress goes ahead as planned.

16.7.5 Fixing Change

Once the change has been implemented it is needed to make the transformation stick to ensure that no one falls back on the change journey, letting go of old identities. To perform health-checks assures that the transformation is sustainable and that old customs are not reverted to bewilderment times, is very important to establish a new beginning with clear instructions on how to proceed from now on. Tools such as 1-1 interviews, surveys, focus groups or direct feedback from health professionals let us know if the change has been finally adopted.

If derived from the new change, it is identified the need for a new research process related to IPM, then activities will go back to the Adaptation and Adoption phase.

16.8 Conclusion

Any change in an organization requires special care to minimize its impact on performance. There is a multitude of psychological theories that guide health experts through the process of change, but that depend much on the person's abilities. In addition there are many emotional aspects that need to be considered, which leads to a long way of a successful implementation of a change. From assessing the current state until obtaining a plan that defines steps to follow, there is a great valley that is hampered by the lack of tools that facilitate this process automatically and objectively. In this regard, the proposed IPM-based solution is framed in a context in which the best of both worlds creates a synergy. While IPM offers understandable, objective and explorative visual representations (Interactive Process Indicators) that allow the organization's data to be interpreted with the minimum effort, it takes advantage of the available methods and the scientific evidence, in an orderly manner, to guide through the change process. As first step, this is an approach presented under a clinical point of view which might be highly valuable for medical teams. However, the truth is that the idea of providing value to patients is still a utopia. Once they left the hospital, patient journey is unclear. Outside the hospital processes can not be measures like in a medical environment, and there is no clue about patients' adherence to treatments, and how it affects the efficiency of the followed interventions. Thus, there is still a lot of work until it can be considered the patient experience, his/her behaviour and other personal circumstances as input data of technologies as IPM is for the application of real personalized medicine.

References

1. Albliwi S, Antony J, Lim SAH, van der Wiele T. Critical failurefactors of lean six sigma: a systematic literature review. Int J Qual Reliab Manag. 2014;31(9):1012–30.
2. Allen B. Effective design, implementation and management of change in healthcare. Nurs Stand. 2016;31:58–71.

3. Allen J, Jimmieson NL, Bordia P, Irmer BE. Uncertainty during organizational change: managing perceptions through communication. J Change Manag. 2007;7(2):187–210.
4. Alshehri S, Benedicenti L. Ranking approach for the user story prioritization methods. J Commun Comput. 2013;10:1465–74.
5. Armstrong M, Murlis H. Reward management: a handbook of remuneration strategy and practice. Kogan Page Publishers; 2007.
6. Armstrong M, Stephens T. A handbook of employee reward management and practice. Kogan Page Publishers; 2005.
7. Austin J, Bentkover J, Chait L. Leading strategic change in an era of healthcare transformation, vol. 9. Springer; 2016.
8. Balushi S, Sohal AS, Singh PJ, Al Hajri A, Al-Farsi Y, Abri R. Readiness factors for lean implementation in healthcare settings–a literature review. J Health Organ Manag. 2014;28(2):135–53.
9. Beatham S, Anumba C, Thorpe T, Hedges I. Kpis: a critical appraisal of their use in construction. Benchmark Int J. 2004;11(1):93–117.
10. Berwick DM, Nolan TW, Whittington J. The triple aim: care, health, and cost. Health Aff. 2008;27(3):759–69.
11. Bodenheimer T, Sinsky C. From triple to quadruple aim: care of the patient requires care of the provider. Ann Fam Med. 2014;12(6):573–6.
12. Buchanan DA, Fitzgerald L, Ketley D. The sustainability and spread of organizational change: modernizing healthcare. Routledge; 2006.
13. Cameron E, Green M. Making sense of change management: a complete guide to the models, tools and techniques of organizational change. Kogan Page Publishers; 2019.
14. Chakravorty SS, Shah AD. Lean six sigma (LSS): an implementation experience. Eur J Ind Eng. 2012;6(1):118–37.
15. Daneva M, Van Der Veen E, Amrit C, Ghaisas S, Sikkel K, Kumar R, Ajmeri N, Ramteerthkar U, Wieringa R. Agile requirements prioritization in large-scale outsourced system projects: an empirical study. J Syst Softw. 2013;86(5):1333–53.
16. Davies HTO, Nutley SM, Mannion R. Organisational culture and quality of health care. BMJ Qual Saf. 2000;9(2):111–9.
17. De Koning H, Verver JPS, van den Heuvel J, Bisgaard S, Does RJMM. Lean six sigma in healthcare. J Healthc Qual. 2006;28(2):4–11.
18. Dingsøyr T, Nerur S, Balijepally V, Moe NB. A decade of agile methodologies: towards explaining agile software development; 2012.
19. Fernández-Llatas C, Meneu T, Traver V, Benedi J-M. Applying evidence-based medicine in telehealth: an interactive pattern recognition approximation. Int J Environ Res Public Health. 2013;10(11):5671–82.
20. George ML, Maxey J, Rowlands DT, Upton M. Lean six sigma pocket toolbook. McGraw-Hill Professional Publishing; 2004.
21. Gill R. Change management–or change leadership? J Change Manag. 2002;3(4):307–18.
22. Halligan M, Zecevic A. Safety culture in healthcare: a review of concepts, dimensions, measures and progress. BMJ Qual Saf. 2011;20(4):338–43.
23. Hayes J. The theory and practice of change management. Palgrave; 2018.
24. Hendy J, Barlow J. The role of the organizational champion in achieving health system change. Soc Sci Med. 2012;74(3):348–55.
25. Hiatt J, Creasey TJ. Change management: the people side of change. Prosci; 2003.
26. Holden RJ, Karsh B-T. The technology acceptance model: its past and its future in health care. J Biomed Inform. 2010;43(1):159–72.
27. Johansson-Sköldberg U, Woodilla J, Çetinkaya M. Design thinking: past, present and possible futures. Creat Innov Manag. 2013;22(2):121–46.
28. Kelley TA. International consortium for health outcomes measurement (ichom). Trials. 2015;16(3):O4.

29. Kitchen P, Daly F. Internal communication during change management. Corp Commun Int J. 2002;7(3):46–53.
30. Klein SM. A management communication strategy for change. J Organ Chang Manag. 1996;9(2):32–46.
31. Kübler-Ross E, Wessler S, Avioli LV. On death and dying. JAMA. 1972;221(2):174–9.
32. Leape L, Berwick D, Clancy C, Conway J, Gluck P, Guest J, Lawrence D, Morath J, O'Leary D, O'Neill P, et al. Transforming healthcare: a safety imperative. BMJ Qual Saf. 2009;18(6):424–8.
33. Liedtka J, Ogilvie T. Helping business managers discover their appetite for design thinking. Des Manag Rev. 2012;23(1):6–13.
34. Lluch M. Healthcare professionals' organisational barriers to health information technologies—a literature review. Int J Med Inform. 2011;80(12):849–62.
35. Lukas CVD, Holmes SK, Cohen AB, Restuccia J, Cramer IE, Shwartz M, Charns MP. Transformational change in health care systems: an organizational model. Health Care Manag Rev. 2007;32(4):309–20.
36. Miller HG, Mork P. From data to decisions: a value chain for big data. IT Prof. 2013;15(1):57–9.
37. Milne P. Motivation, incentives and organisational culture. J Knowl Manag. 2007;11(6):28–38.
38. Myers IB. The Myers-Briggs type indicator: manual. Consulting Psychologists Press; 1962.
39. Nerur S, Mahapatra R, Mangalaraj G. Challenges of migrating to agile methodologies. Commun ACM. 2005;48(5):72–8.
40. Parmenter D. Key performance indicators: developing, implementing, and using winning KPIs. Wiley; 2015.
41. Paton RA, McCalman J. Change management: a guide to effective implementation. Sage; 2008.
42. Plsek PE, Wilson T. Complexity, leadership, and management in healthcare organisations. BMJ. 2001;323(7315):746–9.
43. Porter ME, Teisberg EO. Redefining health care: creating value-based competition on results. Harvard Business Press; 2006.
44. Proctor T, Doukakis I. Change management: the role of internal communication and employee development. Corp Commun Int J. 2003;8(4):268–77.
45. Raghupathi W, Raghupathi V. Big data analytics in healthcare: promise and potential. Health Inf Sci Syst. 2014;2(1):3.
46. Roberts JP, Fisher TR, Trowbridge MJ, Bent C. A design thinking framework for healthcare management and innovation. In: Healthcare. vol. 4. Elsevier; 2016. p. 11–4.
47. Rogers EM. Diffusion of innovations. Simon and Schuster; 2010.
48. Sato S, Lucente S, Meyer D, Mrazek D. Design thinking to make organization change and development more responsive. Des Manag Rev. 2010;21(2):44–52.
49. Schwenk CR. Linking cognitive, organizational and political factors in explaining strategic change. J Manag Stud. 1989;26(2):177–87.
50. Scott TIM, Mannion R, Davies HTO, Marshall MN. Implementing culture change in health care: theory and practice. Int J Qual Health Care. 2003;15(2):111–8.
51. Sikka R, Morath JM, Leape L. The quadruple aim: care, health, cost and meaning in work; 2015.
52. Simoes PMM, Esposito M. Improving change management: how communication nature influences resistance to change. J Manag Dev. 2014; 33(4):324–41.
53. Skinner BF. Science and human behavior. Simon and Schuster; 1965.
54. Snee RD. Lean six sigma—getting better all the time. Int J Lean Six Sigma. 2010;1(1):9–29.
55. Tannenbaum SI, Yukl G. Training and development in work organizations. Ann Rev Psychol. 1992;43(1):399–441.

56. Testani MV, Ramakrishnan S. The role of leadership in sustaining a lean transformation. In: IIE annual conference. Proceedings. Institute of Industrial and Systems Engineers (IISE); 2010. p. 1.
57. Todnem By R. Organisational change management: a critical review. J Change Manag. 2005;5(4):369–80.
58. Waddell D, Sohal AS. Resistance: a constructive tool for change management. Manag Decis. 1998;36(8):543–8.
59. Weiner BJ. A theory of organizational readiness for change. Implement Sci. 2009;4(1):67.

Chapter 17
Interactive Process Mining Challenges

Carlos Fernandez-Llatas

17.1 Introduction

Healthcare domain is facing to the new age of digital transformation. The new challenges that digital health is proposing are dragging the medical community to a new way to care for patients. Digital Transformation does not mean to make the same actions with new tools. It means to leverage the presence of Information and Communication Technologies (ICT) for changing the way of acting [28]. Digital transformation requires a deep change in the protocols, methodologies, and, even, in the mind of users to provide real effective and efficient use of technology.

This deep change is not easy to achieve. Usually, it is thought that resistance to change of human stakeholders is one of the main barriers that Digital Health transformation is facing [21]. But, this is only the top of the iceberg. Health is a very ancient discipline that has changed during aeons and it is focused mainly on the interaction with the patient. Digital Technologies are proposing a new, efficient and effective way of making things that, sometimes, are contrary to this simple human principle [8]. The dehumanization of health is one of the main accusations that traditional health community are reproaching to digital transformation promoters [7]. The loss of human contact in medical visits, the excessive computer dependence of health professionals, or the globalization of health, that decrease the personalization of cares [30] are only examples of the main barriers that digital health transformation is founding in their path to their implantation on the medical community.

C. Fernandez-Llatas (✉)
Process Mining 4 Health Lab – SABIEN – ITACA Institute, Universitat Politècnica de València, Valencia, Spain

CLINTEC – Karolinska Institutet, Sweden
e-mail: cfllatas@itaca.upv.es

© Springer Nature Switzerland AG 2021
C. Fernandez-Llatas (ed.), *Interactive Process Mining in Healthcare*, Health Informatics, https://doi.org/10.1007/978-3-030-53993-1_17

Despite the fact the digitization of health is considered unavoidable, the health professional is blindly accepting the digitization thesis and is applying healthcare making the same things whit different tools, changing the paper by the computer. This is because the computer is not considered a new actor in the system. The computer is considered only a tool. Interactive paradigm [11], and Interactive Process Mining, in particular, are promoting the interactions between the expert and the intelligent system to not only to provide the benefits that computerized systems are providing to society but also, present the computer as a new actor for interacting, counselling and understanding the real behaviour of the diseases and patients. This gives the role of the intelligent system to a new paradigm that humanizes the presence of the computer in the consultation considering it, not only a tool but also an actor in the health process.

The objective of this chapter is to analyze the barriers that are hindering the interaction between medical experts and intelligent systems and highlight the new challenges that we should face up to achieve a more adequate digital health transformation.

17.2   Engage Health Professionals

The indeterminate behaviour of the diseases, depending not only in itself but also in the involvement, attitudes and beliefs of patients, require a *human touch* for gathering intangible information for selecting the best treatments in each specific case. The medical staff acts as an *artist* for selecting the best treatment possible according to their intuition, experience and know-how. Health is not engineering. Although there are wide attempts to create protocols and guidelines that automatize at the maximum the care processes [33], health domain requires always the running knowledge of medical doctors.

The appearance of Machine Learning solutions, prediction models, and other decision support systems has attracted the attention of health managers and researchers for detecting the best practices and measuring the value chain of the patient to offer an effective, efficient and quality care. However, these systems require not only the acceptance of policymakers but also requires the involvement of the data generators. The quality of data is crucial for obtaining precise data-driven models [20].

To engage all the links of the health chain, these methods offer a solution in all its strata. The weakest link in this situation is those professionals that are in charge of collecting the precious data without adequate motivation, the general practitioners, nurses and other auxiliary staff working at health centres. These professionals can see the data collection process as an increased burden in their daily practice [22, 31]. This is because they don't see the direct support of these methods in their daily work, that is mainly focused on providing better care to the patient.

A clear example of that is the coding of diagnosis. There are lots of efforts in health management for providing a standard that allows the classification of known diseases. International Classification of Diseases (ICD) [32] is a worldwide attempt for standardizing how the diseases are coded. This standard is continuously in improvement due to the difficulties of define diseases [39]. This makes complex their use by general practitioners that, besides, should deal with the burden that requires the proper selection, annotation a update of diagnosis in the patients Electronic Health Record, selecting the correct code among more than 70,000 diagnoses currently available, in the time of a visit. In this line, Primary Care is one of the main services that is involved in this process. Primary Care usually is in charge to follow all the patients and their diagnosis codification. However, Primary care professionals claim that the computerization of their patients and the use of a computer are increasing their burden [31] and dehumanizing the communication with the patient [22]. For that, the most interesting details of the patient history are usually expressed as free text and the codification are generally avoided. This made that there is some diagnosis that is deficiently coded, like for example obesity [27].

Primary care professionals do not see any advantage for their collaboration in their crucial codification and classification task because they usually have not accessed to population analysis tools that allow the analysis of the flow followed for their patients. Interactive Process Mining solutions can offer a view of the patients that other techniques can not. Involving the general practitioner in the process of co-creation of the treatment optimization that can suppose a better way to improve the adherence of professionals and the adaption of protocols of diseases to real patients.

The approach of professionals to Interactive Process Mining techniques not only allows the better understanding of the behaviour of treatments to their patients but also will allow to these professionals to have feedback for their efforts in classification and coding of diagnosis. This not only requires the engagement of professionals, but also the support of health managers democratizing the use of tools and data among different health professionals in all stages.

For achieving that, it is important to provide one-medical-field solutions that support professionals in their specific daily practice. One-fit-all solutions require usually more adaption time and are not adapted to daily practice. Specific solutions can create the best tools for supporting the professionals minimizing the increased burden to health professionals [26].

17.3   Look for the Best Representation Languages

With the arrival of the standardization culture, the appearance of languages and models for defining processes with different capabilities, expressiveness and complexity have appeared in the literature [41]. Create an adequate process model is not a trivial task [2]. It is necessary to select the proper tool, with adequate expressiveness and complexity, and in the case to enable interaction, this understandability is crucial.

As medicine is not engineering, medical doctors are not engineers [17]. Representation languages that have been used perfectly in industrial environments have not to sense in the medical domain. Health professionals have different ways to observe, think and act [29].

This not means that medical doctors can not use representation languages for defining their own processes. From the appearance of the Evidence-Based Medicine paradigm [35], there is an increasing culture of defining processes and protocols for reusing and disseminating best practices among the clinical community. These protocols, called usually Clinical Pathways [15], are thought for representing the process in a human-understandable way. Also, there are Computer Interpretable Guidelines [33] that are though for representing these Clinical Pathways in a computer understandable way to facilitate its automation.

Despite the huge work made in this field, the creation, implantation and evaluation of processes have not achieved the expected impact in the clinical community. If the language selected is not adequate, instead to be facilitators in the application of Clinical Pathways, it can become an insurmountable barrier [9]. Process languages should be expressive, flexible, automatable, with no uncertainty nor ambiguity, but above all, it should be easily understandable by health professionals. In another case, there is a high probability of failing in their implantation [9].

In the case of Interactive Process Mining, the problem is obvious. If there is not understandability, there is no interaction. It is critical to provide the correct language that not requires intermediates in the definition and understanding of the processes. The expert should understand the model to allow the connection between the real process and its running knowledge, not only for understanding the process behaviour behind the model but also to produce the proper adaptions of the process and evaluate the decisions taken.

17.4   Interactive Data Quality Assessment

One of the clearest problems, that are appearing in the application of Machine Learning technologies to health care is Data Quality. The excessive burden of health professionals, the necessity of better training in the use of new technologies or the lack of engagement of health professionals, among several other factors, are behind the cause of the low quality in most of the clinical databases. For that, there is an increasing interest in creating methods and methodologies for Data Quality Assessment [42].

As defined in previous chapters, there are several dimensions in the Data Quality problems. Incompleteness, due to missing information; Inconsistency, for the discrepancies among the different sources of data; Inaccuracy, caused by the inexactitudes in the data collection process, etc, are examples of syntactical problems that we can consider in the analysis of the quality in a clinical Data Base [6].

This not only affects directly to the veracity of the information, making that the result achieved and the models inferred have limited confidence but also to the artificial variability added to the existing one, due to those errors. Finally, this supposes a clear decrease in the value of the data and, therefore, to the results that we can provide to professionals [40].

For that, it is necessary to provide algorithms, frameworks and tools that can support professionals not only in the assessment about the data quality to evaluate the validity of the models presented to professionals, but also to understand and correct the data collection process [6].

Classical *black boxed* Machine Learning solutions are difficult to understand, and for that is it's very usual to denoise logs by removing non conforming traces to have cleaner data. However, this produces a bias in the log suppressing the patients that are different, that are those that need more intensive care. Interactive solutions can support health IT professionals in the process of data collection improvement [25]. The use of Process Mining techniques can support in the real understanding of flows and IT and Clinical experts can detect special situations and decide if those are due to errors in the collection process, that can be improved, or due to special characteristics of the patient, that should be treated differently. In any case, this advantage of Interactive paradigm can support the improvement in the process, even in noisy environments.

17.5   Data Protection Laws Barriers

In the last decades, privacy and security laws have been hardened. The development of artificial intelligence and the use that some organizations are giving for acquiring and process information for its benefits in detriment of the privacy of the individual [24], are changing the rules of the world [1].

In the era of Big Data, there are available lots of algorithms, methodologies and tools for providing better support to healthcare professionals not only in their daily practice, but also, for providing a way to improve significantly the medical research giving to us better treatments, diagnosis methods, and medical technologies thanks to current information computing capabilities. Despite there is a huge amount of academic experts in the world claiming for the use of data for creating better medical models and the quantity of data available in hospitals are increasing, the accesses to the data is very difficult for the data scientist.

The current legal frameworks are not adequate for research. The research community can help in the development of a new way to acquire real evidence. For that, it is crucial that governments, legislators and citizens accept a middle term for creating an suitable breeding ground that facilitates the use of artificial intelligence in benefit of all of us. Initiatives like Open Data paradigms [16] can be the solution to start sharing knowledge between the medical community and Data Scientist in a way that can incredibly boost medical research.

17.6 Dealing with Medical Data

The special characteristics of medical data require special tools and methodologies for dealing with it. Medical information systems are usually formed by a constellation of tools, system and databases intended to provide fluid access to the data in a health centre. Hospital Information Systems (HIS), that provides access to data available at hospitals in form of different Electronic Health Records (EHR) available on the hospital or in primary care centres; Radiology Information Systems (RIS), Laboratory Information Systems (LIS), and even, Personal Health Records that stores the Patient-Reported Outcomes. All of this information is segmented and distributed logically and geographically by all the health centres. In addition to that, there is very interesting information available from other sources not only directly related with the health of the patient, like pharmacies but also those related with the patient lifestyle like health apps, gyms and supermarkets that can provide a real and valuable picture of the patient. In this line, the patient is reaching a big source of information. Patient-Reported Experience Measures (PREMs) and Patient-Reported Outcomes Measures (PROMs) [4] are becoming an indicator of great interest in the measurement of the health services impact over the patient. In this line, International Consortium for Health Outcomes Measurement (ICHOM) [19] promote the integration of this data in the Health Information Systems to enable a real assessment of health services based on Value-Based Healthcare paradigm [14].

The different health systems have distinct methodologies and databases existing that has diverse technical strategies that can be incompatible among themselves. This obstructs the interconnection of the databases making difficult their interaction. For that, there are some initiatives for ensuring the interoperability among heterogeneous Databases to build a way for exchanging information, for ensuring a holistic way, and for building complete data sets that include all the information available from the patient. Standards like HL7 FHIR [3], OpenEHR [18], or ISO/CEN 13606 [23] appeared intending to create models that allow a common way to access to medical data. Also, these systems make use of semantic interoperability techniques [34], that allow not only collect the data based on a direct mapping but also use queries for accessing these data in a semantically unambiguous way by using induction, inference and knowledge discovery techniques.

In this environment, the main challenge in the application of Process Mining techniques is to provide the necessary mechanisms to enable their application in a Process-Oriented way. It is necessary to create Process-Oriented Data Reference models that allow the creation of semantic interoperability models that can leverage the advantages of Process Oriented Philosophy. For that, it is necessary that Health Information Systems can provide their Data standardized as logs to allow feeding Process Mining tools. In this line, it is necessary to establish the guidelines for the creation of specific Health Process-Oriented Data Warehouses that provide information in a Process Mining Standardized way. These systems can provide different granularities, different kind of traces definitions, or different layers of information depending on the medical fields that are requiring the information.

17.7 Validation and Adaption of Best Practices and Clinical Guidelines

According to the Evidence-Based Medicine Paradigm [35], the creation of clinical guidelines can support medical professionals in the selection of the best treatments for each disease. However, these guidelines usually have problems in their deployment due to the lack of adherence [37], and sometimes for the doubts about its validity in their application [38].

Apart from the difficulties in the creation of the guidelines, there are lots of environmental conditions, like the intervention of pharmacological industry, the physician-patient relationship, and the researcher's conflicts of interest, that cast doubts the cost-effectiveness of the clinical guidelines developed [13].

So, the question is, are Clinical Guidelines valid for the scenario in which they are being applied?. Recent studies are trying to define methodologies for assessing their validity [36]. But, it is necessary not only to provide validity measures for clinical guidelines but also, solutions that help professionals in the understanding of the adherence problems and propose clues for adapting the guidelines to the problem in which the new protocol is deployed.

Interactive Process Mining Paradigm is a very powerful tool for supporting professionals in the application of clinical guidelines in their daily practice. This is not only because it enables the discovery of the real patient journeys based on the event data collected from patient contacts, but also because Process Mining techniques can offer a continuous view of the follow up of the protocol application effects in a specific context. If these capabilities are applied interactively and iteratively, a better convergence can be achieved in less time [11]. After the deployment of a specific protocol or guideline and based on literature or defined by the experts' groups, Interactive systems offer a human-understandable view of the status of the process. In this way, the current guideline is applied and continuously validated. In each iteration the system shows the differences and the experts detect the inefficiencies and bottlenecks and correct them, proposing a new guideline that is iteratively improved [11].

Process Mining domain is plenty of process-oriented tools and algorithms that can support in medical improvement of clinical guidelines. Some tools can infer clinical pathways using specific Process Mining Discovery algorithms [12]; algorithms that offer suggestions of change in the models for *repairing* them according to the observed reality [10]; or paradigms, like Concept Drift [5], that takes into account the evolution change to discover and measure it, among others. The challenge in the application of these techniques in the health domain resides in the acceptance of the special characteristics of the health care domain for their adequate application in daily practice. Algorithms and tools that used not adequate and medical understandable models, does not take into account the real questions of clinicians or made an excessive denoise of the logs, can be rejected by professionals.

17.8   Conclusions

In the current conjuncture where the Digital Health Transformation is increasing their presence in hospitals, there is a priceless opportunity for data scientist for providing Decision Support Systems solutions to help health professionals in daily practice. Healthcare is a challenging field. The solution is not to provide the most accurate data science models at whatever price. There is a need for creating medical evidence, but there is no medical evidence if they are not understandable by health professionals. In this scenario, Interactive Process Mining methodology supposes a clear advantage over other data science methodologies due to their capability to discover, and present the real medical information in a human-understandable way. However, to leverage this advantage it is crucial to provide the correct tools, algorithms and frameworks to deepen in the necessities of health professionals providing effective solutions in daily practice. For that, it is critical to engage health professionals, not only in the understanding of the results provided but also in the interaction with them. In this line, it is fundamental a multidisciplinary work that involves Data Scientist, Health managers, and clinicians. This scenario requires to use the selection of the best graphical languages in each case, ensuring a fluid communication between the algorithms and health professionals, and reducing at the maximum the need of a Data Scientist that act as a translator between them. In the translation, crucial information might be lost reducing significantly the efficacy of the Data Science system. In addition to that, it is necessary to take care of health data. Data is the basis for the creation of the models. Inaccurate data, produces inaccurate models that provide erroneous information to experts, leading them to wrong decisions. Interactive Data curation, not only provides a better way to achieve cleaner data, but also, make professionals aware of the precision of the data and, then, allow them to estimate confidence on the models and evidence discovered. Without forget, the necessity to cover data protection laws, and providing new tools for connecting medical databases to process mining systems to allow a fluid communication inside Health information systems. Finally, Interactive Process Miners should provide a holistic service to health care professionals not only in the discovery of the processes but also in the continuous validation and adaption of their processes to their patients. These challenges require the integration of several technical and medical technologies and the collaboration of different professionals from several disciplines that usually have different ways to communicate and work. For that, this gap is being filled with the appearance of mixed professionals, like biomedical engineers, that can act as a bridge in the use of these technologies. Until that happens, Data Scientists should create solutions that solve the medical questions according to their needs. We are in an incredible scenario full of opportunities that can lead us to a new age of health.

References

1. Albrecht JP. How the gdpr will change the world. Eur Data Prot Law Rev. 2016;2:287.
2. Becker J, Rosemann M, Von Uthmann C. Guidelines of business process modeling. In: Business process management. Springer; 2000. p. 30–49.
3. Bender D, Sartipi K. Hl7 FHIR: an agile and restful approach to healthcare information exchange. In: Proceedings of the 26th IEEE international symposium on computer-based medical systems. IEEE; 2013. p. 326–31.
4. Benson T. Measure what we want: a taxonomy of short generic person-reported outcome and experience measures (proms and prems). BMJ Open Qual. 2020;9(1):e000789.
5. Bose RPJC, van der Aalst WMP, Žliobaitė I, Pechenizkiy M. Handling concept drift in process mining. In: International conference on advanced information systems engineering. Springer; 2011. p. 391–405.
6. Botsis T, Hartvigsen G, Chen F, Weng C. Secondary use of EHR: data quality issues and informatics opportunities. Summit Transl Bioinform. 2010;2010:1.
7. Cuchetti C, Grace PJ. Authentic intention: tempering the dehumanizing aspects of technology on behalf of good nursing care. Nurs Philos. 2020;21(1):e12255.
8. Diniz E, Bernardes SF, Castro P. Self-and other-dehumanization processes in health-related contexts: a critical review of the literature. Rev Gen Psychol. 2019;23(4):475–95.
9. Evans-Lacko S, Jarrett M, McCrone P, Thornicroft G. Facilitators and barriers to implementing clinical care pathways. BMC Health Serv Res. 2010;10(1):182.
10. Fahland D, van der Aalst WMP. Model repair—aligning process models to reality. Inf Syst. 2015;47:220–43.
11. Fernandez-Llatas C, Meneu T, Traver V, Benedi J. Applying evidence-based medicine in telehealth: an interactive pattern recognition approximation. Int J Environ Res Public Health. 2013;10(11):5671–82.
12. Fernandez-Llatas C, Valdivieso B, Traver V, Benedi JM. Using process mining for automatic support of clinical pathways design. In: Fernández-Llatas C, García-Gómez JM, editors, Data mining in clinical medicine. Methods in molecular biology, vol. 1246. New York: Springer; 2015. p. 79–88.
13. Garrison LP Jr. Cost-effectiveness and clinical practice guidelines: have we reached a tipping point? – an overview. Value Health. 2016;19(5):512–5.
14. Gray M. Value based healthcare. BMJ. 2017;356. https://www.bmj.com/content/356/bmj.j437
15. Hipp R, Abel E, Weber RJ. A primer on clinical pathways. Hosp Pharm. 2016;51(5):416–21.
16. Janssen M, Charalabidis Y, Zuiderwijk A. Benefits, adoption barriers and myths of open data and open government. Inf Syst Manag. 2012;29(4):258–68.
17. Jordan VS. Discussion on "doctors are not pilots and patients are not airplanes: quality improvement in medicine". Qual Eng. 2019;31(1):16–20.
18. Kalra D, Beale T, Heard S. The openehr foundation. Stud Health Technol Inform. 2005;115:153–73.
19. Kelley TA. International consortium for health outcomes measurement (ICHOM). Trials. 2015;16(3):O4.
20. Kerr KA, Norris T, Stockdale R. The strategic management of data quality in healthcare. Health Inform J. 2008;14(4):259–66.
21. Liebler JG, McConnell CR. Management principles for health professionals. Jones & Bartlett Publishers; 2020.
22. Linder JA, Schnipper JL, Tsurikova R, Melnikas AJ, Volk LA, Middleton B. Barriers to electronic health record use during patient visits. In: AMIA annual symposium proceedings. vol. 2006. American Medical Informatics Association; 2006. p. 499.
23. Lozano-Rubí R, Carrero AM, Balazote PS, Pastor X. Ontocr: a CEN/ISO-13606 clinical repository based on ontologies. J Biomed Inform. 2016;60:224–33.
24. Manheim KM, Kaplan L. Artificial intelligence: risks to privacy and democracy. Yale J Law Technol. 2018;37. https://papers.ssrn.com/sol3/papers.cfm?abstract_id=3273016

25. Martin N, Martinez-Millana A, Valdivieso B, Fernández-Llatas C. Interactive data cleaning for process mining: a case study of an outpatient clinic's appointment system. In: International conference on business process management. Springer; 2019. p. 532–44.
26. Martinez-Millana A, Lizondo A, Gatta R, Vera S, Salcedo VT, Fernandez-Llatas C. Process mining dashboard in operating rooms: analysis of staff expectations with analytic hierarchy process. Int J Environ Res Public Health. 2019;16(2):199.
27. Martinez-Millana C, Martinez-Millana A, Fernandez-Llatas C, Martinez BV, Salcedo VT. Comparing data base engines for building big data analytics in obesity detection. In: 2019 IEEE 32nd international symposium on computer-based medical systems (CBMS). IEEE; 2019. p. 208–11.
28. Matt C, Hess T, Benlian A. Digital transformation strategies. Bus Inf Syst Eng. 2015;57(5):339–43.
29. McGrath BM. How doctors think; 2009.
30. Meskó B, Drobni Z, Bényei É, Gergely B, Győrffy Z. Digital health is a cultural transformation of traditional healthcare. Mhealth. 2017;3(9). http://mhealth.amegroups.com/article/view/16494/16602
31. Nápoles AM, Appelle N, Kalkhoran S, Vijayaraghavan M, Alvarado N, Satterfield J. Perceptions of clinicians and staff about the use of digital technology in primary care: qualitative interviews prior to implementation of a computer-facilitated 5as intervention. BMC Med Inform Decis Making. 2016;16(1):1–13.
32. World Health Organization et al. ICD-11 for mortality and morbidity statistics. Retrieved June. 2018;22:2018.
33. Peleg M. Computer-interpretable clinical guidelines: a methodological review. J Biomed Inform. 2013;46(4):744–63.
34. Pileggi SF, Fernandez-Llatas C. Semantic interoperability issues, solutions, challenges. River Publishers; 2012.
35. Sackett DL, Rosenberg WMC, Gray MJA, Haynes BR, Richardson SW. Evidence based medicine: what it is and what it isn't. BMJ. 1996;312(7023):71–2.
36. Shi Q, Rodrigues PP. Monitoring the effectiveness of clinical guidelines: is the recommendation still valid? In: 2018 IEEE 31st international symposium on computer-based medical systems (CBMS). IEEE; 2018. p. 304–9.
37. Slade SC, Kent P, Patel S, Bucknall T, Buchbinder R. Barriers to primary care clinician adherence to clinical guidelines for the management of low back pain. Clin J Pain. 2016;32(9):800–16.
38. Steinhoff MC, Khalek MKAEI, Khallaf N, Hamza HS, El Ayadi A, Orabi A, Fouad H, Kamel M. Effectiveness of clinical guidelines for the presumptive treatment of streptococcal pharyngitis in egyptian children. Lancet. 1997;350(9082):918–21.
39. Tanno LK, Casale T, Papadopoulos NG, Sanchez-Borges M, Thiens F, Pawankar R, Calderon MA, Gómez M, Sisul JC, Ansotegui IJ, et al. A call to arms of specialty societies to review the who international classification of diseases, eleventh revision terms appropriate for the diseases they manage: the example of the joint allergy academies. In: Allergy and asthma proceedings. vol. 38; 2017. p. 54.
40. Thorpe JH, Gray EA. Big data and ambulatory care: breaking down legal barriers to support effective use. J Ambul Care Manag. 2015;38(1):29.
41. van Der Aalst WMP, Ter Hofstede AHM, Kiepuszewski B, Barros AP. Workflow patterns. Distrib Parallel Databases. 2003;14(1):5–51.
42. Weiskopf NG, Weng C. Methods and dimensions of electronic health record data quality assessment: enabling reuse for clinical research. J Am Med Inform Assoc. 2013;20(1):144–51.

Index

© Springer Nature Switzerland AG 2021
C. Fernandez-Llatas (ed.), *Interactive Process Mining in Healthcare*, Health
Informatics, https://doi.org/10.1007/978-3-030-53993-1